TEARS FOR MY SISTERS

Tears for My Sisters

The Tragedy of Obstetric Fistula

L. LEWIS WALL, MD, DPhil

JOHNS HOPKINS UNIVERSITY PRESS
BALTIMORE

Johns Hopkins University Press
2715 North Charles Street
Baltimore, Maryland 21218-4363
www.press.jhu.edu

Library of Congress Cataloging-in-Publication Data

Names: Wall, L. Lewis, 1950–, author.
Title: Tears for my sisters : the tragedy of obstetric fistula / L. Lewis Wall.
Description: Baltimore : Johns Hopkins University Press, [2018] | Includes bibliographical
    references and index.
Identifiers: LCCN 2017012955| ISBN 9781421424170 (hardcover : alk. paper) |
    ISBN 1421424177 (hardcover : alk. paper) | ISBN 9781421424187 (electronic) |
    ISBN 1421424185 (electronic)
Subjects: | MESH: Vaginal Fistula—complications | Obstetric Labor Complications |
    Reconstructive Surgical Procedures | Maternal Health Services | Health Services
    Accessibility | Socioeconomic Factors | Africa
Classification: LCC RG701 | NLM WP 250 | DDC 618.5—dc23
    LC record available at https://lccn.loc.gov/2017012955

A catalog record for this book is available from the British Library.

*Special discounts are available for bulk purchases of this book. For more information, please contact
Special Sales at 410-516-6936 or specialsales@press.jhu.edu.*

Johns Hopkins University Press uses environmentally friendly book materials, including
recycled text paper that is composed of at least 30 percent post-consumer waste, whenever
possible.

In memory of Leonard A. Wall, MD

(1921–2013)

Father, physician, mentor, friend

CONTENTS

The story I tell in this book is multifaceted and complex, spanning thousands of years in time and thousands of miles in space. It is a story that requires multiple voices, for the narratives, personalities, contexts, cases, and the ethical, moral, and political issues with which it is interwoven are vast, complicated, and multidimensional. The problems presented are compelling, heart-wrenching, and disgraceful, but they are also solvable, given adequate political will. The subject of this book is obstetric fistula, a catastrophic complication of childbirth in which the tissues that normally separate the bladder from the vagina are destroyed by prolonged obstructed labor, leaving the victim perpetually soaked in urine, psychologically damaged, physically wretched, and often socially isolated. Once common in the Western world, these injuries have vanished from public consciousness among the world's affluent populations due to the widespread availability of skilled obstetric care, but they remain a major public health problem among the world's poorest women, a preventable cause of much human misery that can, and should, be eliminated.

In chapter 1, I reconstruct the story of the world's oldest known fistula case: the ancient Egyptian Queen Henhenit of the Eleventh Dynasty. Her story is similar to that of millions of women who have sustained these awful childbirth injuries over the thousands of years since *Homo sapiens* first emerged in northeastern Africa. Although an ancient tale, Henhenit's story continues to resonate throughout much of the world today.

Chapter 2 explains the process of obstructed labor, the life-threatening condition that occurs when a fetus will not fit through the birth canal during labor. Obstructed labor is usually fatal for the fetus and catastrophic for its mother under "natural" conditions where medical intervention does not occur. The end result of this process (if the woman survives) is often the destruction of much of her vagina and the creation of a fistula.

Chapter 3 tells the story of how the problem of obstructed labor was finally overcome. For hundreds of years midwives and surgeons made valiant (and generally futile) efforts to help these women trapped in obstructed labor when they could not deliver by themselves. These efforts to aid laboring women were often heroic—and often quite ghastly, characterized by frightful suffering and dismal outcomes. It was not until Cesarean section became a safe operation toward the end of the nineteenth century that women in obstructed labor could expect to survive, intact, and have a living child as well. The result of this triumph of obstetric surgery was the gradual elimination of obstetric fistula as an important public health concern in the industrialized world, where it became (on those rare occasions when it occurred) only an exotic medical curiosity.

But what about the women who had a fistula? Prior to the nineteenth century, an obstetric fistula was an injury that could rarely be cured. The unfortunate woman who sustained a fistula while giving birth was doomed to a life of misery. Chapter 4 tells the story of the frustrating attempts over several hundred years by surgeons to find a way to repair these injuries. Aside from occasional serendipitous successes, the attempts at surgical cure were usually disheartening failures that extracted a great price from the patients who endured them; but life with a fistula was so utterly miserable that women repeatedly subjected themselves to these operations in hopes of finally becoming dry. The path to success was discovered in the middle of the nineteenth century by an obscure Alabama surgeon named J. Marion Sims. His success, and that of his collaborator and successor Thomas Addis Emmet, opened the way for the development of reconstructive gynecological surgery, a specialty that thrives today.

Today in poor nations women do not have access to lifesaving technologies such as Cesarean delivery or to the surgical procedures that can repair their injured organs if they develop a fistula. In poor nations, poor women usually have grim reproductive lives. Obstetric fistula remains a pressing public health problem throughout most of sub-Saharan Africa and other impoverished parts of the world. Chapter 5 explores a part of the world that I know well: the Hausa-speaking communities of northern Nigeria and southern Niger. In this area of West Africa maternal mortality is high and obstetric fistulas are common. I argue that maternal death and obstetric fistula are both reflections of the way in which this particular society devalues women, but the circumstances found there are by no means unique to that part of the world. Wherever poverty is widespread and the status of women is low, obstetric fistulas are likely to be abundant.

Chapters 6, 7, and 8 explore in more detail how lack of resources, the low status of women, and faulty infrastructure combine to produce high rates of maternal death and childbirth injury among the "bottom billion" of the world's women. I use the perspective of the "three delays" to emphasize these points. Obstetric fistulas occur when labor is obstructed and a woman is not delivered in a timely fashion. Most severe maternal childbirth injuries and maternal deaths occur because a complication (such as obstructed labor) is not treated quickly enough. The "three delays" that lead to such awful outcomes are: (1) delay in deciding to seek help when complications arise; (2) delay in arriving at a suitable healthcare facility after the quest for care begins; and (3) delay in receiving needed medical care once a woman arrives at a hospital, health center, or clinic. In a country like the United States where there are plenty of hospitals, organized ambulance services, and few economic barriers to the receipt of emergency obstetric care, these problems may seem minimal, but for poor women in poor countries where the infrastructure is bad and women's health is not a high priority, these delays are as common and as catastrophic as they are unjustifiable.

Chapter 9 explores the values that must be embraced to reverse this situation. I argue that every woman has the right to emergency obstetric care, which should be delivered with compassion, respect, and fairness (justice). The failure to deliver comprehensive emergency obstetric services to the world's women is a direct reflection of the way women are valued in those societies where maternal death and childbirth injuries are common. We have known for at least 75 years how to prevent the major causes of maternal death and severe maternal morbidity. The technologies needed are neither expensive nor complicated. The failure to provide such services to all women is a failure of values and of political will that should not be tolerated.

Chapter 10 tells the remarkable story of Drs. Reginald and Catherine Hamlin, who arrived in Ethiopia in 1959. After encountering the obstetric fistula problem firsthand, they devoted the rest of their lives to treating this condition and working to eradicate it in their adopted country. It is through the work of "fistula champions" like Reg and Catherine Hamlin that this ancient scourge of childbirth will ultimately be eliminated around the world.

I have tried to write simply, but I have occasionally used medical terms that may not be familiar to those without professional training. Therefore, I have appended a glossary of some of the more important terms that occur in this book to help the reader who wishes some assistance. I have also tried to write without encumbering the text with footnotes. The bibliography at the end is extensive and all references mentioned in the text can easily be identified, along with the sources of all quotations.

TEARS FOR MY SISTERS

Confronting Childbirth Injury among the World's Poorest Women

The death of a pregnant woman is a great tragedy. The very existence of our species and the continuity of human society depend upon successful reproduction, as each new generation arises from its predecessor. When a woman dies while pregnant or shortly after the delivery of a child (which may be stillborn itself), families and communities are wracked with grief. Everyone understands why: a death like this raises important existential questions about life, justice, meaning, and the future, while simultaneously creating immediately painful tasks related to burial, the rearrangement of social relationships, family turmoil, and personal sorrow.

The risks of human reproduction are borne exclusively by females. Women are the childbearers in whose wombs the next generation grows and is nourished. Whatever else may divide us, we all have this in common: each one of us was born. Each one of us made the slow and often hazardous journey out of our mother's womb. Some of us had easy births; for others it was more difficult. Some of us were born spontaneously; others required outside intervention: the application of obstetrical forceps or a vacuum extractor, or even the creation of a new birth pathway made through a surgical incision in our mother's abdomen and uterus so that a helping obstetrical hand could guide us into the light. Some of us were born with injuries sustained within the womb; most of us were born healthy and have continued to thrive.

In the West, good obstetric outcomes are the norm. We take reproductive success for granted. On those rare occasions when some form of reproductive misadventure occurs, we demand explanations and file lawsuits that attempt to pin the blame upon those we hold responsible. We dismiss biology and seek redress, justifiable or not. Over 90 percent of American obstetrician-gynecologists have been sued at least once. Most of these obstetric lawsuits involve claims related to injured newborns or stillbirths. The notion that pregnancy and childbirth create unavoidable risks for women is largely absent from public discourse, yet the risks are real: 15 percent of pregnancies—even the "lowest-risk" pregnancies—will develop serious complications that, if not managed promptly and properly, can become life threatening.

At the turn of the twentieth century, maternal mortality in the United States was approximately 600 maternal deaths per 100,000 live births, roughly the situation that prevails throughout most of sub-Saharan Africa today. In the 1920s, Josephine Baker of the New York Department of Health could write, "The United States comes perilously near to being the most unsafe country in the world for the pregnant woman, as far as her chance of living through childbirth is concerned." By midcentury these circumstances had been radically transformed as technology advanced and as access to competent emergency obstetric services improved dramatically. In 2015, the maternal mortality ratio in the United States was 14 deaths per 100,000 live births, and an American woman had a lifetime risk of 1 in 3,800 of dying from a pregnancy-related complication. By contrast, in the African nation of Chad nearly 1 percent of all pregnant or newly delivered women die, and the cumulative risks of reproducing are sobering. There, a woman's likelihood of dying during the course of her reproductive life is 1 in 18. This two-hundred-fold discrepancy (or greater) in women's reproductive health statistics is repeated around the world: maternal mortality and childbirth injury rates are lower than they have ever been among the rich, while the threats of death and disability perpetually stalk the lives of childbearing women in the "bottom billion" of the world's poor. Only 1 percent of maternal deaths occur in affluent countries. The vast majority of maternal deaths occur in South Asia and in sub-Saharan Africa, where the situation is particularly dire. Although Africa holds only 13 percent of the world's people, it nonetheless accounts for two-thirds of the world's maternal deaths.

The women who die in childbirth are gone, and often they are forgotten by their communities as life, of necessity, moves on; but the lingering consequences of reproductive misadventure are most obvious among women who survive a difficult birth experience. For every woman who dies from a complication of pregnancy or childbirth, at least 30 will suffer serious injuries. The most devastating of these injuries is an obstetric fistula, a complication of delivery that destroys the pelvic tissues that separate the vagina from the bladder or rectum. When these tissue barriers are destroyed, urine and feces flow through the vagina to the outside world in an uncontrollable, unrelenting stream. The physical, social, and psychological consequences are dreadful. Wet, soiled, offensive and stinking, deeply ashamed, distraught by the death of her child (who almost invariably succumbs to the travail of prolonged obstructed labor), often unable to comprehend why this has happened to her, over time the woman with a fistula may be abandoned by her husband and those around her, who can't cope with the hygienic catastrophe that has engulfed her. Women with fistulas may be forced to the margins of society, where they dwell in unremitting misery. Even when she can hide her struggle to control her bodily wastes, the psychological trauma produced by a fistula is long lasting, and the damage to her body image is dramatic and profound.

A fistula by itself is rarely fatal, but once established it will not heal on its own. Cure requires surgical intervention. Considering these facts together, it is not uncommon to meet African women who have lived with this condition for 30 or 40 years. Unless they can find a surgeon to repair their injuries and close the defects in the bladder or rectum, these women remain trapped in hideous circumstances for the rest of their lives. But because lack of access to timely surgical care (Cesarean section or instrumental delivery) during childbirth produced the problem in the first place, and because surgical services are so poorly developed throughout the sub-Saharan region, the chances that these women will find relief is small indeed. It is estimated that there are hundreds of thousands—perhaps a million or more—unrepaired fistulas on the African continent, with thousands of new cases each year. The total surgical capacity in Africa to treat these patients is probably no more than 10,000 operations per year, so the overall calculus of suffering indicates a continuing accumulation of avoidable human misery.

Obstetric fistulas are caused by obstructed labor. Labor is obstructed when the baby will not fit through its mother's birth canal. Unless she gets help, the woman whose labor is obstructed may linger in agonizing pain for days with the fetal head impacted in her pelvis, her vulnerable soft tissues crushed by the relentless pressure of her contracting uterus. Fetal death occurs in more than 90 percent of the cases in which labor is obstructed in this way, and the resultant damage to the woman herself can be breathtaking in its scope and severity. In the affluent world, where all women have access to competent emergency obstetric care, an obstetric fistula is a case report, a medical curiosity, the exotic relic of a bygone era, rather than a pressing public health problem. However, for childbearing women in resource-poor nations, the possibility of an obstetric catastrophe like a fistula is an omnipresent threat.

Women with obstetric fistulas are the innocent victims of faulty obstetrical mechanics. They bear no personal blame for their condition, even though they often live in societies that tell them otherwise. A woman in obstructed labor is no more to blame for her predicament than she is for the process of human evolution that reengineered her pelvis to permit bipedal locomotion. She is collateral damage from what Sherwood Washburn has called the "human obstetrical dilemma": the need to deliver large babies with big brains through a narrow, constricted pelvis. The consequences of these biological constraints are amplified by the social settings in which fistulas generally occur. Obstructed labor is more common in parts of the world where girls grow up undervalued and malnourished, marry early, commence childbearing before they achieve full pelvic growth, and deliver babies without skilled birth attendants, functioning healthcare systems, or comprehensive emergency obstetric care. Because fistula sufferers are female and tend to be young, poor, illiterate, and concentrated in rural areas, they lack access to the levers of power that control their societies. They are unknown, unwelcomed, voiceless, and neglected.

In recent years an international movement has developed calling for more resources to be devoted to "neglected tropical diseases": a list of infectious conditions found almost exclusively in tropical countries, most of which are unknown to the general public. These are exotic conditions, with strange, convoluted names like dracunculiasis, lymphatic filariasis, onchocerciasis, schistosomiasis, trichuriasis, Buruli ulcer, and the like. All of these conditions are highly stigmatizing and predominantly affect the poor and dispossessed. All of these conditions are treatable or preventable using low-cost, proven technologies, but they continue to exist only because the resources necessary to treat or prevent them have not been mobilized in the societies where they are prevalent. They persist because of a failure of political will, not because the problems they present are insurmountable.

Like these other exotic conditions, obstetric fistula is a "neglected tropical disease"; it persists because the nations in which it is common lack the visionary leadership, competent management, and political will to create effective maternal healthcare infrastructures. Obstetric fistula persists because the international community has yet to grapple with the grotesque gender inequities that persist throughout the world. Obstetric fistula persists because the world has yet to acknowledge that every woman has a fundamental right to competent obstetric care, no matter where she lives.

This book tells the story of obstetric fistula: what it is, how it develops, why it persists, how it can be treated, how it can be prevented, and, ultimately, how it can be eradicated. In societies where women are valued only because they are childbearers and where they often have little choice about when and with whom they have sex, or when and with whom (or even whether) they become pregnant, maternal death and reproductive injury are common. This lack of respect for women as persons who are worthy in their own right—not simply for their reproductive capacities—is reflected in the paltry investments such societies make in maternal healthcare and in the lack of attention to women's health that is reflected in national health policies and political agendas. That obstetric fistula still exists in the twenty-first century is a mark of shame on the world's medical community. This situation must be changed.

CHAPTER 1

The Tragedy of Queen Henhenit

There was a quiet knock, and the door opened.

"Professor Derry?"

A slim man with a neatly trimmed moustache looked up from his desk, which was piled high with papers, a microscope in the corner. "Yes?" he replied.

"The mummy that Mr. Winlock sent you has arrived. Would you care to examine it?"

"Yes, indeed. Let's go now."

Douglas Derry was a graduate of the University of Edinburgh Medical School, where he had developed a passion for the study of anatomy. After holding the distinguished Crichton research scholarship and teaching practical anatomy to medical students, he left the cold Scottish winters behind to take up a position in Egypt at the Government School of Medicine in Cairo (now the Qasr el-Aini Medical School), where he became fascinated by the anthropology and archaeology of ancient Egypt. Before long, Derry was an institution himself within the medical and scientific community. A man of charm and vision, a delightful host, a willing tour guide, and a raconteur full of stories, he was also a diligent researcher with a passion for mummies. It was he who unwrapped the mummy of Tutankhamen—the famous "King Tut"—after Howard Carter discovered it in the 1920s. If you wanted an anatomical opinion on an ancient Egyptian mummy, Derry was your man. He was known for his keen interest in unusual anatomy and remarkable examples of pathology. That's why Winlock wanted him to examine the mummy of Henhenit.

"Did it arrive in good condition?" Derry asked.

"It was only in reasonable shape. It was stored at the Metropolitan Museum for seventeen years. Winlock packed it carefully, but part of the left side of her face appears to have been damaged in the voyage back home."

The mummy of Queen Henhenit had been discovered by Edouard Naville during his excavation of the temple of Pharaoh Nebhepetre Montuhotep II at Deir el-Bahri in the early years of the twentieth century. Her mummy and its sarcophagus had been given to American Egyptologist Herbert Winlock of the Metropolitan Museum in New York. Winlock and Derry knew each other well. Winlock had consulted with Derry on many occasions about interesting or unusual anatomical specimens (most notably a remarkable cache of bodies of slain soldiers that he found at Deir el-Bahri not far from where Henhenit's mummy was recovered). Now he wanted Derry to examine the mummy of the dead young queen and had returned her to her native Egypt for a final medical consultation.

"Here she is, then. Queen Henhenit. Let's have a look."

They quietly set to work examining the mummy, unwrapping limbs, making measurements, taking notes, exchanging a few words here and there as they pored over the fragile remains.

"Slender woman. Probably was rather petite."

"Not the highest quality embalming for a Middle Kingdom mummy, is it? There's no flank incision."

In the highest standard of mummification practiced in ancient Egypt, most of the internal organs were removed through an incision in the flank, after which they were embalmed and interred separately in special receptacles called canopic jars. The abdominal cavity of the mummy was then often packed with bandages soaked in resin.

"No. They must have embalmed her with an injection through the anus. Look. See how it protrudes."

A common alternative method of mummification involved injecting the intestines through the anus and rectum with a mixture of turpentine and juniper or cedar oil to help dissolve the internal organs prior to packing the body in natron—the embalming salt that removed all of the moisture from the body, mummifying it so that it would be preserved for all eternity.

"Let's open the abdomen."

The scalpel moved slowly through the desiccated tissues, exposing the abdomen and pelvis of the ancient queen.

"The vagina is very dilated. Unusual."

"Abdomen and pelvis, too."

"Is that the bladder? My word. . . ."

There was silence for a few moments, then Derry spoke.

"What an awful thing. How she must have suffered!"

The bladder seemed to fill the pelvic cavity. On close inspection a great rent could be seen in the bladder leading directly into the vagina. Derry picked up a blunt probe and inserted it. The probe passed easily through the vagina into the bladder, clearly demonstrating the presence of a vesico-vaginal fistula, the earliest known example of

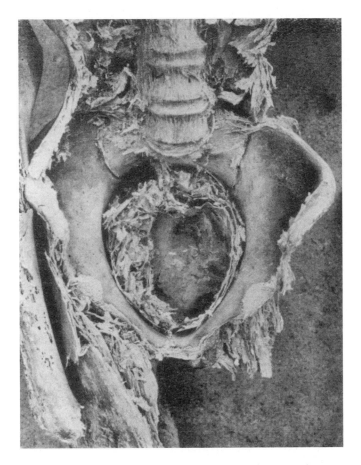

FIGURE 1.1. The mummy of Queen Henhenit, showing a large vesico-vaginal fistula. *From D. E. Derry, "Note on Five Pelves of Women of the Eleventh Dynasty in Egypt,"* Journal of Obstetrics and Gynaecology of the British Empire *42 (1935): 490–495, figure 2.*

such an injury. The story that these tissues told, even in their dry and friable state, was clear, convincing, and tragic (figure 1.1).

"Slim woman. Odd pelvis. Look at the measurements. The transverse diameter is only 104 millimeters from side to side. Very long pelvis. The anterior-posterior diameter is 130 millimeters. I don't see how a baby could get through a pelvis like this and live. It must have taken forever. My God, how she must have suffered. She must have been in labor for days. What an injury! Just look at the damage. The whole bladder base is almost gone. Imagine what it would have been like to live with an injury like that, even as a queen of Egypt."

"Professor Mahfouz sees obstetric injuries like this all the time in peasant women from rural villages. He's written lots of papers on it. It's terrible. Have you ever seen him operate?"

"My God, how she must have suffered."

An Ancient Egyptian Setting

Henhenit lived around 2025 BC at the beginning of what historians refer to as the Eleventh Dynasty, the start of the ancient Egypt's Middle Kingdom. After the death of Pharaoh Pepi II around 2184 BC—an aged man who reportedly had ruled for 94 years—the centralized government of the pyramid-building Old Kingdom fell apart. The power of the capital at Memphis declined, and competing dynasties formed in Egypt's north (at Herakleopolis) and south (at Thebes). For almost 150 years petty local rulers pushed, shoved, and elbowed each other as they competed for power and prominence, none gaining significant advantage over the others and none extending his influence much beyond the confines of his own local domain. While each claimed to be king and pompously outfitted himself with grandiose titles, none had the power to assert his authority as ruler of the whole land of Egypt.

In the southern city of Thebes, however, the situation started to change. A family of local nobles variously named Inyotef and Montuhotep began consolidating power around 2125 BC, expanding Theban influence in Upper Egypt. The local god was Montu, a falcon-headed solar divinity whose importance grew in proportion to the success of his local champions. The name Montuhotep means "Montu is satisfied," and the rulers who bore this name did their best to make sure that this was true.

The power of Thebes increased, gradually encroaching upon the territories of Herakleopolis. When Inyotef III died around 2055 BC, he was succeeded as ruler of Thebes by Nebhepetre (Son of Re) Montuhotep II. This local strongman took the auspicious throne-name of S'ankhibtawy, which means "He who breathes life into the heart of the Two Lands," a rather explicit claim to the title of sole king of both Upper and Lower Egypt. Could he prove it?

An audacious and politically astute ruler, Montuhotep consolidated his local power base (dutifully taking care to satisfy the needs of Montu and his priesthood). He patiently waited 14 years before he finally struck, but when he did, he was unstoppable. He marched north with his army and defeated the "pretender" who ruled at Herakleopolis to become the one true pharaoh of Egypt. To his titles he now added the new name of Sematawy, "He who unifies the Two Lands." Egypt was whole again, and Montuhotep grasped it with both hands.

Succeeding generations of historians regard Nebhepetre Montuhotep II as the founder of the Middle Kingdom (ca. 2030–1640 BC), the truly classic period of Egyptian civilization in which literary, architectural, and artistic styles were set for future generations. Montuhotep II, now with the power of the whole land of Egypt at his disposal, flexed his military muscles and launched expeditions to the north and west against the nomadic peoples living in what today would be modern Libya and against the Nubians to the south. He consolidated power throughout the country, expanded trade, pushed the nomadic marauders out of the Sinai Peninsula, and established safe and orderly caravan and trade routes. The land grew in prosperity, power, and influence.

Montuhotep II was also a prolific builder and an important architectural stylist. The crowning architectural achievement of his long (almost 50-year) reign was the splendid mortuary temple and tomb he carved for himself out of the western hillside along the Nile close to Thebes at Deir el-Bahri. This temple was erected on a rectangular platform nearly 205 feet long from north to south and 151 feet wide, chiseled out of the underlying bedrock. The base of a structure (possibly a small pyramid), surrounded by a colonnade, lies in the middle of the temple complex. This columned ambulatory is surrounded by a wall decorated with carved reliefs, beyond which was another (now ruined) colonnade. One approaches the platform of the temple and pyramid by a long ramp on the eastern side, which originates on a lower level with its own colonnade. The farther, western end of the complex narrows into the rocky cliffside behind the pyramid and the surrounding ambulatory, where it descends into another colonnaded court within which is the great sanctuary for the soul (*ka*) of the king with its accompanying transverse hypostyle hall and a small sanctuary. The entire temple complex is surrounded by a high wall of limestone. The wall reliefs were originally surmounted with a frieze of stars, a strip of alternating red and blue squares, and ornamental figures similarly painted red and blue.

Between the tomb-sanctuary and the pyramid on the western side are a series of subsidiary chapels and rock-cut shaft-tombs in which some of Montuhotep's queens were buried, priestesses of the goddess Hathor. In these subsidiary chapels—with their gaily colored cornices and green lily-pillars—offerings were made to the spirits of these royal women after their deaths. Archaeologist H. R. Hall, writing in Edouard Naville's 1907 excavation report, called it "a sort of XIth Dynasty Westminster Abbey; the king's courtiers and officials were buried not merely in the court, but actually in the outer colonnade of his temple." After her tragic death, Henhenit would ultimately come to rest in one of these tombs.

The Tragedy of Henhenit

Henhenit was a priestess of the goddess Hathor, a divinity of special prominence at the court of Montuhotep. An ancient deity, even for Egypt, Hathor was the Guardian of the Mountain of Kurn, the great hill rising above the cliffs of Deir el-Bahri. She was a loving mother figure, a protectress, a goddess of fertility and childbirth, but also the patroness of music, dance, and wine. She was the Golden One, the Mistress of the Sycamore, the sun-eye, the embodiment of divine order (*maat*), as well as the muse of sexuality and erotic pleasure. The later Greeks and Romans had no trouble recognizing in Hathor their goddesses Aphrodite and Venus. These attributes made Hathor popular, and popularity in turn brought more adherents. Increasingly, those adherents came from the ruling elite, which amplified the power of her priesthood and temples. These influences reinforced one another in synergistic ways. The influence of the goddess grew at the court of the new pharaoh, particularly among elite women.

Although Montuhotep was linked, by name and origin with the god Montu of Thebes, he realized that reunifying Egypt required ideology and propaganda as much as it required military might. In a polytheistic world, political space could always be created for another helpful deity. Because the goddess Hathor was so firmly linked to the court and the ruling elite, it was politically useful for Montuhotep to portray himself as the son of Hathor, thereby adding genealogical legitimacy to his claim to be pharaoh. In support of this position, prior to the conquest of Herakleopolis, Montuhotep married a number of priestesses of Hathor as a way of strengthening his political base. Henhenit was one of them.

This was astute politics on the part of Montuhotep, but it also carried with it some pleasant fringe benefits. Hathor was a joyful goddess, patroness of dance and wine, both things that were pleasing to the king. One dance song, dedicated to Hathor as the goddess of wine, depicts the pharaoh as an enthusiastic participant in the celebrations in her honor:

The pharaoh comes to dance
He comes to sing (for thee)
> O, his mistress, see how he dances,
> O, bride of Horus, see how he skips,
The pharaoh whose hands are washed,
Whose fingers are clean
> O, his mistress, see how he dances,
> O, bride of Horus, see how he skips
When he offers thee
This *mnw*-urn with wine
> O, his mistress, see how he dances
> O, bride of Horus, see how he skips,
His heart is sincere, his body in order,
There is no darkness in his breast,
> O, his mistress, see how he dances,
> O, bride of Horus, see how he skips.

Like her goddess, Henhenit loved to dance, and she was a lovely woman. She had smooth unblemished skin, sparkling eyes, and a coy smile that gladdened the hearts of those upon whom she bestowed it. She was slender, with full breasts, a tiny waist, and narrow hips, and she walked with an ambulant grace that made the diaphanous linen garments she wore rustle like the fronds of a palm tree caressed by a gentle Nile breeze. It did not take Nebhepetre Montuhotep long to become aware of her. The pharaoh relished reports about beautiful women, particularly if they were members of politically useful families, and when he saw her dancing, her arms raised up toward the sky like the long, gently curving horns of Hathor's sacred cow, swaying in time to the *shush shush shush* of the sistrum, the rattle sacred to the goddess, he wanted her for himself. Not only would this satisfy his personal passion, but it would further cement his reputation as a king who paid attention to the gods and their priesthoods, one who courted their influence—and deserved their support. The pharaoh was assiduous in his courtship of the lovely Henhenit, and when she finally acquiesced, Montuhotep (like his god Montu) was content.

Within a few months Henhenit was pregnant. The early months of her pregnancy passed uneventfully, except for some nausea, but as pregnancy progressed she found it increasingly awkward to get around. Because she was so slim, her gravid belly tended to throw her off balance, and it was difficult to dance gracefully for Hathor when the physics of movement had changed so dramatically. But her demeanor remained calm, her affect was contented, and her eyes still sparkled. Henhenit was happy. She looked forward to producing a child, perhaps a son, possibly a future pharaoh himself. With each passing week her abdomen grew bigger, more rotund and swollen, like an exquisite Nile melon ready for harvest.

Henhenit's water broke just before dawn. Soon after, her labor pains started, gradually increasing in strength and frequency. She fastened a spiral pendant of golden wire around her neck, an amulet sacred to her goddess reminiscent of the bicornuate uterus of the sacred cow. It would assure her protection during birth. Henhenit smiled and murmured to herself the lines from Hathor's sacred hymn, "Come to me, Hathor, my mistress, in my fine pavilion, in this happy hour with this pleasant north wind." Everything would be all right.

By late morning Henhenit was in active labor with hard contractions coming every three to four minutes. There were no drugs to alleviate her discomfort. She felt the full force of each contraction. Her only relief was the support of her female friends, her servants, and the midwives who routinely attended each birth. Because Henhenit was a queen of Egypt, her labor would probably have been more pleasant than that experienced by the common women of the town or countryside. They labored in small, cramped mud-brick huts lighted only by smoky lamps. Henhenit had all the luxuries of the royal place at her disposal, but the physiology of childbirth was the same regardless of her status. Childbirth was a great social leveler, bringing highborn and common women down to the same position: each had to push her child out by herself—or die trying. Her fellow priestesses of Hathor (who was, after all, the goddess of fertility, sexuality, and childbirth) provided her with additional encouragement and support. In the normal course of things, Henhenit could have expected to deliver her baby before sunset when the great god Re descended below the western horizon in his solar boat to begin his nighttime journey through the underworld. By the time Re reappeared in the east to herald a new day, Henhenit should have been recovering comfortably, snuggling her newborn child against her breast and dropping off to sleep— just another young Egyptian mother, tired but happy that everything had passed successfully.

It didn't work out that way.

When morning came Henhenit had not yet had her baby. Her uterus was still contracting hard, trying to push the baby out, but her labor was not progressing. Her slender figure, delicate waist, and narrow pelvis—the very things that had so aroused the ardor of the pharaoh—now became a terrible obstacle. Her child (probably a male, because male babies tend to be larger on average than females) was too big to fit through her birth canal. The baby's head had descended into her pelvis, where it had come to rest against her pelvic bones, but the head was too large and Henhenit's pelvis was too small to allow it to navigate the last few inches into the outside world. Her labor was obstructed. Even though she was queen of Egypt, there was little anyone could do to help her. She was on her own.

The priestesses of Hathor prayed to the goddess for help, but she did not hear them—or if she did, she chose, for her own inscrutable reasons, not to intervene. Physicians were summoned, but their recipes (some of which were truly disgusting) were equally ineffectual. The midwives applied soothing ointments and slippery oils, trying to speed things up. They inserted their fingers into Henhenit's vagina, probing, hoping to find some way to aid her birth, but nothing worked, and the attempts to help only increased her misery. She was drenched in sweat. The delicate golden spirals of her amulet had been twisted grotesquely out of shape where she had desperately clutched them during the spasms of her labor.

With each contraction the baby's head was forced ever more tightly downward, but her pelvic bones were unyielding. With each contraction her baby's head was pushed more and more tightly against the soft tissues of her pelvis, crushing the cervix, bladder, and vagina against her pelvic bones, crushing the muscles, nerves, and blood vessels in her pelvis as well, the uterus relentless but unsuccessful in forcing the baby out.

Henhenit was becoming frantic from the pain, which was intense and increasing. She was dehydrated and weak from the struggle of trying to push the baby out. She desperately needed to urinate, but she hadn't been able pass anything at all for more than 10 hours. She didn't understand why. She had never needed to go so badly in her entire life, yet nothing would come out. The reason for this urinary distress was that the baby's head had pressed her urethra and bladder neck so tightly up against her pelvic bones that the bladder outlet was completely occluded. Nothing could pass this obstruction. If anyone had thought to try (and no one did) the blockage was so tight that even a metal catheter would not have been able to force the bladder open.

Her labor continued throughout the day and into the next night. Each contraction became a fiery trial from which she could not escape. The intensity of her pain grew exponentially, but the baby did not budge. A careful observer of Henhenit's labor would have seen her large, obviously gravid belly but would have also noticed a second bulge expanding above her pubic bone, rising gradually toward her navel. This was her bladder, which was slowly filling with the urine that she could not expel. It was stretching and thinning, all the while battered by her baby's head, which crushed the base of her bladder against the unyielding bones with each uterine contraction.

After more than three days in labor, Henhenit developed a fever. She was weak and had started bleeding. An infection had started in her uterus, and the discharge from her vagina was rank. For two days, she had been squatting on the bricks the midwives used to help support women in childbirth, valiantly straining to push the baby through her pelvis, but her legs had given out. At first they just lost their feeling, but eventually she could not move them at all—the pressure from her baby's had had compressed the plexus of lumbosacral nerves on each side of her pelvis, crippling her. Now she could neither stand nor walk. She fell off the bricks and toppled over onto the floor. Her servants had to carry her to bed.

She became delirious, drifting in and out of consciousness. In the fourth day of her labor, just when those around her had given up hope, something changed. The baby shifted and slipped lower into her pelvis. After a few more contractions, Henhenit expelled it onto the bedding in a gush of blood and foul-smelling dark green fluid. The stench was awful. The baby had been dead for several days.

The tragic death of her child saved Henhenit's life, but it also ruined what was left of it. Her labor had reached an impasse from which there was no happy exit. Many women in her situation died undelivered. In some cases (usually older women who had been through childbirth several times) the uterus ruptured, finally unable to sustain the relentless contractions that could not expel the fetus. The uterine muscle, strained to its breaking point and its fibers shredded by constant stress, would burst, expelling the baby into the woman's abdomen with fatal consequences for both mother and child. Death from hemorrhage would follow relatively swiftly. For other women, death from obstructed labor was a long, slow process, resulting eventually from the combination of infection, hemorrhage, dehydration, and utter exhaustion. Henhenit's baby began to decompose shortly after it died. Because the process of decay was slow, the body remained firm initially. Henhenit continued to labor, trying to expel the small corpse that was still trapped in her birth canal, but as it macerated, the baby's body softened. Two days later its head finally collapsed, the bones of the skull sliding over the liquefied brain. The obstruction was relieved, the body passed, and her labor was finally over.

The midwives cut the baby's umbilical cord with a flint *peseshkef*-knife—an easy task in this case, since the decomposition of the tissues was quite advanced—and took its body away. The placenta separated soon afterward and was dutifully removed. As soon as the placenta was out, the midwives began vigorously to massage Henhenit's uterus, an agonizing procedure after four days in labor with an infection setting in, but it was important to expel the clots and fluid and to make the uterus contract. If the uterus did not clamp down forcefully enough, Henhenit could bleed to death, a common complication in cases where the uterus was exhausted after prolonged labor. Fortunately, her bleeding was not severe.

They carried Henhenit to another room, where they washed her and laid her on a fresh bed. In a few days she was able to sit up and eat soft foods, but she still could not stand or walk. The grief of her child's death compounded her physical misery, but the worst was yet to come.

Henhenit was wet. With some alarm she thought that she was bleeding. She reached down with her hand and touched herself but found only a little blood, nothing unusual for a woman who had given birth a few days before. Oddly, her hand smelled like urine. Henhenit could not remember when last she had urinated, but she knew she was not trying to empty her bladder just then. There was no sensation of bladder fullness. The wetness increased. Her bedding was now sodden with urine. She called out to her servants. They lifted her up, carried the wet linen away, replaced her bedding, and laid her down again.

"Incompetent fools," she thought as she slid her hand over the cloth by her hips. "The bed is still wet." She ordered them to repeat the process, berating them for their negligence. Again they lifted her up, carried away the wet linens, replaced her bedding, and laid her down again. She was still wet.

To her horror, Henhenit realized that the problem was not her servants; it was her. She had no control over her urine. It was dribbling out in a constant stream, but it was not coming out of the urethra as it should have; rather, it was running out of her vagina. Whenever she moved, she caused a trickle of urine. When she raised herself up, the trickle became a gush. Henhenit had developed a vesico-vaginal fistula.

Her labor had been obstructed because her pelvis was too small to allow the passage of her baby. In the lengthy struggle that ensued, the soft tissues of her bladder and vagina had been trapped between her pelvic bones and the fetal skull as the baby was forced deep into her pelvis by the uterine contractions. Like seeds of barley strewn between two millstones, these vulnerable tissues had been crushed by the forces pressing down on them. Unable to void because her outlet was obstructed by the fetal head, Henhenit's bladder had become grossly overdistended. As it stretched, the bladder grew thinner and thinner and progressively more vulnerable to injury. Eventually the pressure from the baby's head cut off the blood flowing through the fragile capillaries supplying the bladder wall and vagina. Deprived of their oxygen supply, these tissues died. Over the next few days these tissues decayed just as had the dead fetus that had been lodged against them. After Henhenit passed her stillborn fetus, the necrotic tissues separating her vagina and bladder also came away, producing a massive hole—a fistula—between these two structures.

As a result of this injury, Henhenit was no longer able to hold urine. Her kidneys continued to function, filtering the waste from her blood to produce a steady stream of urine, but when the urine passed through the ureters into her bladder it simply ran out through the large hole that now existed there. The urine dribbled into her vagina, down her thighs and legs and onto the bedding on which she lay, anxious and fearful. Because urine formation is a continuous process, Henhenit was always wet. Each time the ureters contracted, another pulsation of urine was sent to her injured bladder, where it would splash over the edges of the fistula, across the raw tissues of her vagina, and down her genitals. Over time, her skin was eroded by the constant exposure to the wetness and the irritating organic salts contained in the urine, creating painful ulcers that would not heal. No matter how much she bathed, no matter how often her bedding was changed and she was helped into new clothes, Henhenit could never get dry.

Worse still, she stank. There was no other way to describe it. Living with Henhenit was like living in a latrine. Urine was a constant presence that neither she nor anyone else could control. Perhaps Hapy, the great god of the Nile flood, could have washed the stench away, but he, like Hathor, was unresponsive to her prayers. As a queen of Egypt, Henhenit could get fragrant spices from the land of Punt, but even these were not sufficient to mask the odor that followed her everywhere she went.

When Montuhotep II heard of her terrible ordeal, he was saddened. Henhenit had been one of his favorites, she of the lithe figure and the sparkling eyes. He prayed for her recovery, and on several occasions he even visited her, but he was dismayed by what he found. She could not rise to greet him, and even though she had been dressed in the most elegant of garments, it was obvious that something was terribly, horribly wrong. No amount of padding or incense could mask Henhenit's problem for long.

The pharaoh summoned his senior physician, who had seen every type of battle wound and illness. A wise clinician of vast experience, he understood Henhenit's problem as soon as he saw her. "This is not an illness that can be treated," he told the king. "Try to make her comfortable and pray to the gods. There is nothing we can do."

As a concession to his other wives (who complained about the smell and the wetness), Montuhotep II removed Henhenit and sent her away. He built her a small villa on the west bank of the Nile—the side of the river where the dead were buried—because, for all intents and purposes, Henhenit had departed from the land of the living. A few slaves (who had no choice in the matter) were sent to live with her and to continue the endlessly repetitive daily tasks of bathing her and washing mountains of laundry, but many of them mocked Henhenit behind her back. They may have been slaves, but at least they could control their bladders. Some queen of Egypt!

Her friend and cowife, Kauit, a fellow priestess of Hathor, came to see Henhenit in her now-humble lodgings, but because the distance from the palace was great, these visits were sporadic. Over time, they grew further and further apart; eventually they stopped altogether. The Great Wife Tem, principal queen of Egypt and mother of Montuhotep's presumed heir, was polite but distant. She did not visit Henhenit. In fact, Tem was pleased at the way things had worked out (though she did not state this publicly). Not only was Henhenit's child—a potential rival to her own son—stillborn, but the devastating injuries that she had sustained during labor eliminated her (she of the slender hips and fetching smile!) as a competitor for Pharaoh's affection.

Eventually Henhenit regained enough strength and movement in her legs (the left one was always worse) to walk unsteadily using a stick for support, but she never went out in public. She was always wet, and the chronic sores on her vulva and thighs made it painful to walk any distance. She trailed urine wherever she went, and the slaves made little jokes among themselves about "Henhenit's private River Nile" that, unlike their river, was constantly in flood. She grew accustomed to the smell—what else could she do?—even though others were repulsed by it.

As her health worsened, Henhenit descended into a deep depression. Lonely, abandoned, mocked, and miserable, she often had back and flank pain from the chronic infections that ascended up her urinary tract to attack her kidneys. Gradually her kidneys began to fail, and one night Henhenit lost consciousness. She died the next morning.

Her slaves brought word to the palace that Henhenit was dead. The royal court activated the proper funerary protocols, and Henhenit's body was given over to the embalmers, who washed her body and began to prepare it for burial. First they ran a long metal hook through her nose into her skull so that they could scramble her brain and remove it piece by piece. Then the mortuary priest flushed out her bowels with an enema of turpentine mixed with juniper or cedar oil before packing her body in natron—a desiccating sodium salt mined in the desert—for 70 days to remove the water from her tissues and to complete the process of mummification. It was the first time since her labor that Henhenit had been dry.

Her body was wrapped in linen bandages and carefully placed in a coffin. Montuhotep II granted permission for her to be buried in his mortuary temple, which was under construction at Deir el-Bahri, and a shaft was dug in the colonnaded court to accommodate her body. Although she was royalty, her coffin was rather plain and the tomb itself was rather small. So small, in fact, that her sarcophagus had to be prefabricated. It had been constructed in pieces so that it could be lowered into the tomb chamber and assembled there from its component parts. Her friend and cowife Kauit would eventually be buried in a tomb next to her.

The Archaeologists

Over succeeding centuries, the temple of Nebhepetre Montuhotep II was abandoned. Hatshepsut, the great pharaoh-queen of the Eighteenth Dynasty, would later borrow liberally (both architecturally and, in a few places, physically) from Montuhotep's temple as she constructed her own magnificent mortuary shrine that impinged on the edges of Montuhotep's space. The rubble of centuries gradually accumulated, and Montuhotep's temple was buried in debris. In 1893 an archaeological society called the Egypt Exploration Fund began excavations at Deir el-Bahri, employing 85 eager Egyptian workmen with shovels to reveal the lost works of the Eleventh Dynasty. After a decade of work, they uncovered the remains of Montuhotep's temple.

As the excavation progressed, it reached the colonnaded court on the western end of the temple, a rectangular space some 65 feet wide and 75 feet long, in which were two rows of octagonal columns with eight pillars in each row. As the team excavated and mapped, they uncovered "pit tomb number 11." As the official report by H. R. Hall and E. R. Ayrton described it, "Situated to the south of No. 10, this tomb had originally been under one of the columns of the temple." This was the tomb of Henhenit.

"The pavement had been removed," Hall and Ayrton wrote, "but when we discovered the shaft it had been blocked up by the fall, from the temple above, of a piece of a large sixteen-sided column (XVIIIth Dynasty). The shaft was full of the debris of the temple. The entrance to the chamber had been formerly closed by two large blocks of sandstone, which had been only slightly shifted by the plunderers to allow of the passage of a man's body into the interior." The tomb was not intact, having been robbed in antiquity, a sad but common finding in Egyptian archaeology, but the tomb was not empty.

> Within the chamber was a long limestone sarcophagus of the same type and construction as that of Kauit, with the exception that the long sides, the lid, and the base were each made of two slabs instead of one, which, of course, greatly facilitated its removal, also on the top of the longer side slabs were placed long pieces of stone with the grooves for the lid. It was, however, incomplete since the only ornamentation outside was a line of hieroglyphs painted green, and two uza eyes on the east side without the customary scenes. On the inside was the usual line of hieroglyphs, outlined in black, containing the . . . formula for the ka [soul] of the royal favorite and priestess Henhenit.
>
> The lid had been broken into three pieces, which lay on the rubbish accumulation at the bottom of the chamber.
>
> Fragments of a large square wooden coffin were found in the shaft, with a line of hieroglyphs painted in green on a white ground; this, like the sarcophagus, bore the name of Henhenit, priestess of Hathor, and only royal favorite.
>
> Within the sarcophagus was the mummy of a woman, no doubt Henhenit, lying on the cloth wrappings. Her hands and feet are small and delicately formed, her hair short and straight. It is a very interesting mummy. It and the sarcophagus have been assigned to the Metropolitan Museum of New York.

Seventeen years later, Herbert Winlock, then curator of Egyptian antiquities at the Metropolitan Museum, returned Henhenit's body to Cairo so that it could be examined by D. E. Derry. Upon inspecting her mummy, Derry wrote, "Even in the present dried-up condition of the parts it would be difficult for a foetal head to pass through, and there seems to be every probability that the severe damage discovered was brought about at the time of parturition, with the subsequent death of the woman."

Henhenit, queen of Egypt, priestess of the goddess Hathor, and royal favorite of Pharaoh Nebhepetre Montuhotep II, was an early victim of the human "obstetrical dilemma." Humans have the most complicated obstetrical mechanics of any species of higher primates. When that birth process goes awry, the results may be disastrous—as poor Henhenit's mummy demonstrates.

Henhenit in Context

Henhenit is the earliest known case of vesico-vaginal fistula, that terrible complication of obstructed labor in which the tissues between the bladder and the vagina are destroyed by childbirth. Even though she was a prominent member of Egypt's ruling class, the circumstances of her life—and the tragic nature of her subsequent death—were determined not by her elevated social position but rather by her biology. Biology is no respecter of persons (even if they are queens of Egypt), and the biological burdens of reproduction fall exclusively upon females. The unruly nature of human reproduction means that birth is always fraught with uncertainty. The possibility of a catastrophic outcome lurks inside every pregnancy (even if only a relatively small number actually end disastrously), and every woman faces the risk of disabling illness or injury when she becomes pregnant. If a good outcome is to be salvaged when biological misadventure occurs, there must be ready access to effective obstetric care. Access to skilled attendance in childbirth, blood transfusions, antibiotics and other drugs, anesthesia, Cesarean delivery, and the like is now universally available in wealthy, industrialized countries. The average female citizen of Britain, Scandinavia, or the United States has access to lifesaving technologies that were beyond the wildest dreams of the ancient queens of Egypt, but, sadly, such lifesaving interventions are still beyond the reach of most women in the impoverished countries of sub-Saharan Africa and South Asia today. This book explores the causes, consequences, and remedies of this inequity.

CHAPTER 2

The Human Obstetrical Dilemma and Its Consequences

For a species to survive, it must reproduce successfully. Those that reproduce most effectively will be the most successful species. This simple idea is the principal point of Charles Darwin's often-misunderstood theory of evolution. "Survival of the fittest" simply means survival of those species that reproduce best. Reproduction takes place differently in different classes of animals. An amoeba splits into two "daughters." Most fish spawn eggs into the environment, where they are fertilized externally. The larvae that result develop outside their mother's body, where they are at the mercy of predators and the elements. A hen lays an egg that is fertilized internally but is subsequently covered by a hard protective shell and then expelled, after which it is incubated until it hatches. Mammalian eggs are fertilized internally and then gestate within an internal uterus (except for a few, odd, egg-laying and marsupial species) until the young have matured, at which time they are expelled into the outside world. The process of birth in mammals is called "parturition": the act of bringing forth young. It is neither simple nor straightforward. The clinical term for difficult birth is "dystocia."

Reproduction is never 100 percent successful in any species, including our own, and reproductive misadventure is common. The amoeba may not split properly and dies in the process. Spawned fish eggs may not be fertilized or may drift downstream to be dashed on river rocks. Egg-laying species such as birds, amphibians, and reptiles can suffer from a condition called "egg-binding" in which the egg forms normally but then becomes stuck in the oviduct. This condition is particularly common in small birds such as finches, cockatiels, lovebirds, and budgerigars (although it can affect almost any avian species), and it may lead to life-threatening complications. Unable to pass the egg she has produced, the distraught female suffers intensely in the effort to expel it and may even die from shock, nervous paralysis, metabolic disturbances, and intestinal or urinary tract obstruction. Veterinarians sometimes have to perform a

Cesarean delivery of the entrapped egg to save the life of a bird caught in this predicament.

Mammals also suffer from reproductive misadventure. Human farmers breed animals selectively to enhance traits that we find attractive but that may not be to the natural advantage of the species in question. It was his observations on the results of such experiments that helped Charles Darwin conceive of the idea of natural selection that lies at the heart of his theory of evolution. Large sections of his book *On the Origin of Species* deal with phenomena of this kind. Purebred dogs propagated to achieve aesthetically attractive physical characteristics often have so many reproductive problems that the only way they can reproduce is with human surgical assistance: the Cesarean section rate in purebred Boston terriers, for example, is over 90 percent.

Why Human Birth Is Difficult

Human females may also suffer from difficult labor. So common is this phenomenon that the Hebrew Bible declared it to be an immutable fact of human existence ordained by God. The Hebrew myth of human origins narrated in the book of Genesis lays the blame for difficult parturition squarely upon women themselves. According to the text, dystocia is a punishment visited upon women because Eve disobeyed God's command not to eat of the fruit of the Tree of the Knowledge of Good and Evil and persuaded her husband, Adam, to do the same. God, after discovering her transgression, said to her, "I will greatly increase your pangs in childbearing; in pain you shall bring forth children, yet your desire shall be for your husband, and he shall rule over you" (Gen. 3:16 NRSV). The priestly scribes (all male) who wrote this book therefore validated both the subordinate position of women in their society and set up a huge theological barrier to obstetrical progress that was not overcome until Queen Victoria decided to let John Snow administer chloroform anesthesia to her during the birth of her eighth child (and second son), Prince Leopold, in 1853.

In the worst cases, childbirth is not merely difficult; it is physically impossible. This occurs when there is not enough room for the fetus to pass through its mother's birth canal. Obstetricians refer to this condition as "obstructed labor." Untreated, obstructed labor is a catastrophe that rarely ends happily. If it drags on for days, obstructed labor usually ends with the death of the child and often with the death of the mother. Many women who survive this ordeal develop a fistula, so understanding obstructed labor is the key to understanding the obstetric fistula problem. To understand obstructed labor, we first need to understand the mechanics of normal human labor.

As with all other parts of the body, the shape and structure of the human pelvis is the product of competing evolutionary forces. The main force that has shaped the evolution of the human pelvis is one of our uniquely human characteristics: we walk upright on two legs. In his dialogue the *Statesman*, the ancient Greek philosopher Plato famously defined human beings as "featherless bipeds." Although it is true that we are featherless (Desmond Morris called us all "naked apes"), what is really unique about humans is that we are *obligate bipeds*; that is to say, our normal form of locomotion involves walking around upright on two legs. Other animal species, including knuckle-walking great apes and trained circus dogs, may walk around on two legs for short periods, but their movements are awkward, use great amounts of energy, and cannot be sustained for more than a few minutes. We, on the contrary, move about on two legs smoothly and gracefully. We can cover vast distances using a sustained two-legged pace and do so efficiently, even relentlessly. (We can also go around on all fours, but it is awkward, painful, and inefficient for us to do so, whereas this is not true for a lion or a quarter horse.)

It is not entirely clear just when the ancestors of our genus *Homo* (generally referred to as hominins) first began walking erect, but it seems likely that this occurred around 4 million years ago. Bipedal walking provided numerous advantages to these species, which were emerging in Africa. For example, by raising the head higher, away from the ground, bipedal walking provided better lines of sight in the tall savannah grasses. Bipedal locomotion wasn't fast—these early hominins couldn't outrun a cheetah in a life-or-death sprint—but it was well adapted to covering long distances in a steady, reliable manner, which had important implications for foraging for food. Perhaps the most significant contribution that upright locomotion made, however, was freeing the two limbs of the upper body for other uses: carrying, foraging, gathering—and, ultimately, for the development of tool use. The implications of this change were explosive and revolutionary. This was probably an important factor that also drove the increasing size of the hominin brain (about which more later). Bipedal locomotion incurred certain costs, however. These are seen most clearly in the changes that had to occur in the structure of the pelvis for us to walk upright in an efficient manner.

The pelvis is a bony ring that protects the organs of the lower abdomen: the gut, the urinary bladder, and the reproductive organs. The spinal column attaches to the pelvis at the sacrum, and the lower extremities attach to the pelvis at the iliac bones, which in turn are attached to the sacrum on the right and left sides. This means that the pelvis is the center of an amazing balancing act that keeps the upper body aligned above it while the lower body dances around below, keeping everything upright without falling to one side or the other. Although we take this process for granted during our everyday movements, it is really a complex mechanical problem that required multiple changes in skeletal anatomy to work properly.

Perhaps this is easier to understand if we compare the posture and skeletal structure of humans with that of chimpanzees, our closest biological relatives (figure 2.1). Notice first the differences in the lower limbs. Chimpanzees have shorter lower limbs and longer upper limbs than do humans because they are knuckle-walkers who stoop over while using both the upper and lower limbs for propulsion. As a result, the chimpanzee's center of gravity is different from that of humans. In our case the center of gravity is positioned directly over the pelvis. This allows us to use only the two lower

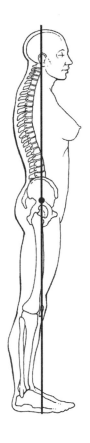
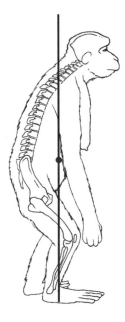

FIGURE 2.1. Differences in posture and center of gravity between humans and chimpanzees. © *Worldwide Fistula Fund, used by permission.*

limbs when we walk. We may swing our arms for balance when we stride, but we no longer support any weight with the upper limbs, as do chimpanzees. You can clearly see that the human center of gravity runs directly through the line of the hips, which are positioned directly under the spinal column and in line with the lower extremities.

Arriving at such an arrangement also required a reconfiguration of the spine. The human spinal column is S-shaped, with lumbar and cervical curves. This also allows for better central balance and a certain "springiness" that helps with locomotion. The chimpanzee spine is shaped more like a flattened C. The foramen magnum (the large hole at the base of the skull through which the spinal cord exits the brain) is also positioned differently in humans. The human skull is centered over the cervical spine, whereas in chimpanzees this articulation lies further to the back, giving the chimpanzee a more drooping head. Again, the difference is the human need to maintain central balance of the body with respect to the pelvis, and having a skull centered directly over the spine helps make this possible. The knees in humans have moved medially, toward the center of gravity, compared with the chimpanzee knee. The human foot has changed as well. We have retained a grasping thumb on our hands, but the prehensile grasping toe (which would be so useful for controlling a television remote control while in your recliner) has vanished in favor of a more locomotor-friendly alignment in the foot.

The biggest changes, however, occurred in the architecture of the pelvis itself. The differences between a human and a chimpanzee pelvis are illustrated in figure 2.2. The chimpanzee pelvis (which is probably similar to the remote ancestral pelvis of all the great apes) is essentially a cylinder, perfectly well suited to knuckle-walking locomotion. Anatomists commonly describe three planes in pelvic anatomy: the pelvic inlet, the midpelvis, and the pelvic outlet. In the chimpanzee pelvis all three planes are of similar size and they are aligned in parallel fashion, forming a cylinder. In humans, this is not the case. In humans the pelvic inlet, the midpelvis, and the pelvic outlet are all of different dimensions, and the planes are not aligned; rather, they are skewed. This is the result of the anatomic trade-offs that were required for bipedal locomotion and balance. These changes are of enormous obstetric importance. They are one of the main reasons that human birth is so difficult, particularly when compared to that of chimpanzees.

So far I have discussed only the evolutionary pressure exerted on the pelvis by bipedalism. If this were the only factor that needed consideration, we wouldn't really have much of an obstetrical problem. But the evolution of human birth has been profoundly affected by another important force that started to influence our early hominin ancestors after they began walking around on two legs. Anthropologists refer to this process as "encephalization," that is, increasing brain size over evolutionary time. The progressive encephalization of hominin species over the past 3.5 million years is shown in figure 2.3. It is easy to see the progressive and dramatic increase in cranial

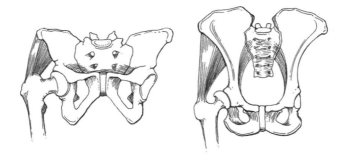

FIGURE 2.2. Differences in architecture between the human pelvis (left) and the chimpanzee pelvis (right). Note the cylindrical shape of the chimpanzee pelvis. © *Worldwide Fistula Fund, used by permission.*

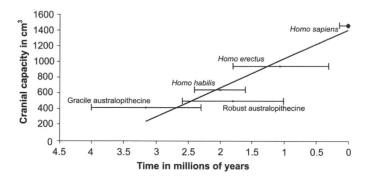

FIGURE 2.3. Progressive encephalization (increasing cranial capacity) in the course of hominin evolution. © *Worldwide Fistula Fund, used by permission.*

capacity that has occurred between early australopithecines and modern humans. Why is this important?

Bigger brains require bigger skulls to contain them. This means that over time hominin species started producing offspring with bigger heads, which they then had to be able to pass through the pelvis during childbirth. This has been a major distinguishing characteristic of members of the genus *Homo*. The evolutionary pressures of bipedalism and encephalization were in conflict: bipedalism required a narrower, tighter pelvis with shrunken dimensions to meet the mechanical requirements of upright locomotion, but at the same time the steady increase in brain size made the fetal head fit ever more tightly into the pelvis as evolution continued. The conflict between these two forces produced what anthropologist Sherwood Washburn famously referred to as the "human obstetrical dilemma," and it is easy to see the problem that resulted: narrow pelvis + big head = difficult labor. Several evolutionary strategies developed to compensate for this problem, involving adaptations in the maternal pelvis as well as compensatory mechanisms in the human fetus and newborn infant. There were also important changes in the actual mechanics of childbirth.

The female human pelvis is built differently than the male human pelvis. This is why a forensic anthropologist looking at the skeleton of a murder victim or an ancient burial can tell whether the body in question belonged to a man or a woman. The differences, which are due almost exclusively to the requirements of childbearing, are shown in figure 2.4. The female pelvis has been under significant evolutionary pressure to change to accommodate the requirements of parturition: women who had larger pelves and easier births would have a selective advantage in reproduction compared to women whose pelves were configured differently. Over evolutionary time this has led a sexual dimorphism in the shape of the human pelvis. The male pelvis is nar-

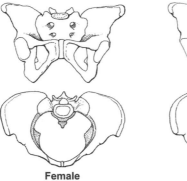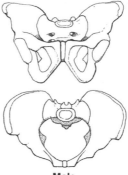

Female	Male
• Wide subpubic angle	• Narrow subpubic angle
• Round pelvic inlet	• Heart-shaped pelvic inlet
• Laterally flaring iliac blades	• Less flared iliac blades
• Larger pelvic outlet	• Smaller pelvic outlet
• Ischial spines more laterally located	• Ischial spines protrude into the outlet
• Wide sciatic notch	• Narrow sciatic notch

FIGURE 2.4. Sexual differences in human pelvic morphology.
© *Worldwide Fistula Fund, used by permission.*

rower and more heart shaped, whereas the female pelvis is more ovoid. The subpubic angle (under which a baby must pass during birth) is sharp and angular in males but wide and more rounded in females. The ischial spines—two bony lateral protuberances at the midpelvis (the plane of least dimensions where childbirth is concerned)—are more prominent and protruding in males but flatter and more lateral—off to the side—in women, where they are more or less out of the way of a fetus descending through the birth canal. The sacrum at the back of the male pelvis projects more anteriorly, whereas the female sacrum "hangs back" a bit, thus giving more pelvic capacity, an advantage in childbirth. All of these changes in the female pelvis serve to increase—even if only marginally—room in the birth canal, making it easier for the fetus to pass; but even small changes may have produced enormous reproductive advantages considering the tight fit between a human baby and the pelvis of its mother.

Two important adaptations in response to these evolutionary pressures can also be seen in the fetus and newborn. The first of these has to do with the sutures of the fetal skull. The cranium, or "braincase," of the skull is made up of eight different bones (one frontal, two parietal, two temporal, one sphenoidal, one ethmoidal, and one occipital). These bones are held together by strong, fibrous elastic tissues known as cranial sutures that are visible on any skull. In the adult, these suture lines are fixed and unyielding; the bones of the skull are fused together. The important adaptation to childbirth is that the sutures of the fetal and newborn skull are not fixed; rather, they are pliable and elastic. This means that the bones of the fetal skull are moveable; the fetal head can accommodate itself to the forces that impinge upon it during childbirth by changing its shape. The sagittal suture that runs along the middle of the top of the head and separates the two parietal bones is particularly pliable. In a difficult labor, these bones may overlap considerably, depending on the disproportion between the size of the fetal head and the size of maternal pelvis (technically called "cephalopelvic disproportion") during labor. When labor is difficult, the skull of a newborn baby often shows the molding produced by the tight fit and difficult delivery, the typical "cone head." The sutures of the skull gradually fuse between 12 and 18 months of life, providing strong, solid, bony protection for the brain, while in the meantime allowing adequate room for the rapid development of the newborn brain.

This process of brain growth outside the uterus—after birth—is another important human adaptation to our obstetric dilemma. This phenomenon is called "secondary altriciality," and it means that, unlike many species that are able to make it on their own after birth, humans require prolonged nurturing and supervision by their mothers in order to develop normally. As anthropologist Robert Martin has written in *The Cambridge Encyclopedia of Human Evolution*, "The special dependence of the human infant on parental care is a by-product of the large size of the adult human brain. Because the mother's pelvis limits the maximum size of the neonate's head, a relatively large proportion of brain growth must take place after birth—a specialization unique to humans. Considered in terms of brain development, human gestation is really 21 months long, with 9 months in the uterus followed by 12 months in the mother's care." In most primate species, brain growth slows down after birth, but in humans brain growth continues at a swift pace, particularly in the first year of life. If the same degree of brain growth took place inside the womb, human birth would be well-nigh impossible.

This leads us to the subject of "obstetrical mechanics," a term that refers to the movements made by the fetus as it passes through the birth canal during delivery. The difficulty of this journey is the heart of the human obstetrical dilemma. The fit between the fetal head and the maternal pelvis in the higher primates is shown in figure 2.5: orangutans (*Pongo*), chimpanzees (*Pan*), gorillas (*Gorilla*), and humans (*Homo*). Among our primate cousins, parturition is comparatively easy because the fetus is relatively small with respect to the size of its mother, her pelvis is capacious, and the three planes of the pelvic inlet, the midpelvis, and the pelvic outlet are parallel and nicely aligned. Under these circumstances, birth is relatively quick and simple; it is essentially a "straight shot" in which the fetus simply drops through the pelvis to be born. Not so in humans: the fit between a human fetus and the pelvis it must traverse is tight. Human labor is long and arduous by comparison. For a human fetus to be born, it must execute a precise series of maneuvers as it descends through

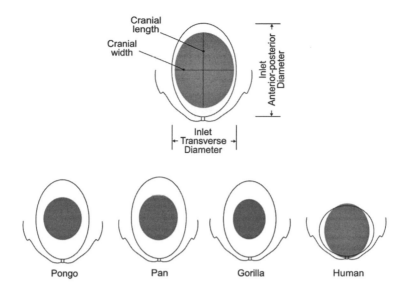

FIGURE 2.5. Relationships between the fetal head and the maternal pelvis in higher primates: *Pongo* (orangutan), *Pan* (chimpanzee), *Gorilla* (gorilla), and humans. Note the extremely tight fit in humans. © *Worldwide Fistula Fund, used by permission.*

the birth canal, driven by the uterine contractions. It must constantly readjust its position in the bony pelvis as it descends, rotating to get through the narrow midpelvis, then realigning itself before it can emerge into the external world.

The mechanism of labor (in a normal presentation with the fetal head the foremost and lowest part down in the birth canal) consists of seven steps, shown diagrammatically in a "time lapse" sequence in figure 2.6. In early labor the fetal head engages, descends into the birth canal, flexes against the fetal chest to reorient itself, rotates internally through the narrowest portion of the pelvis at the level of the ischial spines, extends as it comes down past the midpelvis toward the outlet, rotates externally as the head comes out from under the pubic symphysis, and then is finally expelled from the pelvis at the moment of birth. In first pregnancies, particularly in young mothers, labor is often a long and tedious process, taking many hours to complete. It is not a straight shot through the pelvis as it is in many other species.

Labor can be prolonged for many reasons, including weak, inefficient, or uncoordinated uterine contractions. When the force of the contractions is strong but further progress does not occur, labor is obstructed. The most common cause of obstructed labor is feto-pelvic disproportion: the fetus is simply too large to fit through the available

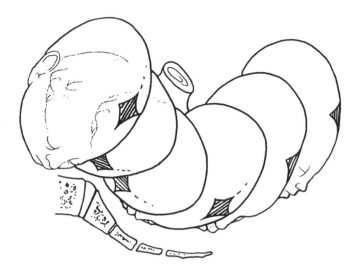

FIGURE 2.6. Rotational birth mechanics in humans, showing the progressive reorientation of the fetal head with respect to the maternal pelvis as it descends during labor. © *Worldwide Fistula Fund, used by permission.*

space in its mother's pelvis. Most commonly this is due to the size of the fetal head, which is the largest part of a baby (thus, "cephalo-pelvic disproportion"). Sometimes the obstruction is caused by diseases or deformities of the fetus, by abnormalities of the maternal pelvis, or by a malpresentation in which the baby does not come down headfirst but rather lies sideways in the pelvis (a transverse lie), comes down hindermost-fore (breech), or is positioned in some other unusual manner such as presenting with the face and chin as the leading part rather than the top of the head. Sometimes the mismatch between the pelvis and the fetus is absolute; in such cases it is physically impossible for the baby to fit through the available space. A case of absolute cephalo-pelvic disproportion, reproduced in figure 2.7, is taken from William Smellie's justly famous eighteenth-century *Sett of Anatomical Tables*. You can see that there is no way for the fetal head to traverse the space between the sacrum and the pubic bone. The head is tightly compressed, the parietal bones have been forced together and are overlapping. In this case, vaginal delivery would be impossible. So what happens then?

In resource-rich countries like the United States, Canada, Britain, or Scandinavia, this problem is solved by Cesarean section (humorously known to obstetricians as "vaginal bypass surgery"). A Cesarean delivery is a surgical operation in which the

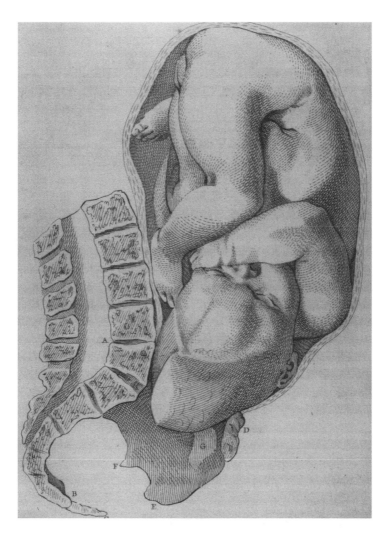

FIGURE 2.7. Absolute cephalo-pelvic disproportion, as depicted in an eighteenth-century obstetrical atlas. The fetal parietal bones are overlapping, and there is no way for the skull to fit through the pelvis. The original caption reads, "Gives a side view of a distorted pelvis . . . with the head of a full grown foetus, squeezed into the brim, the parietal bones decussating each other, and compressed into a conical form. . . . This . . . shews the impossibility in such a case to save the child, unless by the Caesarian operation, which however ought never to be performed excepting when it is impracticable to deliver at all by any other method. Even in this case, after the upper part of the head is diminished in bulk, and the bones are extracted, the greatest force must be applied in order to extract the bones of the face, and the basis of the skull, as well as the body of the foetus." *From William Smellie,* Sett of Anatomic Tables *(London, 1752), plate xxviii.*

normal route of delivery through the vagina is "bypassed" by making an incision in the abdomen and uterus and extracting the fetus (sometimes with a pair of forceps) through this alternate opening. In cases of obstructed labor, Cesarean section is lifesaving for both the mother and her child, particularly when the obstruction is diagnosed early and delivery takes place soon thereafter.

Successful Cesarean section is a relatively recent phenomenon in the history of medicine, however. Prior to the late nineteenth century, Cesarean delivery was usually only carried out on pregnant women who had just died, in a frantic attempt to save the baby after its mother's death. Because anesthesia was not yet known, blood could not yet be transfused, aseptic surgical technique had not been invented, and antibiotics didn't exist, for all practical purposes performing the operation on a living woman was to sentence her to death. Heroic therapy like this would be considered only in the most desperate of circumstances. But the discovery of anesthesia, antisepsis, and asepsis, and the subsequent capability to transfuse blood and administer antibiotics, coupled with more rigorous obstetric training and deepening clinical experience, made Cesarean delivery safe and generally accessible—at least in wealthy nations. This can be seen in the relentlessly rising rates of Cesarean delivery in the United States and other industrialized countries, where one in every three pregnant women now delivers her child by Cesarean and some women are beginning to demand Cesarean birth as a matter of convenience, without a recognized obstetric indication for the operation.

For most of the world's poorest women, however, Cesarean delivery still lies out of reach, even in cases in which it would be lifesaving for mother and child. In West Africa the rate of Cesarean delivery is only 1.3 percent—well below the absolute minimum requirements for preserving maternal life and health—and in extremely poor countries the rate is even lower. Within these societies it is the wealthier, more powerful, and more educated classes who can access such medical services. The rural poor, in particular, are largely abandoned when it comes to emergency obstetric care. What happens to them when labor becomes obstructed?

Obstructed Labor and the Vesico-Vaginal Fistula

Labor is involuntary. Although we still do not understand precisely what triggers the onset of uterine contractions, once active labor begins, it moves at its own pace. Labor can often be augmented or increased, but it is extremely difficult to slow down or to stop. It is not under voluntary control—a woman can't decide that she is too tired to go into labor or postpone it to a more convenient time. Once labor starts, it continues relentlessly until the uterus has been emptied of its contents, the baby delivered, and the afterbirth expelled. Normally, barring complications, this lasts 12 hours or less, but when labor is obstructed the normal mechanics of delivery are deranged. A useful analogy might be to an electric motor whose rotor suddenly becomes stuck. Unless the rotor loosens so that it can begin to spin freely, over time a catastrophe will occur. A careful observer will hear the ominous change in pitch as the motor starts to labor, feel the heat generated by its struggles, and eventually sniff the smoke that is produced before the engine grinds to a halt, catches fire, or explodes.

In obstructed labor, the involuntary and uncontrollable contractions of the uterus run up against an immovable object: the fetus trapped in its mother's birth canal. The uterus labors relentlessly in an attempt to drive the fetus through its mother's pelvis and complete the birth, but forward progress grinds to a halt because there is not enough space for the child to pass. The fetus is driven deeper and more tightly into the pelvis, wedged against the unyielding bones of the pelvis, which block all further progress, and the woman and her baby become trapped—just like the frozen electric motor—in a situation that is likely to end badly without some skillful outside intervention.

As the fetus is squeezed ever more tightly against the obstacle that blocks its exit, the soft tissues of its mother's pelvis are trapped in the bony vise created by the fetal head and her own pelvic bones. The pressure on these tissues increases with the unrelenting force of the uterine contractions, constricting the small blood vessels that keep these tissues alive. Eventually the blood flow is cut off completely, and the soft tissues thus entrapped begin to die.

Each scenario of obstructed labor is different, and the outcome of any individual case depends upon multiple complex and interrelated factors: Was the woman healthy when she went into labor? Is she anemic? Are there other medical conditions present such as diabetes, high blood pressure, or a bacterial infection of the uterus? Is the baby healthy and able to tolerate prolonged and difficult labor? Has the mother had multiple previous births, or is this her first? Has she had a previous Cesarean section? Is she adequately hydrated (an important consideration in hot tropical climate)? Is she able to empty her bladder? Can she eat any food to maintain her strength? Does she have emotional support?

In obstructed labors that last for several days, the fetus usually dies. In many cases the woman herself succumbs to the combination of relentless pain, exhaustion, infection, hemorrhage, and underlying poor health—her "motor" simply burns out. If the uterus is tired and worn down by multiple previous births—or if she has had a previous Cesarean section but is unable (or unwilling) to get to a hospital for emergency care—the uterine muscle may rupture, expelling the fetus and placenta into the abdominal cavity in a terminal hemorrhagic event. In most cases, the fetus dies from asphyxiation, unable to withstand the unremitting pounding of the contracting uterus. After death, the fetal body begins to decay, softening as it macerates. Eventually decomposition will reach a point where the fetal corpse becomes pliable enough to change its conformation in the maternal pelvis, slip past the point of obstruction, and slide out through the vagina as a stillbirth.

The woman's bladder is particularly vulnerable during this process (figure 2.8). The base of the female bladder and the urethra (the tube through which the bladder normally empties) are fused into the tissues of the anterior vaginal wall under the pubic bone. As labor wedges the fetal head deep in the maternal pelvis, these tissues become extremely vulnerable to injury. In many cases the pressure of the fetal head compresses the bladder and urethra up against the pubic bone, effectively closing them off and preventing the laboring woman from urinating. In normal individuals (depending on bladder capacity and fluid intake) the bladder fills and empties about eight times per day (usually more in pregnancy); but, when the fetal head is wedged into this area by obstructed labor, the outlet may be held shut so tightly that passage of urine is impossible. The kidneys do not stop the vital bodily function of producing urine, and so, with each passing hour, the pain of a progressively overdistended bladder is added to the agony of obstructed labor. Many women caught in these circumstances will not be able to urinate at all for three or four days! The bladder expands as the kidneys fill it with urine. As it stretches, the bladder wall becomes thinner and thinner, making it progressively more vulnerable to injury from the unyielding pressure of the

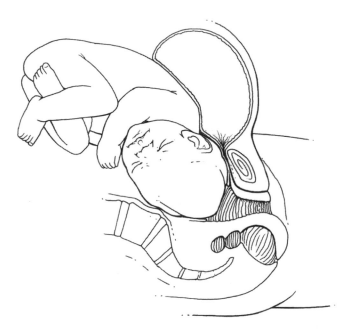

FIGURE 2.8. Impaction of the pelvic tissues during obstructed labor. Note the compression of the bladder base against the pubic bones by the fetal skull and the bladder, which has become overdistended because of the patient's inability to void. © *Worldwide Fistula Fund, used by permission.*

fetal head. Eventually the blood supply to these crushed tissues is compromised, and they die, necrosing and sloughing away. Usually this takes place several days after the birth of the stillborn child, leaving a vesico-vaginal fistula through which urine runs in a continuous and uncontrollable stream (figure 2.9).

There is no absolute duration of time in obstructed labor after which a fistula will form. An obstetric fistula is a crush injury that leads to the death of the compressed tissues, their subsequent sloughing, and formation of a passageway between the bladder and the vagina. The injury results from the interplay of multiple variables (figure 2.10): the degree of feto-pelvic disproportion, the level in the birth canal at which the obstruction occurs, the force compressing the soft tissues, the duration of that compression, and the resilience of the tissues (which is impacted by blood supply, genetics, maternal nutrition, and other factors). Together, all of these factors determine the threshold at which necrosis occurs, leading to the formation of a fistula. In some cases it may take days for this to occur; in other cases it may happen over the course of only a few hours.

The most important existential fact to comprehend about a vesico-vaginal fistula is the relentless nature of the urine loss experienced by the sufferer. To have a fistula is not a matter of being a little bit wet, cleaning up, and then being a little bit wet again a few hours later. Living with a fistula is not an on-again, off-again experience where periods of dryness alternate with intermittent periods of wetness; rather, the

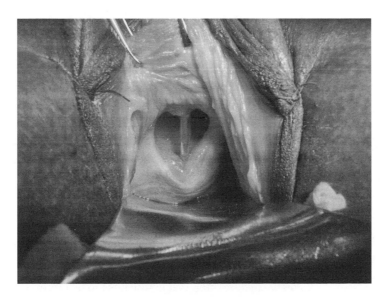

FIGURE 2.9. A vesico-vaginal fistula from obstructed labor. A metal sound has been passed through the urethra and is clearly visible through the defect in the bladder base. *Photo by Andrew Browning.*

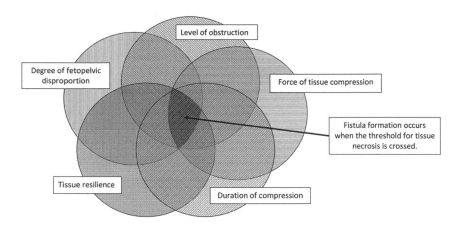

FIGURE 2.10. The multiple factors determining when a fistula will form as the result of obstructed labor. © *Worldwide Fistula Fund, used by permission.*

incontinence produced by a fistula is constant, pitiless, unremitting, and inexorable. There is no escape. There is no exit. The afflicted woman can never get dry. When she walks, the urine trails behind her. When she sits, where she sits is wet (figure 2.11). When she reclines, she lies down in urine. When she sleeps, the bedding is soaked. The urine runs out of her vagina, down her legs, onto her clothes, and onto the floor 24 hours of every day. Most women in Africa and Asia who have a fistula cannot contain this leakage even if they try. The continence pad industry doesn't exist in the impoverished nations where fistulas are a problem, but even if they wanted to use such products, the vast majority of women with a fistula are too poor to afford them. For many reasons which will be discussed later, the women who develop fistulas from childbirth trauma are among the poorest women in the world. Often they have only one set of clothes, which is constantly wet and reduced to rags.

The unremitting leakage of urine creates both physical and psychological problems. When the fistula first develops, many women are initially fastidious and compulsive about their hygiene. Over time, however, they realize they are engaged in a losing battle. No matter how hard they try, they can never stay clean. Even so, they may become obsessed with trying, devoting hours of effort every day attempting to conceal their problem. It becomes the central focus of their existence. The constant wetness starts to break down the skin around the vaginal area. When they sit or lie down, the excoriated tissues are compressed, making them vulnerable to bed sores. Urine contains organic salts, and as the moisture evaporates, a thin crust of these salts is left behind as an irritant on the skin, causing pain and creating a potential opening for secondary infection. The smell of urine in such cases can be pervasive.

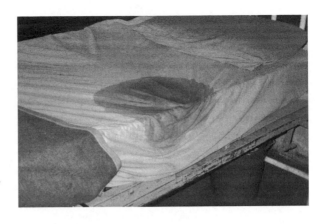

FIGURE 2.11. The plight of the fistula patient. She had been sitting on this bed for only 20 minutes before the photograph was taken. *Photo by the author. © Worldwide Fistula Fund, used by permission.*

One of the hallmarks of adult behavior in all cultures is the ability to control bodily wastes. Micturition and defecation are important recurring physiological events, but they must be performed *only* at socially appropriate times and places. "Potty-training" of one kind or another is an important biobehavioral landmark that separates infancy from maturity, and those who do not attain such developmental goals on the expected schedule cause universal parental anxiety. The loss of bowel or bladder control can be forgiven if it occurs as part of an understandable—if unfortunate—self-limited illness (such as an acute episode of gastroenteritis that produces copious diarrhea or a raging urinary tract infection that causes the bladder to empty involuntarily), but when loss of this normal control is prolonged and repetitive, the affected individuals are reclassified. They are no longer fully functioning members of adult society; they regress to a more infantile state. This has very important social implications: the development of urinary or fecal incontinence is one of the most common factors in industrialized countries that precipitates the decision to admit elderly men and women into nursing homes. In the United States, loss of urinary control often means the concurrent loss of independent living, respect, and personal autonomy as well.

Faced with the aesthetic and hygienic problems created by a fistula, the families of these women react in different ways. It is often impractical for women with a fistula to live in intimate association with their families, so over time they tend to become isolated, living in peripheral parts of the family compound away from the cooking and cleaning and day-to-day social interactions that constitute normal family life (figure 2.12). They can become even more isolated within their communities. They are not regarded as pleasant visitors whose arrival should be cause for joy or celebration; they are a burden to their friends and neighbors. Their unclean state excludes them from religious activities and community social interaction. Over time, their husbands may find them to be intolerable burdens on family life, particularly if all of their time is spent traveling from place to place in search of a cure. (It is not without exaggeration that Dr. Reg Hamlin called these women "fistula pilgrims.") Most studies of

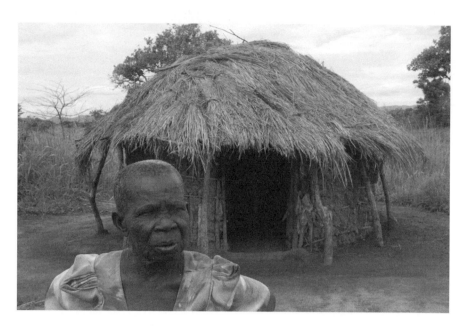

FIGURE 2.12. Josephine, an elderly Ugandan woman with an unrepaired vesico-vaginal fistula, and the hovel in which she lives. *Photo by the author. © Worldwide Fistula Fund, used by permission.*

fistula patients show extremely high levels of divorce or separation, particularly the longer the fistula has been present. Incurable chronic disease puts a similar stress on marriages in Western countries.

And in cultures where the physical cause of the fistula—a disruption of normal obstetrical mechanics resulting in prolonged obstructed labor—is not well understood, rumors of the condition being caused by the presence of an ugly venereal disease, by sexual licentiousness, by other kinds of immoral personal behavior, or by the visitation of divine punishment from God or the ancestral spirits are all too easy to circulate. To the physical stigma of constant urine loss is often added an undeserved moral stigma as well.

It should be no surprise that women with fistulas suffer from loss of self-esteem, poor body image, and depression. Although most fistulas can be closed surgically by skillful hands using low-technology techniques, access to surgical care is generally poor in the countries where fistulas are common (this is part of the reason these women developed a fistula in the first place). Their condition is often regarded as incurable and hopeless, when in fact this is generally not true at all. The World Health Organization estimates that there are 6 million cases of obstructed labor worldwide each year (mainly in developing countries). Thousands of new fistula cases (perhaps as many as 130,000) occur each year. Although many women who develop obstructed labor die during childbirth, the hardier ones survive. If they are unlucky enough to have a fistula, they may live in misery for many years after sustaining their injuries. There are no accurate data on fistula prevalence, largely because these women often live in remote areas and are hidden from view, but the current total capacity for fistula repair in impoverished countries is only about 10,000 cases per year, and it is unevenly distributed across sub-Saharan Africa and South Asia. The worst of these cases have become "dead women walking." It is no wonder that some take their own lives. My friend Dr. Abbo Hassan Abbo, professor of obstetrics and gynecology at the University of Khartoum Faculty of Medicine in Sudan, tells a heart-rending story of group of Somali women with fistulas who chained themselves together and jumped off the dock in Mogadishu in a mass suicide.

Other Consequences of Obstructed Labor

This is all pretty depressing, but the reality is actually often even worse. A vesico-vaginal fistula is only the most obvious of a complex set of injuries that may be produced by obstructed labor. This spectrum of injuries is known by the somewhat cumbersome name of the "obstructed labor injury complex" (table 2.1). With a little explanation, however, it is easy to understand how these injuries occur.

The female pelvis is essentially a bony funnel through which three main organ systems exit, each with its own outlet or orifice: the urinary tract at the top (bladder and urethra), the genital tract in the middle (uterus, cervix, and vagina), and the gastrointestinal tract at the bottom (the sigmoid colon, rectum, and anus). These organs are supported by a complex network of muscles and connective tissue which form the pelvic floor, all supplied by a series of blood vessels and nerves. The major nerve trunks come out of the lumbosacral spine, curve around the sides of the pelvis, and exit to form the nerves that innervate the lower extremities. Gestation occurs in the uterus, from which the fetus is expelled during labor. Because the genital tract lies between the urinary and the gastrointestinal tracts as they exit the pelvis, any or all of these three organ systems may be damaged by the mechanical derangements that occur during obstructed labor, depending upon the location, nature, and degree of the obstruction, and how long labor lasts.

Obstructed labor is implicated in many acute obstetrical injuries. There is often injury to the cervix, which may be trapped between the fetal head and the maternal pelvis. When labor is prolonged, the uterine muscle gets tired, and, after delivery has been accomplished, it may not contract down firmly on the placental attachment site, leading to postpartum hemorrhage. The fetus and placenta are normally wrapped up inside a sac filled with sterile fluid (the amniotic membranes and fluid). This sac ruptures during delivery (the breaking of the waters), and when it does, the sterile contents of the uterus are now exposed to the external environment. The longer labor continues without delivery of the fetus and the placenta, the greater is the likelihood

Table 2.1. *Spectrum of injuries in the obstructed labor injury complex*

Acute Obstetric Injury
Hemorrhage, especially postpartum hemorrhage from uterine atony
Intrauterine infection and/or systemic sepsis
Deep venous thrombosis
Massive vulvar edema
Pathological uterine retraction ring (Bandl's ring)
Uterine rupture

Urologic Injury
Genito-urinary fistulas (vesico-vaginal fistula and complex combinations of injuries)
Urethral damage, including complete loss of the urethra
Bladder stone formation
Urinary stress incontinence
Acute and chronic ureteral injury (hydro-uretero-nephrosis)
Acute and chronic urinary tract infection (chronic pyelonephritis)
Kidney failure

Gynecologic Injury
Cessation of menstruation (amenorrhea)
Vagina scarring and narrowing, leading to loss of sexual capability
Damage to the cervix, including complete loss of the cervix
Pelvic inflammatory disease
Infertility and childlessness

Gastrointestinal Injury
Recto-vaginal fistula
Scarring and narrowing of the rectum
Anal sphincter injury and anal incontinence

Musculoskeletal Injury
Inflammation and injury of the pubic bone
Diffuse trauma to the pelvic floor

Neurological Injury
Foot drop
Neuropathic bladder dysfunction

Dermatological Injury
Chronic excoriation of the skin from maceration by urine and feces

Fetal/Neonatal Injury
Over 90% stillbirth rate with a high death rate among living newborns
Neonatal asphyxiation, infection and birth injuries (such as scalp damage, nerve palsies, bleeding in
 the brain, etc.)

Psychosocial Injury
Social isolation
Separation and divorce
Worsening poverty
Malnutrition
Posttraumatic stress disorder
Depression, sometimes leading to suicide

that an infection will set in. Prolonged labor—particularly when well-meaning birth attendants have been examining the woman or attempting to manipulate the intrauterine contents—sets the stage for a uterine infection (chorioamnionitis and endomyometritis), which may spread beyond the confines of the uterus to produce life-threatening systemic sepsis. The constant straining and pushing during labor may produce massive edema of the external genitalia and increases the risk (which is already increased by the simple fact of being pregnant) of a potentially fatal blood clot in the pelvis or lower extremities. In some cases of difficult or obstructed labor, the uterus actually goes into a peculiar kind of muscular spasm, producing something called a Bandl's contraction ring, which constricts the uterus, prevents delivery, and may actually injure the fetus if fetal parts are trapped within the muscular ring itself. In the worst cases, the uterus simply gives way and ruptures, producing a surgical emergency as the fetus and placenta are expelled into the abdominal cavity.

I have remarked already on genito-urinary fistula as the most prominent urological injury caused by obstructed labor. Obstetric fistulas usually form between the bladder and the vagina, but any part of the lower urinary tract may be involved. Given the right circumstances, quite complex fistulas may result. For example, a patient may develop a compression injury to the ureter (the tube that brings urine down to the bladder from the kidney) that produces a uretero-vaginal fistula. In these cases the bladder is intact, but there is a hole in the "pipe" carrying urine to the bladder. Diagnosis of this problem may be tricky and the treatment more complicated. In other cases the crush injury primarily affects the urethra, the tube through which urine normally passes out of the bladder during voiding. These injuries are particularly difficult to repair because the entire urethral tube may be destroyed and it is often difficult to reconstruct a functioning conduit that also maintains normal continence. In some cases (often if a Cesarean delivery has been performed) the fistula may exit the bladder and enter the uterus itself, so that urine runs from the bladder into the uterine cavity and out through the cervix into the vagina. Countless complex combinations of injuries may be produced, depending on the particular circumstances that developed during labor.

Sometimes a stone forms in the bladder along the edge of the fistula or on a foreign body (such as a surgical suture) that protrudes into the bladder. The urine salts encrust the object, growing as a stalagmite does on the floor of a cave. Bladder stones are extremely irritating and very painful (Benjamin Franklin was tormented by a huge bladder stone—although not a vesico-vaginal fistula—toward the end of his life), and bladder stones are often associated with chronic infections. Successful fistula repair requires removal of the stone, allowing the bladder to heal, prior to attempting surgical closure.

The combination of chronic urinary tract infection, ureteral compression, and scar tissue formation often obstructs the drainage of the kidney, leading to chronic infection of the upper urinary tract and, over time, can cause death from kidney failure.

When the fistula from obstructed labor is huge, the bladder may be almost completely destroyed and the injury so large that it is impossible to close. In other cases, the fistula can be closed successfully by surgery, but the bladder that remains is so tiny—perhaps with a capacity of only 2 ounces—that urination must take place two or three times an hour. Such unrelenting urinary frequency is little better than a fistula. In some cases the urethral stump becomes completely detached from the damaged bladder (a so-called circumferential fistula) so that not only is there a fistula that must be closed but the urethra must also be reattached to the bladder that remains. In other cases the fistula may be closed successfully, but, because there has been so much damage to the urethra, the normal closure mechanism is completely broken. In these cases the unfortunate woman remains incontinent because even the slightest rise in abdominal pressure—from a cough, a sneeze, or picking an object up off the floor—forces urine out through the damaged urethra. This situation is really no better than a fistula and is often very difficult to treat.

Other parts of the female reproductive tract may be horrifically damaged by obstructed labor. The uterus may be infected after a prolonged and difficult labor and delivery; in some cases the walls of the uterine cavity scar together (a condition known as Asherman's syndrome), preventing both menstruation and future conception. In prolonged labors—especially labors accompanied by postpartum hemorrhage (a common phenomenon after obstructed labor, when the uterus is too exhausted to contract properly)—the woman may suffer a stroke that destroys her pituitary gland. This condition (known as Sheehan's syndrome after the Scots physician who first described it) can occur because the changes to the pituitary gland during normal pregnancy make it vulnerable to sudden massive changes in circulating blood volume. The pituitary gland enlarges markedly during pregnancy, in part because of the normal increase in blood volume and in part because of the increasing hormonal demands created by pregnancy. The pituitary is nourished by a delicate network of capillary blood vessels, but when a massive hemorrhage occurs after delivery, the rapid loss of blood that may result can produce a precipitous drop in pressure inside these delicate vessels that leads to a "pituitary stroke": infarction of the gland, tissue death, and loss of pituitary function. The result (if the woman survives the hemorrhage and the acute endocrinologic changes that may develop) is a failure to lactate normally, loss of menstrual periods, infertility, loss of adrenal stress hormones, and a wide range of other endocrinologic side effects, some of which may be subtle but debilitating. This condition is now extremely rare in industrialized countries. Today Sheehan's syndrome is found almost exclusively in areas where obstetric care is poor or nonexistent—the places most affected by obstetric fistula.

Pressure necrosis of the genital tissues is common after obstructed labor. The same process that leads to the formation of a genito-urinary fistula can also damage wide swaths of the vagina, depending on what is compressed and for how long. When a fistula forms, the normal tissue that separates the bladder from the vagina dies and sloughs away, but in many cases the area of necrosis is surrounded by badly injured tissues that somehow manage to survive. In the course of healing, dense scar tissue often forms at the site of injury, usually surrounding the fistula itself. During surgical repair, this tissue must be released or cut away. In some cases the vagina has been so heavily damaged that it shrivels away almost entirely, leaving only a small scarred and foreshortened lumen that will barely admit the introduction of a little finger, much less a husband's penis. When this happens normal sexual functioning is impossible, and infertility is almost certain. In other cases the cervix—which plays an important role in conception and which also must dilate and thin out to allow the birth of a child—is often badly damaged during obstructed labor, and in some cases it is entirely destroyed. Future fertility is almost impossible when this occurs.

There is normally a continuous, open pathway in the human female genital tract between the vagina and abdomino-pelvic cavity. The vagina is open to the outside world. The cervix opens into the vagina and connects the vagina with the uterine cavity. The Fallopian tubes exit from the uterine cavity into the pelvis, where they lie in close proximity to the ovaries. When ovulation occurs, an egg is released from the ovary, grasped by the fimbriated end of the tube and taken inside, where it is fertilized. The fertilized egg then descends into the uterus, where it implants and gestates, eventually to begin the process of parturition at the end of pregnancy. But this open anatomy also means that the female genital tract is highly susceptible to ascending infection if pathogenic bacteria from the vagina manage to gain entry into the cervix and uterus. When such an infection occurs, it may lead to scarring of the uterine lining and particularly to scarring and damage to the tubes, which become blocked. This infection (pelvic inflammatory disease) causes acute pain, abscess formation, and subsequent "tubal factor" infertility (because there is no longer free passage of egg from above or easy entry of sperm from below). The result may be acute life-threatening infection in severe cases and chronic pain and infertility afterward. Women who have suffered from obstructed labor are at high risk for these complications.

It is easy to see, then, how this combination of injuries leads to infertility and subsequent childlessness. The pattern is often repeated. Obstetrician-gynecologist Andrew Browning has written, "Obstetric fistula patients invariably have dreadful obstetric histories. The antecedent delivery usually ends in a stillbirth and even multiparous patients often have previous histories of multiple stillbirths and neonatal deaths." In a series of 899 patients with fistulas seen at Evangel Hospital in Jos, Nigeria, Wall and colleagues found a stillbirth rate of 92 percent for the index pregnancies in which the fistula occurred. Of the 75 live births that resulted from these pregnancies, there were an additional 14 neonatal deaths, usually within a week of delivery. The past reproductive history of these women was indeed dreadful. As a group, these 899 women had given birth to a total of 2,729 children, of whom only 819 (30 percent) were still alive.

Andrew Browning evaluated a series of 49 patients who became pregnant after successful fistula repair surgery and for whom clinical records were available. As a group these women had had 115 deliveries prior to development of a fistula but only 33 live births (28.7 percent). Of the 49 pregnancies Andrew followed after fistula surgery, five patients had a planned elective Cesarean delivery prior to labor, all with a live birth. Forty-one patients had emergency Cesarean sections, two following premature rupture of their membranes, the rest in early labor. One patient had a set of live-born twins, one patient had a stillbirth when her operation was unexpectedly delayed. Three other women had vaginal deliveries: one precipitously, resulting in a live birth; one extremely prematurely at 26 weeks and complicated by severe malaria, ending in a neonatal death; the last also premature, resulting in a neonatal death. Over the same period, an additional 24 women who had had a successful fistula repair operation returned to the hospital with a another fistula that resulted from obstructed labor in a subsequent pregnancy. All of the babies involved were stillborn.

The gastrointestinal tract exits the pelvis behind the vagina, so it is also potentially subject to the same kinds of compression injuries during obstructed labor as those that affect the urinary tract. A recto-vaginal fistula is a fistulous connection between the rectum and the vagina. Because the human pelvis opens posteriorly, there are fewer bony obstacles there than in the front. Recto-vaginal fistulas are less common in obstructed labor than are vesico-vaginal fistulas, but they still occur, often in combination with a genito-urinary fistula. Women with combined recto- and vesico-vaginal fistulas are especially miserable. To the misfortune of constant urine loss is added the wretchedness of continual loss of gas and stool. The resulting skin problems are compounded, and the offensiveness of her condition is greatly multiplied in these circumstances. Successful repair of combined fistulas is often more difficult than repair of an isolated urinary or rectal injury, and in the worst cases there is scarring and stricturing of the rectum to contend with as well.

Not all anorectal injuries in newly delivered women are the result of tissue compression during obstructed labor. The bony arch of the pelvis rises anteriorly, blocking exit of the fetus in that direction, but in the posterior vagina only muscle and soft connective tissue lie in the way of the fetal head as it is delivered. In difficult deliveries, this soft tissue may tear, ripping through the perineum and anal sphincter into the rectal lumen itself. The anal sphincter is unique because it is a circular muscle that normally remains contracted all the time, unlike other muscles, which are activated intermittently. Muscles contract by shortening their fibers, so when the circular anal sphincter muscle is torn, it retracts. This may open the anal outlet so completely that retention of any stool is impossible. When an obstetric recto-vaginal fistula occurs today in an industrialized nation, it is almost always due to an acute laceration of the sphincter (often associated with forceps or an unsupervised precipitous delivery) rather than from the pressure necrosis that occurs during prolonged obstructed labor. These are outlet injuries from acute delivery trauma rather than the crush injuries from obstruction, which tend to occur higher up in the vagina during obstructed labor, but even partial tears of these muscular structures may have a lifelong impact on women's pelvic health.

One of the most devastating injuries from obstructed labor is foot drop. In this condition the nerves to the lower extremity are damaged, leading to loss of muscle function in the foot (figure 2.13). The injury is usually caused by compression of the lumbosacral nerve plexus in the pelvis by the fetal head, but it may also occur in the limb itself by injuring a peripheral nerve as the woman squats and pushes for hours trying to get the baby to come out.

A woman with foot drop is unable to dorsiflex her foot, meaning that she is unable to raise her foot normally during walking. Because of the nerve injury, the foot hangs down limply from her ankle. In order to walk she must therefore adopt a high-stepping gait on the affected side, raising her entire leg up into the air to move forward. Not only is this an extremely inefficient way to walk, which requires an increased expenditure of energy, but it also puts the foot itself at risk for trauma from being knocked against rocks, roots, and other obstacles.

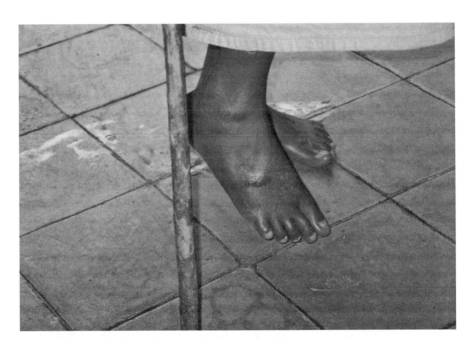

FIGURE 2.13. Foot drop due to compression of the lumbosacral nerve plexus by the fetal head during labor. Note how this patient must walk using a stick for support. Note also the trail of urine that follows her everywhere. *Photo by the author.* © *Worldwide Fistula Fund, used by permission.*

Most women with foot drop can manage to get around only with the aid of a walking-stick. Fortunately, many women who develop this condition (known in the older medical literature as "obstetric palsy") will recover spontaneously over time, but in the worst cases both sides of the body are affected and the unfortunate woman is unable to walk at all. When this occurs she will likely spend most of her time lying down, swaddled in urine-soaked bedding, an emblem of complete human despair. Unable to move without assistance and lacking adequate physical activity, she will gradually develop limb contractures and become a complete invalid. These are among the most heart-rending cases of obstetric fistula.

The cumulative effects of such injuries are overwhelmingly tragic, particularly since many of these devastated women are still only children themselves. Barely past puberty, they are suddenly confronted with a cataclysmic change in their life circumstances. Rather than entering into their much-anticipated and highly desired status as new mothers (and therefore, as fully adult members of society), their life prospects have instead turned to ashes. They are left not only with the grief of a dead baby but also with a profoundly altered body image, a degrading and stigmatizing affliction that is difficult to understand, and a future that will likely be dominated by social isolation, separation and divorce, childlessness, poverty, depression, and despair.

Adverse events of this kind are difficult to comprehend. What is obstructed labor like in the real world, in clinical circumstances where those in charge lack the resources, skill, knowledge, and understanding to deal with such complications? Perhaps the most moving description of a case comes from the pen of Dr. Naguib Mahfouz. Dr. Mahfouz, who was mentioned in passing in chapter 1, was the first native Egyptian to qualify as an obstetrician-gynecologist. In 1966 he wrote an autobiographical memoir called *The Life of an Egyptian Doctor*. In it he recounted the event during his medical school career that prompted him to choose obstetrics as his specialty.

The Ordeal of Dr. Mahfouz

When he was a medical student in Alexandria, Egypt, at the turn of the twentieth century, it was customary for members of the medical school faculty to eat lunch with the medical students. Mahfouz remembered that one day Dr. Shoukry, who was the assistant director of the government hospital in Alexandria, missed lunch but joined the students for dinner later, looking very worried. He explained to Mahfouz that he had a case of difficult labor and asked him whether he would like to help out. Mahfouz, who was only a teenager himself at the time and had no experience at all in matters of reproductive medicine, jumped at this unexpected opportunity. At this point in his medical career, he had never even seen a normal delivery, much less a complication or a case of obstructed labor. He recounted what happened next:

"I went with him to his clinic and there found on the operating table a lady whom they had tried, unsuccessfully, to deliver with forceps without anaesthesia." Consider what it would be like to have undergone multiple failed attempts at instrumental delivery without any pain relief. Mahfouz, who as yet was still only a lowly medical student, was nonetheless put into service as an anesthetist. He wrote, "I began to administer the anaesthetic and reassured the patient, saying, 'Rest assured your labour will soon end successfully.'" She answered, as he later recalled, "In your hands I am not afraid for your face gives me courage." Thereafter, they struggled.

"For two hours Dr. Shoukry tried, unsuccessfully, to deliver the head with forceps but it would not come down. He then asked me to change places with him and try to do a podalic version and bring down a foot as my hand and arm were thinner than his." An internal podalic version is an old operative technique in obstetrics in which a hand is inserted into the uterus past the fetal head, the baby is grabbed by the feet, turned into a breech presentation, and then, using the legs for traction, the baby is pulled out backward. Attempting an internal podalic version would have been a heroic, difficult, last-ditch obstetric maneuver, and Mahfouz was justifiably appalled at being asked to attempt this himself at the very first delivery he had ever witnessed. He modestly demurred, writing, "I declined, saying that I had no experience whatsoever in deliveries."

But there was no alternative. Dr. Shoukry took over and made the attempt. "Dr. Shoukry tried to pull down a foot and it took him a whole hour before he succeeded." This was desperate obstetrics indeed. Had Mahfouz been unsuccessful in administering the anesthetic, the agony the poor woman went through would have been unimaginable.

Finally, Mahfouz wrote, Shoukry "and his assistant were able to deliver the body of the foetus up to the shoulders only but the head would not come down." They had successfully turned the baby into a breech and had delivered the legs and trunk, but now the head was trapped, stuck inside the birth canal. Undaunted, "they went on pulling the shoulders until the body of the foetus was severed from the head." Seeing the headless body of the newborn baby before him, Mahfouz was horrified. In shock and disbelief, he stammered out his suggestion that the patient be taken "to the Government hospital or else calling an obstetric surgeon into consultation. They replied that among all the Egyptian and foreign doctors in Alexandria there was not one who was an obstetrician." There were no qualified obstetricians in the entire city of Alexandria, once the wealthiest, most important, most cosmopolitan city in the world. Mahfouz staggered out of the room and ran away, shaken and stunned.

The following day, he found Dr. Shoukry and asked him about the lady's condition. He was told that she had died during the night with the head of her baby still entrapped in her uterus. This was stunning news to Mahfouz; he was completely unhorsed by these events. "I was deeply distressed," he wrote, "and could not eat all that day nor sleep a wink all night. I even took a hypnotic [sleeping pill] but still I could not sleep. The moment I began to doze the vision of the headless baby thrown on the ground and the mother lying on the table with the child's head still in her womb haunted me."

So deeply was he affected by this that for two days he was incapable of functioning. "On the third day," he recounted, "I knelt down and fervently prayed to God to save me from my insomnia and help me to devote my life to the relief of patients in difficult labour. Strange to say, I had hardly finished my prayers when I felt a sudden calm. That night I slept without hypnotics. It was then that I resolved to do everything in my power to study obstetrics and gynaecology and to dedicate my life to help women suffering from difficult labour."

At the time Mahfouz wrote, Cesarean section was not yet a common operation, and obstetrics was not a well-developed branch of medicine, particularly in poor countries like Egypt. Today, in most parts of urban Egypt (and certainly in Alexandria), obstructed labor would be diagnosed early and a Cesarean delivery would be performed before circumstances reached such an awful climax. In much of sub-Saharan Africa, however, obstructed labor is not diagnosed in a timely fashion, and the resources to deal with it simply do not exist. Likewise, the lack of surgical resources means that a woman who suffers from a vesico-vaginal fistula often cannot get an operation to cure it.

Obstetric fistulas from obstructed labor are no longer the public health problem in wealthy countries that they were at the beginning of the nineteenth century. Obstetric fistulas have been virtually eliminated from the United States and other industrialized nations by the development of safe, effective treatments for obstructed labor. The most important technologies that made this possible were the obstetrical forceps and safe, reliable techniques for Cesarean delivery. The conquest of obstructed labor was long and difficult, lasting into the twentieth century; but its accomplishment was triumphant.

CHAPTER 3

The Conquest of Obstructed Labor

Difficult labor—dystocia—develops because of abnormalities in one or more of the three key elements of childbirth. Obstetricians refer to these factors as the "Three Ps": the powers (the expulsive forces, primarily uterine contractions, but also maternal "pushing" in the second stage of labor), the passenger (the fetus and the way it is positioned in the birth canal), and the passageway (the birth canal itself). Resolving difficult labor requires identifying abnormalities in the Three Ps and correcting them. In times past, midwives had very few tools with which to do this. While it is true that women have been having babies for thousands of years, it is also true that obstetric problem solving was extremely difficult and often ineffective in the past. Many times there were no good solutions to the problems that arose, and many women died during labor, often in horrible circumstances. This chapter reviews the treatment of obstructed labor from the earliest interventions to the rise of safe Cesarean section at the end of the nineteenth century. Cesarean section is now the treatment of choice for most cases of obstructed labor. Under the right conditions Cesarean delivery is safe, effective, and lifesaving. Ready access to safe operative obstetrics is the reason that obstetric fistulas have vanished as a public health problem in the industrialized world.

In obstructed labor, where the fetus is stuck in the pelvis, unable to pass through the narrow straits between the pelvic bones, there were few effective treatments available before modern obstetric techniques began to be developed toward the end of the seventeenth century. When such cases arose, only three options were available: (1) augmentation of the expulsive forces to push the fetus out of the pelvis, (2) making the fetus smaller (a bloody and gruesome matter that killed the child if it was still living), or (3) increasing the size of the birth canal (also a bloody and gruesome matter, which often killed the mother). All three options were fraught with uncertainty, and all were difficult to accomplish successfully and safely under the circumstances that then prevailed.

In theory, the expulsive forces could be increased by making the uterus contract more vigorously by using a drug. A fungus that grew on stored grain—ergot of rye—was found to be a uterine stimulant. It was powerful, but it was also unpredictable. Not only was it difficult to prepare in a standardized manner, but it was also tricky to administer. There was no reliable dose-response curve, so the results were haphazard. It was a matter of "let's give ergot of rye and see what happens." If labor was absolutely obstructed—as it would have been in the worst cases of feto-pelvic disproportion—administration of a uterine stimulant would only have rammed the fetus more tightly into the pelvis, further crushing the woman's soft tissues and worsening the condition of both mother and child. Additionally, there was no antidote. Once ergot was given, it could not be "called back"; you were committed to whatever happened. Attempts to push the fetus out (by pummeling, shoving, or even jumping on the contracting uterus) could easily exhaust the mother or rupture the uterus, both with catastrophic consequences. Attempts to pull the fetus out through the vagina required suitably designed instruments and detailed knowledge of both pelvic anatomy and obstetrical mechanics, all of which were late arrivals to clinical practice.

Diminishing its bulk to allow the fetus to pass unobstructed—a procedure euphemistically called "lessening the fetus" or "lessening the head"—was often successful in treating obstructed labor, but this procedure required destruction of the fetus and its piecemeal removal from the vagina and uterus in a grisly attempt to save the laboring woman's life. This was physically demanding and emotionally exhausting, as well as dangerous. It carried the risk of fatal injury to the mother's internal organs if not expertly done, and usually it was undertaken only after the fetus was already dead and the woman herself was sinking fast from her laborious ordeal.

Attempts to enlarge or alter the birth canal were heroic interventions that were often fatal to the laboring woman. They required cutting through the already injured soft tissues of the vagina and pelvis, sawing through bone (as in the operation of symphysiotomy in which the pubic bones were transected to break the bony pelvic ring and expand the birth canal), or opening the belly and uterus to create an altogether new transabdominal passageway for fetal delivery by Cesarean section. The risk of infection was ubiquitous, and before the discovery of anesthesia such operations produced unimaginable suffering that could only be borne through the most formidable determination and stoicism on the part of the woman involved.

Considering these options, it should be no surprise that in most cases of obstructed labor the most commonly adopted course of action was procrastination. People simply waited in hopes that nature would somehow spontaneously put things right and that the woman would eventually deliver, unaided, by herself. Sometimes this actually did happen, if the pelvis was not excessively narrow and the fetus was not too large. If the uterine contractions remained vigorous, the child was sometimes born spontaneously (and occasionally alive), albeit with profound molding of its malleable head, and some women recovered thereafter without undue incident. In many cases, however, the fetus was asphyxiated during its ordeal, and days later the woman would pass her stillborn child after it had started to decompose and had softened enough to slide between the obstructing bones. These were the women who developed obstetric fistulas. Other women in obstructed labor simply died—from uterine rupture, from hemorrhage, from uncontrolled infection, or simply from sheer exhaustion, their vital forces utterly expended in the fruitless attempt to deliver their child.

The Obstetrical Forceps and Instrumental Vaginal Delivery

It is often said that when obstetrics is good, nothing is better, but when it goes bad, nothing is worse. These sentiments were certainly true in Europe and the United States in the eighteenth and nineteenth centuries. Although most women delivered their babies successfully and recovered from childbirth tolerably well, if obstetrics went bad—as it most often did in cases of obstructed labor—things could be grim indeed.

For most of Western history, midwifery was the exclusive domain of women. Males were involved in childbirth only in rare circumstances—usually when the delivery had gone very bad and the life of the laboring woman was at stake: cases in which an arm instead of a head presented in the vagina and delivery was impossible, for example, or cases in which a fetus had died in the uterus from obstructed labor and instruments were required to remove the decaying fetal corpse in a desperate attempt to preserve the woman's life.

This started to change toward the end of the seventeenth century, first in France, then across the Channel in England and Scotland, as well as in other European countries. Men began to take a practical interest in obstetrics. The most prominent of these "man-midwives" was a French obstetrician named François Mauriceau, who trained midwives and carried on a clinical practice at the famous Hôtel-Dieu in Paris. The term that we commonly use for such practitioners today—"obstetrician"—is a later invention; in his day Mauriceau preferred to call himself an *accoucheur*, a sophisticated (some would have said "pretentious") occupational title derived from the Old French verb *accoucher*, meaning "to give birth to a child." An *accoucheur* was a high-priced, socially elite, and fashionable male birth attendant, a man-midwife. *Accoucheurs* like Mauriceau were soon all the rage in Paris, particularly among wealthy women of high social status. Mauriceau also wrote the first high-quality textbook of obstetrics in European history.

In 1683 Mauriceau's obstetrical textbook was translated into English by Hugh Chamberlen as *The Diseases of Women with Child and in Child-bed*. Chamberlen was a well-known man-midwife, descended from a long line of successful male obstetric practitioners (themselves originally French) who had fled to England to escape religious persecution in the sixteenth century. Hugh Chamberlen had originally planned to write his own treatise on practical midwifery but decided to translate Mauriceau's work instead, including in this English edition marginal notes pointing out where he disagreed with the clinical practice of his French colleague. A translation of this kind would not have been particularly noteworthy except for the curious remarks that Chamberlen made in his preface to the book. Writing specifically in disagreement with Mauriceau's comments in chapter 17 of book 2, which described removal of a fetus trapped in obstructed labor using hooks, Chamberlen declared that horrible practices like this were no longer necessary "because my father, brothers, and my self (tho none else in Europe that I know) have, by God's blessing, and our industry, attained to, and long practiced a way to deliver women in this case, without any prejudice to them or their infants." Thus, in one of the cheesiest examples of self-promotion in the history of medicine, Chamberlen declared that he and his family possessed a secret for delivering women in difficult labor that would save their lives and the lives of their babies—if only women would come to them for help. He declined to provide details or to share his secret with the wider world.

The "secret instrument" to which Chamberlen referred was the obstetrical forceps, a surgical instrument that could grasp the fetal head to effect delivery without destroying the child in cases in which vaginal delivery would otherwise have been impossible (figure 3.1). As far as historians can tell, the Chamberlens were the first to have invented a pair of forceps like this, and they managed to keep it a closely guarded family secret for more than a century. Once Chamberlen announced his "secret," however, it wasn't long before others ferreted out the details and began to construct their own versions of the forceps. Soon the floodgates of operative delivery were opened, for both good and ill.

The forceps were a pair of (relatively) atraumatic graspers—rather like a pair of salad tongs—that were introduced into the vagina along each side of the fetal head. After the blades were passed separately, they were locked together to form a single unit. With a firm purchase on the fetal head, the operator could then apply substantial force to pull the fetus through the birth canal and into the outside world. This technique undoubtedly saved the lives of countless women and many of their children; when misapplied, however, the forceps can do enormous damage.

How did the availability of the forceps affect the treatment of obstructed labor? In cases of absolute cephalo-pelvic disproportion, where it was physically impossible for the head of the fetus to pass between the pelvic bones, the forceps were of little use. But in cases where the disproportion was relative rather than absolute, ratcheting up the expulsive forces through strategically applied traction was a true game changer.

One of the first persons to become expert in the use of forceps was a London man-midwife named William Giffard, who in 1734 published (posthumously) a book entitled *Cases in Midwifry*, which described 225 deliveries, the circumstances of each case, what he did, and the outcome. Two of his cases illustrate the extreme challenges faced

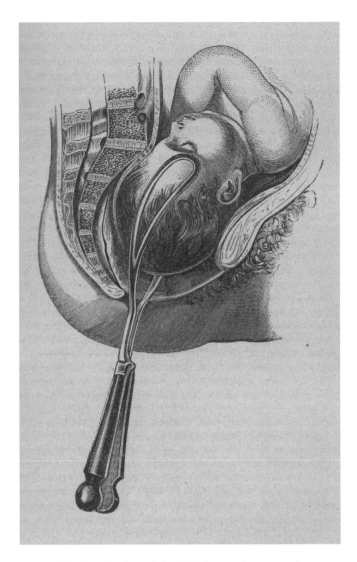

FIGURE 3.1. Application of the high forceps in a case of cephalo-pelvic disproportion. *From Francis Henry Ramsbotham, The Principles and Practice of Obstetric Medicine and Surgery (Philadelphia: Blanchard and Lea, 1859), plate 41.*

by obstetric practitioners in the early eighteenth century and what could (and could not) be achieved with the new operative technology at their disposal.

Giffard's case 59 took place on February 18, 1728, when he was called to see "a poor woman, the wife of a coachman near St. Martin's Lane," who was in labor. Giffard examined her and found her cervix incompletely dilated. She was still in the first stage of labor. The fetal head was sunk down deep and pushed back closely against her sacrum at the back of the pelvis. Her contractions were feeble, and the intervals between them were long. He gave her an enema in hopes of stimulating her labor (the enema being referred to rather picturesquely as a "carminative clyster"). He also gave her "an opiate draught," which was undoubtedly more pleasant. Both the enema and the opium were to be repeated in eight hours if she was not making any progress in labor.

Giffard returned to see his patient the following day. She had made slow progress. The fetal head was farther down in the pelvis, and her cervix was almost fully dilated. She again received a carminative clyster and a draught of opium.

On February 20 he returned again. She had now been in labor for at least 48 hours. In spite of enemas and opium, she had still not delivered. Her cervix was completely dilated, and he could readily pass his fingers between the cervix and the fetal head, which he found "was closely locked between the bones that form the pelvis." Her "pains" (contractions) were weak, and so was she. Giffard "thought it advisable to attempt her delivery, judging her not to have strength sufficient to force the child forwards, so that the life of both mother and infant might have been lost, if labour had been longer delayed." He passed his forceps (which he called his "extractor") through the cervix and over the fetal head, and "fixed it on the lower part of the occiput [bone at the back of the fetal head] near the neck. I now advised the poor woman to bear strongly down, I pulling at the same time with my extractor." After several efforts, he was able to pull the fetal head down to the vaginal opening. He then disengaged the instrument and delivered the head using his hands. "The shoulders," he reported, "stuck a little, but I soon loosened them," and "the rest of the body readily followed." The midwife who was present tied the umbilical cord and cut it, after which Giffard reached up and extracted the placenta by hand. To his delight, "the child proved a very lively and lusty boy; it had no other mark but a slight bruise near the ear, and was entirely well in two or three days." To Giffard, this case was "further proof that an infant presenting with the head, and sticking in the passage, may be brought out whole and alive, without hooks, or lessening the head." Considering what probably would have happened had he not used his "extractor" or what probably would have been done to the woman and her child less than a generation before, this was an obstetrical triumph. Yet not all cases concluded so successfully.

A little less than 18 months later, Giffard was called to another delivery involving the wife of a journeyman tailor, in Angel Court, Drury-Lane, which he described as case 71. The patient had been in labor for 30 hours, and her membranes had been ruptured for 20 hours before the midwife called for help. The baby was still so high in the pelvis that the midwife could not even tell Giffard whether it was headfirst. A course of enemas had not helped move the delivery along.

That the head had not descended after so long a time was ominous; such cases portended obstruction at the pelvic brim. An obstruction to labor this high in the pelvis never ended happily. On examination, he found the cervix fully dilated but the pelvis extremely narrow, with the sacrum tipping quite far forward toward the pubic bone. Nonetheless, her pulse was strong and her strength seemed good. She said that she was willing to persevere, so he let her be, hoping that the uterine contractions would return in force strong enough to "drive the child forwards." Giffard well knew that time and patience were usually obstetrical virtues. Many cases made unexpected progress even after many hours, and, because the fetal skull is so malleable, the combination of strong uterine contractions and molding of the fetal head might yet produce a happy result. He ordered enemas and opium, to be repeated in eight hours if no progress was made.

The following morning he "found matters just as they were the preceding day." More enemas and opium were prescribed. "About three a'clock in the afternoon," he wrote, "I met the midwife, who told me that the woman remained in the same condition; so I desired if there was no change in the evening, she would let me know; and accordingly about ten that night, a woman came and desired me to go with her, telling me that the poor woman's strength sunk apace." He hurried back to his patient. He found her exhausted and making no progress at all after at least three days in labor. An attempt at forceps delivery was necessary. What he described thereafter was an ordeal whose difficulty can scarcely be imagined, occurring as it did during a home delivery, by candlelight, without anesthetics, under unsterile conditions, and with no additional expert assistance or help.

He first passed one side of his extractor up behind one ear and attempted to use it as a lever to dislodge the fetal head (a not uncommon obstetrical maneuver then, but one that would never be attempted today). He was unsuccessful. He then passed the other half of the forceps along the other side of the head over the ear and fixed the blades in place. "I pulled with all my strength," he wrote, "but could not find it move in the least, the passage between the bones being so very strait [narrow]. . . . My instrument, in pulling, slipped off several times, the upper part of the head giving way to the pressure made upon it; wherefore, as I could not by this expedient bring the head forward beyond the bones, I judged there was but one way left to bring out the child . . ."— that was "lessening the head."

This was an alternative he was reluctant to embrace, since previously he had always been successful in drawing out a fetal head stuck in the pelvis like this, but, no matter what he did, it would not budge. The woman's pelvis was just too narrow. This was a case of absolute cephalo-pelvic disproportion (figure 3.2). The laws of physics decreed that the head could not pass through the available space. There was no alternative: "As the passage between the bones in this woman was so very strait [narrow], and the head large, I was put under the necessity of lessening the head of the child, to deliver the woman; for otherwise she must have died with the infant remaining in her."

"Lessening the head" meant collapsing the fetal skull so that it could be extracted through the narrow pelvic passageway (figure 3.3). Under the best of conditions it

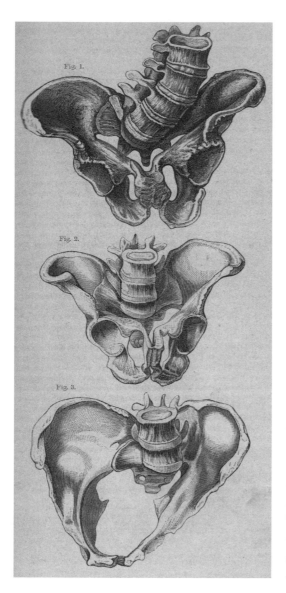

FIGURE 3.2. Deformed pelves of the kind that often produced absolute cephalo-pelvic disproportion in the eighteenth and nineteenth centuries. The pelvic diameters were so distorted that no fetus could pass through them. The middle pelvis is that of Jane Foster, who underwent the first Cesarean section in England in which the patient lived, in 1793. *From Francis Henry Ramsbotham,* The Principles and Practice of Obstetric Medicine and Surgery *(Philadelphia, Blanchard and Lea, 1859), plate 8.*

was a grisly task, even when its use was compelled by the situation. Giffard opened the fetal scalp with the tip of his scissors and drove the blades into the brain (figure 3.4).

> By this means I was able to get in two fingers, with which I enlarged the opening, and squeez'd out the brains; and taking hold of the skull and outer teguments, I drew towards me with all my strength; but yet it would not move, the bones of the head giving way, and breaking off, so that I brought out at divers times several pieces of the skull. I then passed

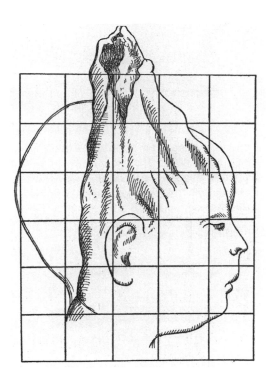

FIGURE 3.3. Illustration of a fetal head that has been "lessened" by the use of a cranioclast, demonstrating the reduction in size necessary for vaginal delivery in cases of obstructed labor. *From J. Whitridge Williams,* Obstetrics: A Text-Book for the Use of Students and Practitioners *(New York: D. Appleton, 1903), figure 406.*

up a hook, and endeavoured to fix it below the ear; but by pulling, the membranes and bones gave way; yet I had this success, the head advanced so far that I was able to get a finger into the mouth, and there bending it, I with much labour and pains brought it out by the chin. I was then in hopes I had surmounted my greatest difficulty; but I found it stuck again at the shoulders. I pulled several times at the neck with all my strength, but to no purpose, the shoulders not advancing in the least; I therefore endeavoured to pass a blunt hook into the arm-pit, but by pulling, the parts tore away; yet I had this advantage, the other shoulder advanced into the passage: I was able to pass two fingers into that arm-pit, by which I extricated both shoulders, and the remaining parts then readily followed.

He was then able to extract the placenta by hand, along with some clots of blood and a portion of the fetal membranes.

The delivery finally concluded, his attention returned to the poor suffering woman. "I put warm and soft cloths to the parts, as well to defend them from the cold air, which is very prejudicial, as to receive the impurities which flow from the womb after delivery. I ordered her at first a little wine diluted with water to refresh her after so great a fatigue, and that she should be kept quiet and still; and after an hour to be put to bed."

He coated her bruised and injured genitals with emollients liberally prepared with whale oil. The woman was so battered from her labor and delivery that at first she was unable to pass urine, but, fortunately, this soon resolved without the need of a catheter.

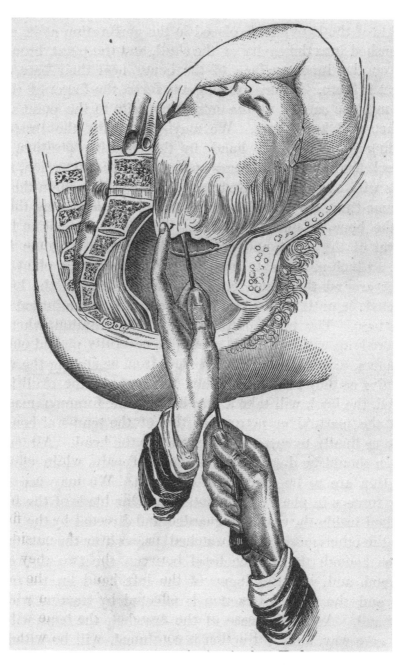

FIGURE 3.4. The technique of craniotomy to "lessen the fetal head" in cases of obstructed labor. *From William H. Byford,* A Treatise on the Theory and Practice of Obstetrics *(New York: William Wood, 1870), figure 131.*

He continued applying compresses of warm oil to the internal and external parts, and over time she gradually recovered. "The next day I found her pulse regular and soft," he noted, "very little thirst, her cleansings in good order, no pain or uneasiness in making water, and in every respect better than I could have expected . . . and on the third day all her complaints vanished."

This patient was lucky. Although she lost her child (this was the inevitable outcome of these cases at that time), she herself survived. She was fortunate to have been attended by an *accoucheur* as skilled as William Giffard. In lesser hands she might have been killed by the errant slip of an instrument wielded by a clumsy surgeon reaching up inside her uterus in an attempt to disarticulate the fetus trapped inside—a fetus that was assuredly dead after four days of hard obstructed labor. Perhaps even more importantly, this exhausted woman seems to have recovered without developing an obstetric fistula, which was a common occurrence in such labors.

The Prevalence of Obstetric Trauma

How common were traumatic deliveries like this? It is difficult to obtain accurate statistics and even more difficult to compare them with similar data from our own time when conditions are so different from those of the 1700s. The Scotsman William Smellie, probably the most skilled man-midwife of the eighteenth century, stated in his *Treatise on the Theory and Practice of Midwifery* (1752) that "difficult cases do not frequently occur," estimating that in 1,000 deliveries only 10 children "shall be born without any other than common assistance," and that "not above three, six, or eight shall want extraordinary assistance" with the use of instruments. Most women then, as most women today, delivered without extraordinary difficulty and with generally favorable neonatal outcomes. (Although what was acceptable then was vastly different from what we would consider acceptable today.)

How often did disastrous childbirth outcomes occur? How many women developed a vesico-vaginal fistula from prolonged labor in the eighteenth century? These are difficult questions to answer with any surety. In the absence of effective biological interventions the chance of dying from childbirth complications was high, perhaps as much as 1 percent of women in any given pregnancy. Looked at over the course of a reproductive lifespan in an era when effective contraception did not exist and a woman might have 12 or 15 pregnancies, her lifetime risk of dying from a childbirth complication would likely have been as high as 1 in 8 or 1 in 6. Until fairly recently, this was the risk of maternal mortality in many parts of sub-Saharan Africa, and this was also largely the case in most parts of western Europe and the United States at the beginning of the twentieth century.

Perhaps the best evidence concerning maternal morbidity and mortality for the period considered here comes from a paper by Robert Bland, the "physician-man-midwife" of the Westminster General Dispensary in London. "Lying-in" (maternity) hospitals began to appear in London in the middle of the eighteenth century as charitable institutions providing delivery care to the lower classes of society. In 1781 Bland sent a letter to the Royal Society in which he gave obstetrical statistics for the Westminster General Dispensary between 1774 and 1781. He reported the outcomes of 1,897 deliveries over that period, something less than 300 deliveries per year—a small number indeed, but the best information available. According to his statistics, 1 in 30 women had "unnatural labors," by which he meant some sort of fetal malpresentation (mainly varieties of breech presentation or transverse lie), and 1 in 111 had "laborious labors," by which he meant prolonged childbirth. Eight of these required "lessening of the head" (1 in 236 deliveries), a reliable statistic for estimating absolutely obstructed labor. In 9 additional cases forceps were used (either a single blade or both blades) to effect delivery. Nine women (1 in 210) had a uterine hemorrhage before or during labor, and one-third of these women died. Of the five women who developed an infection ("puerperal fever"), 80 percent died. One woman developed a combined vesico-vaginal and recto-vaginal fistula after labor, and another woman sustained a severe laceration of the anal sphincter. Adding it all up, he concluded, "105 of these [1,897], or 1 in 18 [5.5 percent], had preternatural or laborious births, or suffered in consequence of labour. Of this number of cases, 43, or 1 in 44, were attended with particular difficulty or danger; and 7 only, or 1 in 270, died."

Based on these statistics and using extremely conservative criteria, we may assume four cases of obstructed labor due to absolute cephalo-pelvic disproportion for every 1,000 deliveries and 1 percent of labors needing some form of operative interference. Bland's figures give a maternal mortality ratio of 330 maternal deaths per 100,000 births, which is worse than the current estimates for the modern "developing world" as a whole but roughly equivalent to the current maternal mortality ratios in West Africa. Since many maternal deaths occur in the six weeks following delivery, there is little doubt that if Bland had longer-term follow-up, his statistics would be much worse. By comparison, data from the MOMA study, a population-based prospective study of severe maternal morbidity carried out in six major West African cities, showed an overall uterine rupture rate of 1.2 per 1,000 deliveries and a vesico-vaginal fistula rate of 1.0 per 1,000 deliveries. In rural areas (where healthcare is generally much worse than in urban centers) the fistula rate was 12.4 per 1,000 deliveries. Bland's London would appear to have had an obstetric profile similar to that of modern West Africa.

The Conservative Reaction to Instrumental Obstetrics

By the end of the eighteenth century there was a conservative reaction to the obstetrical interventionism that had characterized the initial introduction of the forceps, particularly in Britain. The most influential clinical writer was Thomas Denman, the leading obstetrician of his day. Denman understood well the suffering produced by obstructed labor, writing at one point, "The distress and pain which women often endure while they are struggling through a difficult labour, is beyond all description, and seems to be more than human nature is able to bear under any other circumstances," but he was unconvinced that, in the vast majority of cases, anything other than watchful waiting was necessary. "The far greater part of those labours which are rendered difficult by the distortion of the pelvis, only require a longer time for their completion," he wrote. In his opinion, only absolute necessity could justify operative intervention. In fact, Denman was so conservative that he formulated this rule of obstetrical practice, which held sway in Britain for decades: "The head of a child shall have rested for six hours, as low as the perinaeum . . . before the forceps are applied," even if the woman's contractions have ceased. Nobody was going to accuse *him* of premature intervention (but imagine pushing for six hours with the fetal head actually at the vaginal opening and doing nothing about it).

Denman's influence permeated obstetrical thinking well past the midpoint of the nineteenth century through the writings of his successors James Blundell, Francis Henry Ramsbotham, and others. In reading the former author in 1840 or the latter in 1859, one finds almost no differences in philosophy or approach compared to Denman in 1790. Consider Blundell: "We ought to give fair trial to the full efforts of the uterus for four-and-twenty hours after the discharge of the liquor amnii [amniotic fluid];—abstaining, as long as may be, from the use of instruments;—for they are great evils; and meddlesome midwifery is bad." Or consider the astonishing statement of Ramsbotham, more than a decade after the discovery of ether and chloroform anesthesia: "I unhesitatingly declare my conviction, that the treatment of rendering a patient in labour insensible through the agency of anesthetic remedies . . . is fraught with extreme danger; and that it will at no very distant time, unless, perhaps, in some exceptional cases, be banished from the practice of the judicious obstetric physician."

Ramsbotham was a resolute anti-interventionist in obstetrics, who wrote, "If you must err, then, take my advice; and err rather by the neglect or rejection of instruments, than by their too frequent use." He steadfastly refused to consider the use of anesthesia "even where instruments are required to finish the delivery"; rather, he would rely upon the fortitude of laboring women to bear the burdens thrust upon them by childbearing, believing that "as women possess, perhaps, a larger share of passive courage than men, we may, I believe, generally trust to their fortitude." This would have been small comfort after three days in labor, however.

Women required a great deal of "passive courage" indeed if they were to withstand a long "laborious labour." Ramsbotham knew what the clinical course of unrelieved obstructed labor was like, because he described it in his textbook, *The Principles and Practice of Obstetric Medicine and Surgery* (1859). Although most women recovered "tolerably well" after the fetus had delivered, he noted that some developed "very bad symptoms" as "the consequence of depression from loss of power, excitement, or injurious pressure." Women who had endured prolonged obstructed labor could progress from "exhaustion," to "inflammation of the pelvic viscera," and finally to "deep collapse." At this end stage of the process, "the system falls into a state of exhaustion, from which it never rallies": "The mental and bodily powers are completely worn out; the pulse flags; the extremities become cold; there are excessive weariness of the limbs, vomiting, sunken features, and a hollow eye; probably no pain is complained of, and the expression of the face is sufficient to indicate the danger." The treatment was "domestic stimulants, nourishment, cordial medicines, opium, Aether, and ammonia," which were "the best and only means to restore the ebbing vitality." In reality, these women would recover on the basis of their own fortitude, or they would die.

When inflammation set in, the patient was approaching the point of crisis. "This state is known by shivering, general fever, and local pain," he wrote, "by a quick pulse, white tongue, thirst, heat and dryness of skin, deficient secretion of milk, and by the lochia [postpartum vaginal discharge] being suppressed, or scanty and of bad odour; and there is pain on pressing the lower part of the belly." Pain to palpation in the lower abdomen was usually an early sign of localized peritonitis, which often spread explosively through the abdomen and ended fatally as "puerperal fever."

When the patient reached the state of "deep collapse," her condition was ominous. Deep collapse occurred after "extensive contusions and subsequent mortification" of the injured tissues from prolonged labor. At this stage the patient would exhibit "entire prostration of strength, . . . muttering delirium and watchfulness, . . . cold clammy extremities, . . . quick, weak, tremulous and often irregular pulse," harbingers of the crisis that would resolve "after hovering on the brink of destruction" either with her death or with a slow return to health.

If such patients survived, they would often develop "sloughing" of the vagina with varying degrees of tissue destruction: a vesico-vaginal or recto-vaginal fistula or, even worse, both. "Occasionally," Ramsbotham wrote, "the bladder, rectum, and all the coats of the vagina, will become gangrenous; the three cavities will be thrown into one; and if the patient survive, of which there will then be little chance, most miserable indeed must be the remainder of her life." "Little can be done by medicine under this unfortunate condition," he thought. Rather, he recommended local care with fomentations and dressings of lint soaked in turpentine and oil, after which, the patient should be secluded. "As soon as the patient is able to be removed, she should be sent into the country; a change from the close atmosphere of the town to a more healthy air has often given a fillip to the constitution, has renovated the sinking powers, and put an immediate check to some of the worst symptoms." Getting the patient with a vesico-vaginal fistula out of the way in this manner, however, would also seclude her from view—a condition in which she would likely spend the remainder of her life, miserable, alone, and rejected by polite society.

The intensely conservative reaction that followed the introduction (and subsequent abuse) of the obstetric forceps, was summarized passionately by James Blundell, who wrote, "Beware of impatience and violence! Beware of lacerations! Have mercy upon the patient! Again I say, have mercy upon her! Remember that a thrust of the hand here, is as fatal as a thrust of the bayonet! Wounds more dreadful were not inflicted on the bloody field of Waterloo! Wombs and women are not to be taken by assault!" Yet fear of using instruments in vaginal delivery when they were absolutely indicated ruined many women's lives and led to the unnecessary deaths of their children.

Why Not Cesarean Section?

If opposition to the use of obstetric forceps was so adamant, how much more vehement was the rejection of Cesarean section in cases of obstructed labor. Women could undergo a forceps delivery and still survive even botched procedures, but until the end of the nineteenth century Cesarean section was almost assuredly a sentence of death for women. There were many reasons for this high case fatality. Foremost was that Cesarean delivery was regarded as the operation of last resort, so women undergoing it were almost dead before it started, and this was hardly conducive to favorable outcomes. There was no conception of aseptic or even antiseptic surgical technique at this time, and, in any case, most women who underwent the operation had been in labor for several days and the uterus was already infected as a result. The incision in the uterus through which the fetus would be extracted would have allowed blood and infected amniotic fluid to pour into the abdominal cavity, resulting in generalized sepsis and death in fairly short order. Errors in technique could cause massive intraoperative bleeding. Also, (as described later) there was as yet no good way to close the uterine incision, which guaranteed both continued bleeding and continual drainage of infected fluids into the abdominal cavity. The intestines could be entrapped in the unsutured uterine incision, resulting in death, and almost any other surgical misadventure that could be imagined could happen in the hands of unskilled, nervous surgeons working in bad conditions. In 1790 Thomas Denman declared starkly, "In every case in which the Caesarean operation has been performed in this country the patients have died." Although anecdotal reports of successful Cesareans had appeared dating back to the Renaissance, and numerous medieval texts illustrate miraculous Cesarean births, the practitioner who attempted Cesarean section for any reason other than absolutely desperate necessity faced withering criticism from the medical profession—and possibly worse from society and the law. The medical profession was adamantly against such brutality.

For François Mauriceau, the leading obstetrician in eighteenth-century France, Cesarean section was "damnable policy" undertaken only "to satisfy the avarice of some people, who care not much whether their wives die, provided they have a child to survive them." He doubted that it was possible for a woman to survive the procedure, writing lividly, "If they say, to render the fact less horrible in appearance, that it [Cesarean section] must never be undertaken but when the woman is reduced to the utmost extremity; to that I answer, that a woman often recovers beyond hope or probability: and, if they object that she may likewise escape after this operation; I do utterly deny it, by the testimony of the most expert chirurgeons [surgeons] that have practiced it, who always had bad success, all the women ever dying in a short time after." To Mauriceau, if you did a Cesarean, you killed the mother. There was no medical justification for cold-blooded murder.

The Irish obstetrician Fielding Ould, writing 50-some years after Mauriceau, was equally scathing in his denunciation of Cesarean delivery, referring to it as "this unparalleled piece of barbarity," "this detestable, barbarous, illegal piece of inhumanity," an operation which "must necessarily destroy the mother." Even a century after Ould, in 1840, James Blundell refused to countenance any attempts at Cesarean delivery even in cases of transverse lie, in which the fetus is positioned crossways in the uterus with an arm or shoulder foremost in the birth canal—a presentation in which vaginal delivery is physically impossible. (Today a transverse lie is recognized as an absolute indication for Cesarean section anywhere in the world.) So strong were Blundell's fears about Cesareans that he wrote, "But if we once admit the obstetric principle, that the Caesarean operation may be performed in transverse cases as a substitute for turning [repositioning the fetus in the uterus and extracting it by the feet], there would, I fear, be no end to the abusive adoption of this operation by the rash and adventurous; and the greatest mischief might ensue. Against such use of the operation, therefore, in the present state of knowledge, I feel it a duty to raise my voice."

Dr. William Simmons of Manchester, England, was a committed "anti-Cesareanist." In 1798 he reviewed the history of Cesarean section in a pamphlet entitled *Reflections on the Propriety of Performing the Caesarean Operation*. By his account—the prevailing one of his day—Cesarean section was dismal, unnecessary, unwarranted, and never indicated under any circumstances whatsoever. He wrote, "I hope that in future all trace of the Caesarean operation will be banished from professional books; for it can never be justifiable during the patient's life, and stands recorded only to disgrace the art [of obstetrics]." Near the beginning of his essay, Simmons noted that he had been drawn to the subject of Cesarean delivery "by a late occurrence," by which he obviously meant an instance of Cesarean section that had been performed locally. Simmons's little pamphlet initiated one of the most rancorous, vituperative, and long-winded professional squabbles in the history of obstetrics.

Dr. John Hull, recently arrived in Manchester, was the surgeon involved in the "late occurrence" of a Cesarean section referred to by Simmons. Hull took great personal offense at Simmons's pamphlet and responded personally, indignantly, and at length (229 pages) in a book entitled *A Defence of the Cesarean Operation*, directed against Simmons. The late eighteenth century was a rollicking, unfettered, pamphleteering age in which authors routinely attacked each other with gusto about whatever topic was at issue. Hull accused Simmons of being "actuated by invidious and malicious motives," and wishing "to destroy the character of a man," namely himself, Dr. John Hull. The arguments rocked back and forth between the two doctors (and the two camps they represented) for two years, becoming increasingly personal, defamatory, and unbalanced.

Hull's main point—which was that you could hardly expect anything other than bad outcomes in Cesarean sections if you waited until the patient was exhausted and dying rather than intervening early in the course of hopelessly obstructed labor—would eventually be proven right, but few other people were courageous enough to say so and to do so in such cases. In his book *The History of Caesarean Section*, J. H. Young states, "The general opinion amongst British obstetricians, with a few exceptions, . . . was that Caesarean section was not justified if the child could be extracted by any other method." Until the end of the nineteenth century, British obstetric practitioners would do almost anything to avoid Cesarean delivery: the use of high forceps, manual attempts to turn the fetus in the uterus and extract it by the feet, or destructive procedures such as that performed by John Giffard on the poor coachman's wife in St. Martin's Lane. For a brief period, however, there was a flurry of interest in another operative intervention in obstructed labor called symphysiotomy.

Symphysiotomy

In 1597 French surgeon Severin Pineau attended the autopsy of a woman who had been hanged for an unspecified crime only 10 days after giving birth. Pineau was struck by the fact that when her body was examined after death, her pubic bones were freely moveable, one even riding up higher than the other. Why not, he thought to himself, cut the bones of the pubic symphysis apart (symphysiotomy) in cases of difficult labor to open up the constricted passageway and permit a more sure and speedy delivery? If the bones appeared to do this themselves in certain circumstances, surely surgical intervention would be simple, timely, and lifesaving. There is no evidence that Pineau (or anyone else) actually tried this procedure on a living woman, but in 1655 J. C. de la Courvee tried it experimentally on the corpse of a woman who died in labor with the fetus still inside her.

Almost 170 years later, in 1768, a brash young surgical student named Jean-René Sigault declared to the French Royal Academy of Surgery that surgical division of the pubic bones should be introduced into practice as a substitute for Cesarean section. Sigault said that he had seen cases of spontaneous rupture of the pubis during labor (a relatively rare event). Why not do it yourself as the standard operation for difficult or impossible deliveries? Surgical ethics being somewhat more relaxed in the eighteenth century than they are today, Sigault asked the academy to give him a condemned criminal upon whom he might conduct such experiments. The academy wisely rejected his proposal.

This rejection left Sigault humiliated, and he slunk away to lick his wounds, but he did not give up. In 1772 he wrote a treatise that argued (without any actual clinical evidence) that symphysiotomy would be a safer, surer, and more rapid operation than

Cesarean section. The main argument on his behalf was the fact that Cesarean section was still a virtual death sentence for the woman who underwent one. He waited for an opportunity to prove his case (figure 3.5).

On October 1, 1777, a favorable opportunity arose. Sigault was called to consult on the fifth delivery of a soldier's wife, named Madam Souchot. Madam Souchot was a classic case of obstructed labor: She was 30 years old and a dwarf—only 3 feet 8.5 inches tall—who also had rickets and a deformed pelvis (see figure 3.2). Her obstetric history was grim. She had had four previous stillbirths, all of which required operative assistance by "internal version and extraction" to remove the dead fetuses. Internal version and extraction was a common—but difficult and dangerous—obstetrical maneuver in which the operator inserted his hand into the uterus, turned the fetus around, grabbed it by the feet and extracted it—often with considerable effort—as a breech delivery (figure 3.6). This procedure would have been unbelievably agonizing in the days before anesthesia, yet Madam Souchot had suffered through this four times before. Her previous delivery had been attended by the famous French obstetrician Andre Levret, who reportedly measured the diagonal conjugate of her pelvis (the distance between the pubic bone and the sacrum) at only 2.5 inches—certainly enough room to become pregnant, but not enough room for a baby to get out!

In the company of his friend and fellow obstetrician Alphonse Leroy, Sigault performed his first symphysiotomy, at night, by the light of a candle held by a female

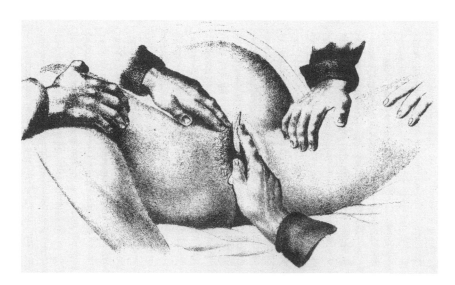

FIGURE 3.5. The technique of symphysiotomy, cutting through the cartilaginous union of the pubic bones in an attempt to widen the birth canal to allow vaginal delivery in cases of obstructed labor. *From J. P. Maygrier,* Midwifery Illustrated *(New York: Harper and Brothers, 1834), plate 52.*

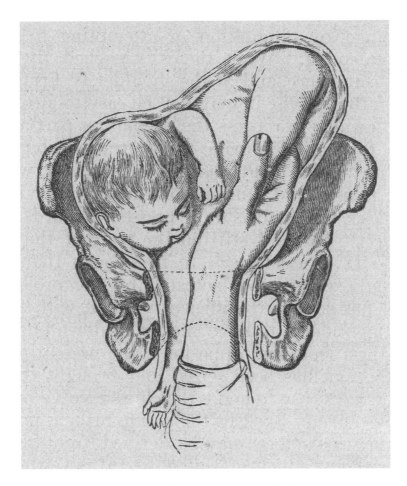

FIGURE 3.6. The technique of internal version, in which an attempt was made to reposition the fetus in the uterus, turn it into a breech, and extract it by the feet. This was difficult to do and absolutely agonizing for the laboring woman. *From William S. Playfair,* A Treatise on the Science and Practice of Midwifery *(Philadelphia; Henry C. Lea, 1876), figure 147.*

assistant. Using a long narrow-bladed surgical knife called a bistoury (more commonly used for draining abscesses), Sigault cut through the skin and fat over Madam Souchot's pubic bone, split the pyramidalis muscles, and sawed through the cartilage of her pubic symphysis. The bones split apart immediately, separating by 2.5 inches (and injuring her urethra in the process). Sigault immediately ruptured the fetal membranes, grabbed the baby's feet, and delivered the child by breech extraction. His operation of symphysiotomy worked!

Even better for Sigault was the fact that the monthly meeting of the Faculty of Medicine was to be held the day after this delivery. He attended the meeting, full of self-importance, and rendered a dramatic account of the difficult delivery he had accomplished successfully just the night before. His audience was impressed; but it should be noted that this was a meeting of the Faculty of *Medicine*, not *Surgery*. These physicians—(who would be referred to as internists today)—had little or no knowledge of either obstetrics or surgery and would have been a much softer audience for Sigault to impress than a roomful of battle-hardened surgeons. This was by no means the Academy of Surgery, which had snubbed him eight years before. Sigault persuaded the Faculty of Medicine to appoint a committee of inquiry to follow this case and to issue a report about it in due course.

On December 3, 1777, only nine weeks after her delivery, Madam Souchot herself appeared before the Faculty of Medicine. The committee of inquiry presented its report, and Sigault read another paper on the case. Madam Souchot had been able to sit up in bed six weeks after delivery, and to walk a few steps on postpartum day 46. Although she had problems with urinary incontinence from her urethral injury, she could stand alone for short periods and walk with assistance—all noteworthy but not unexpected complications of a surgically induced fracture of the pelvis (which is what the operation of symphysiotomy amounted to). The healing of her wound was hampered by the constant curious prodding of the members of the committee of observation— but Madam Souchot was clearly alive and ambulatory, which was more than many surgeons had expected when Sigault made the case for his operation nine years before.

The Faculty of Medicine was impressed. It recommended that Sigault's two papers be published (in Latin and in French), that Madam Souchot be awarded a small pension, and that Sigault and his assistant Leroy be awarded silver medals inscribed with their names in recognition of the substantial contribution to medicine they had made. Sigault's operation of symphysiotomy had been officially endorsed by a prominent medical body.

The Faculty of Surgery remained unhappy. There is an old adage in surgery that "it is better to be lucky than good." To the surgeons, Sigault's operation was a matter of luck, not prudent surgical technique, and a public controversy soon erupted, with books, pamphlets, and letters to newspapers arguing both for and against this radical new operation. The facts about Madam Souchot's pelvic capacity were disputed, and the necessity for her being delivered in this manner was questioned. As is often the case with new surgical operations, however, many people jumped on Sigault's symphysiotomy bandwagon before any significant experience had been acquired. He had been lucky in his first case, but many others who followed him were not so lucky when they tried their hands at it. A series of cases soon followed, and many of them turned out badly. Sigault's opponents took full advantage of these (predictably) poor outcomes, using them as cudgels with which they beat him both mercilessly and with enthusiasm.

Sigault's most ferocious critic was Jean-Louis Baudelocque, the most eminent obstetrician in Paris. Baudelocque was rightly concerned that the enthusiastic adoption of an unproven operation for obstructed labor could produce serious complications. He was particularly concerned about the belief (then growing, perhaps as a matter of wishful thinking) that symphysiotomy could replace Cesarean section in every case in which labor was obstructed. Baudelocque thoughtfully undertook anatomical studies on cadavers and showed that whereas the transverse diameter of the pelvis could be widened by dividing the pubic symphysis and separating the bones, most of the obstructions that occurred during labor did not involve this particular plane of the pelvis. The obstructions that really mattered were anterior-posterior (front-back) obstructions at the pelvic brim (the "superior strait"), not obstructions of the transverse plane. If you separated the pubic bones 2.5 inches, you would enlarge the anterior-posterior pelvic plane only one-third to one-half an inch—hardly enough to make a difference in a case of obstructed labor with a severely deformed pelvis.

Baudelocque soon had plenty of information about the kinds of injuries symphysiotomy could produce in the women who underwent it. Thoughtful observers immediately understood the kinds of complications that could arise, whereas enthusiasts who, in Baudelocque's words, were "seduced by the charms of the new operation," tended to overlook them in their hurry to perform the latest fashionable surgical procedure. The iliac bones articulate to the sacrum at the back of the bony pelvic ring. If that ring is broken in front and the pubic bones are separated sideways, by mechanical necessity this outward movement will be carried back to the sacroiliac joints, which could potentially be ruptured themselves. The bladder is also directly beneath, and the urethra is directly attached to, the pubic symphysis. Both organs could be injured by cavalier manipulations of these bones. If you understood, as Baudelocque did, that transverse separation of the bony ring would only marginally expand the anterior-posterior diameter at the pelvic brim, then in some cases of severe pelvic contracture you might be no better off after sawing through the pelvis at the pubic symphysis than you were before you started. This would be a horrific position in which to find yourself.

Baudelocque described several cases that vividly illustrated these complications. In one case a woman who was only three feet tall developed obstructed labor. It took three men to saw through her pubic symphysis. After they had done so, they managed to separate the pubic bones to a distance of about two fingerbreadths. Forceps were applied to deliver the fetal head and, while doing this, the separation between the bones suddenly widened to four fingers, accompanied by "a remarkable noise of tearing," as the stillborn child emerged. The woman died six days later after having been literally ripped in half.

In another case a symphysiotomy was performed, but the procedure only succeeded in producing a separation of 1.5 inches between the bones. The fetus was dead, but even then it could not be extracted through the available space. Failure to get the fetus out would have ensured the death of the patient. "Everything that art could suggest was tried," Baudelocque wrote, "but all in vain. They first pulled off the left leg [of the fetus], and pushed back the dismembered thigh into the uterus, in order to clear the way to the other extremity which they could not bring down, though M. Guerard and two other accoucheurs labored at it one after the other." Finally, it seemed like the head was starting to descend, so they waited to see whether the woman would expel it by herself, but no progress was made. They were finally forced to open the fetal head and extract the brain, in hopes of collapsing the skull so that it would pass through the severely narrowed pelvis. Eventually they applied both the forceps and the crotchet—an obstetrical hook—in attempts to extract the skull, but, he wrote, "They could only get away some pieces of it with a sort of nippers, and the rest appeared immoveable." With great effort, the fetus was eventually expelled. "This operation, begun at one o'clock in the afternoon, was not finished till about nine in the evening," he remarked. The woman died 11 days after her delivery.

In still another case a symphysiotomy was performed in an attempt to deliver a dead fetus. The symphysiotomy incision extended internally, and the woman also sustained a deep perineal laceration in the course of the manipulations to try to extract the fetus. The woman survived but was "overwhelmed with infirmities which proceeded from the operation." She was bedridden at home for two months, and, destitute, she was sent to the poorhouse, where she spent another month in bed. Her pubic bones never healed, remaining separated by more than half an inch. She also developed a prolapse of the bladder and uterus "as big as a fist." But, worst of all, the bladder and vagina were "destroyed by a gangrene" developing from the obstructed labor, the surgical injury, and the resultant infection "from whose surface the urine continually distils by two openings which seem to be those of the ureters." The result of the operation was the traumatic delivery of a dead child, pelvic instability from a nonhealing union of the pubic bones, utero-vaginal prolapse, and a vesico-vaginal fistula that could never be closed. Surely this woman would have preferred to die than to live in such a state of constant misery.

In spite of such cautionary cases, certain Italian surgeons took up the operation of symphysiotomy with enthusiasm and even tried to expand its utility beyond the limits of reason. Professor Galbiati of Naples conjured up the operation of "bipubiotomy," which he tried upon a poor pregnant dwarf on March 30, 1832. This woman was only 3 feet 6 inches tall, and the space between her pubic bone and sacrum was only one inch. Nonetheless, Galbiati tried to deliver her vaginally. According to the American obstetrician Robert Harris, Galbiati "devised the plan of opening her pelvis by a subcutaneous section with an Aitkin chain-saw, cutting the horizontal and descending rami" of the pubic bones on either side (figure 3.7). With the pubic bones completely severed, Galbiati thought he would simply be able to lift up the poor woman's pelvis in the front (rather like opening the top of a steamer trunk) and the baby would slide out beneath it. As Harris noted, "He succeeded in delivering the woman of a dead foe-

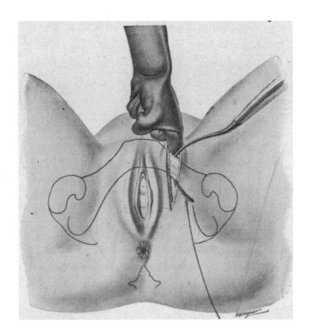

FIGURE 3.7. Pubiotomy. An alternative method to attempt enlargement of the birth canal during obstructed labor by sawing through the pubic bone itself. *From E. E. Shears and George Peaslee Shears,* Obstetrics, Normal and Operative *(Philadelphia: J. P. Lippincott, 1917), figure 396.*

tus, but such was the injury produced by stretching the tissues over the severed bones, that she died in agony on April 3d, four days later, her vagina, vulva, and surrounding tissues being all gangrenous." The operation did not generate any enthusiasm elsewhere.

In France, Baudelocque's assault on symphysiotomy withered the early enthusiasm that had developed for it. The obstetrically conservative English never really adopted it, and early bad experiences in Germany prevented the practice from taking hold there as well. Americans did not take it up, either. There was more enthusiasm for the operation in Belgium, Holland, the Italy, but for all practical purposes symphysiotomy never became a standard obstetrical practice anywhere. Today the operation is almost never used in affluent countries, but it is sometimes used with advantage in resource-poor parts of the world if surgeons understand its limitations and proper operative technique.

Cesarean Section

J. Robert Wilson has aptly remarked that "the early history of cesarean section is based principally on mythology." In ancient times there were undoubtedly numerous "experimental" Cesarean operations carried out as atrocities of war upon pregnant women who were unlucky enough to live in a town or village that was overrun by their people's enemies, but such instances (if and when they occurred) did nothing to advance legitimate medical practice. The ancient Romans, among others, had laws that forbade the burial of a woman who died while pregnant with her fetus still inside her. This was known as the Lex Regia or "King's Law," and so the dead child would be cut out of its dead mother and buried separately. Kingship among the Romans did not last long (neither did the republic), and when Rome became ruled by an emperor, the law became known as the Lex Caesarea, or "Caesar's Law." It is popularly believed that the Caesarean operation is so named because Julius Caesar was born in this manner. Definitive proof that this was *not* the case comes from the fact his mother Aurelia lived into her 60s—hardly likely if she had been subjected to this procedure.

Although common today, in ancient times to have been delivered by Cesarean section would have been miraculous. In the ancient world it was believed only fitting and proper that those who became great later in their lives should have their future greatness heralded by the miraculous nature of their births—and so their biographies were written to conform to this tradition. (The most conspicuous example of this ancient thought habit is the miraculous stories surrounding the birth of Jesus of Nazareth found in the Gospels according to Matthew and Luke in the New Testament, but there are many other instances of this phenomenon). This cultural pattern of describing the birth of eminent or holy men as occurring through a miraculous Cesarean delivery continued in western Europe throughout medieval times—but, again, it did nothing to advance surgical science.

During the Renaissance surgery began to take tiny steps forward toward a more secure, scientific foundation, and the invention of the printing press allowed thoughtful surgeons to start circulating new ideas. Obstructed labor had posed a problem as old as humankind but without the appearance of any satisfactory solution. In the late sixteenth century a few pioneers struck out boldly in their attempts to aid women who found their labors obstructed. Tradition declares (with scant evidence to support it) that Jakob Nufer, a Swiss pig-gelder, performed the operation on his own wife when her labor became arrested. She is said to have survived, and to have delivered five more children (including a set of twins), while her firstborn lived to be over the age of 70. The historical accuracy of this story (which was not written down until almost a century after it was alleged to have occurred) is highly suspect.

What can be verified is an increasing interest in the theoretical (if not the practical) solution to obstructed labor by abdominal delivery in the century following Nufer's supposed surgical triumph. Scipione Mercurio was an Italian physician who, in 1596, published a work (illustrated by woodcuts) in which he described Cesarean delivery as a remedy for pelvic contraction and obstructed labor. He recommended that the operation be performed only by skilled anatomists (he decried the practice of barbers operating on people) and stated that the operation should be done only if there were no alternative, beginning a centuries-long tradition of Cesarean section as a last resort.

To perform the operation, Mercurio wrote, the surgeon would need at least three "strong and courageous" young men or young women, two of whom were tasked with holding the arms and shoulders of the patient while the third pinioned her thighs and legs together. In the days before anesthesia, this was an essential component of the operation. Two or three more assistants should be ready to hand the surgeon whatever he requested. He recommended marking the line of the incision with ink, as well as cross-hatching it to show where sutures ought to be placed at its conclusion. Invoking the name of God, the surgeon then cut down to the rectus muscle and the peritoneum, incised the uterus (lightly, so as not to injure the child inside), removing the fetus along with the placenta (figure 3.8).

Once the child had been removed, the surgeon was then instructed to cleanse the uterus inside and out with a special decoction made for this purpose, consisting of "artemisia, agrimony, betony, mallow, leaves or flowers of pomegranate, and dried roses on the one hand, and on the other hand birthwort, sedge, and sweet-smelling bulrushes; this decoction is made in sour black wine, using enough to consume two pounds; it is then strained and to the filtrate are added two pounds of that water which blacksmiths use to extinguish glowing irons; it is then boiled again." The decoction was then used to moisten the incision inside and out, thereby stopping the flow of blood. This done, the uterus could be dropped back into the abdomen (nothing was done to close the uterine incision), and the abdomen could be sewn up again. This

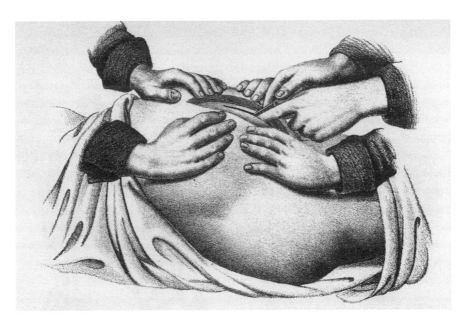

FIGURE 3.8. The traditional technique for Cesarean section using unsterile technique, with unwashed hands and fingers probing the incision and holding the patient down on the table. The mortality was high. *From J. P. Maygrier,* Midwifery Illustrated *(New York: Harper and Brothers, 1834), plate 61.*

required an assistant to push the intestines back inside while the stitches were applied.

The surgical aftercare was "the same as for other wounds, namely digestive remedies, purges, and consolidants," combined with a regimen of intrauterine herbal enemas designed to clean out the uterine cavity, followed by a regimen of vaginal suppositories made from rose oil and egg yolks.

Though Mercurio writes with confidence, there is no indication that he ever performed this operation himself, and it is even more doubtful that a patient could have survived his regimen of aftercare without dying an agonizing death within a few days from rampaging peritonitis and pelvic sepsis hastened by his intrauterine injections.

A better contemporary treatise on Cesarean delivery was written by the Frenchman Francois Rousset in 1581. Rousset's treatise was 228 pages long and consisted of detailed instructions on how to perform the operation, along with case reports of successful Cesarean sections, many of which he had personally tried to authenticate. This small book was destined to be the standard work on Cesarean delivery for several hundred years. Rousset's book, like that of Mercurio, gives no indication that he had ever performed a Cesarean section himself, but he was forceful in advocating that the operation be performed early when no other alternative means to delivery presented itself.

In the prefatory sonnet that he wrote to his treatise, Rousset referred to obstructed labor as the obstetrical Gordian knot. According to classical legend, the Gordian knot was an extraordinarily elaborate knot that tied an ancient oxcart to a post in the city of Gordium in ancient Phrygia. When Alexander the Great passed through Phrygia during his conquest of the Persian Empire, he was told that whoever could untie the knot would become the ruler of Asia. Alexander pondered the complex knot for a few moments, then raised his sword and split it in half with one swift blow. Having thus "untied" the knot, Alexander fulfilled the prophecy.

Rousset advised his readers to "be also like Alexander: provide more humane, less cruel, and safer assistance. Asia never brought this great man as much glory as the world will grant you for performing caesareans—the joy of knowing that you have saved the lives of mothers and their children." Brave words, which, due to the extremely high mortality associated with the operation, were rarely heeded, in spite of the extraordinary suffering experienced by the woman in obstructed labor that (in his words) "could scarcely fail to horrify even the most barbaric people in the world."

Cesarean Section Comes to America

The first successful Cesarean section in England was performed by James Barlow of Lancashire in 1793 upon Jane Foster, a 40-year-old woman from the village of Blackrod who had several living children. She had had the misfortune, when returning from the market in Wigan, of falling off a fully loaded cart, which rolled over her pelvis, crushing her pubic bone and confining her to bed for six weeks. She became pregnant shortly after her recovery, but when it came time for her to deliver, her labor was obstructed by the distortion of her pelvis from her accident (see figure 3.2, middle pelvis). After several days in labor, Barlow was sent for. When he examined her, he reported, he "was extremely surprised to find that I could barely pass my finger between the ossa pubis [pubic bone] and the last lumbar vertebra, so great was the narrowness at the brim." He believed it was impossible to deliver her vaginally, by any means. He told the assembled family that the only option was Cesarean section; they refused.

After another night spent in the agony of obstructed labor, Jane Foster consented to surgery the following morning. She was lifted out of bed and placed on a table, after which Barlow made an incision from the navel to the pubic bone, opened the abdomen and uterus, and extracted a dead fetus along with the placenta. Her abdominal incision was closed with seven sutures, and she was put back to bed and "passed a good night." Rather miraculously, she recovered completely and lived another 28 years, though she never again became pregnant.

The first well-attested case of successful Cesarean section for obstructed labor in the United States in which the mother survived was performed by Dr. John Lambert Richmond of Newton, Ohio, in 1827. A graduate of the Medical College of Ohio (where he had previously worked as a janitor), he was called in April 1827 to see "Miss E.C.," who had been in labor some 30 hours, attended by two unhelpful midwives. The midwives were unable to give Dr. Richmond any meaningful account of the case except, as he related, that "she had fits [seizures]" and that "the pains did no good" as far as moving her labor along. The seizures suggest that Miss E.C. was probably suffering from eclampsia, a deadly complication of pregnancy-induced hypertension, as well as obstructed labor, making her situation incredibly dire. Dr. Richmond believed his first priority was trying to manage her convulsions, but he had little to work with. "I was seven miles from home," he wrote, "and had but few medicines with me." He treated her with opiates (laudanum) and sulfuric ether (which likely would have had an anesthetic effect), applied hot flannels moistened with alcohol to her feet, and did the best he could. He requested that they send for help, but unfortunately none could be obtained "on account of high water in the Little Miami [River] and the darkness of the night." All he had was a set of "pocket instruments" at his disposal.

His patient was critically ill, seizing periodically, and her labor was not progressing. There was nothing else to do: "I was convinced that the patient must die, or the operation be performed," but the conditions were grim indeed. It was one o'clock in the morning, and he was in a cabin in the middle of nowhere, cut off from communication and all medical help. "The house," he wrote, "was made of logs that were green and put together not more than a week before. The crevices were not chinked, there was no chimney, nor chamber floor." It was a foul and stormy night, with high winds blowing into the cabin through the chinks in between the logs so hard that his assistants "had to hold blankets to keep the candles from being blown out." There was no real anesthesia, but perhaps the combination of sulfuric ether and loss of consciousness from her seizures sufficed to give her some relief.

The operation was difficult. He made a vertical incision from her navel to just above the pubic bone and then cut downward. When he reached the uterus, he cut through it in a similar fashion. Unfortunately, the placenta was attached to the anterior wall of the uterus, right underneath the point where he made his incision. He cut into it, precipitating a hemorrhage, which filled the abdominal cavity. He wiped out what he could and tried to deliver the child. Again, it did not go well. The fetus "was uncommonly large," "the mother very fat," and, he lamented, "having no assistance I found this part of my operation more difficult than I had anticipated." The placenta was lacerated and soon separated from the uterus. He found that he could not get the baby out. He could not raise the fetal head out of the pelvis where it was deeply wedged after over 34 hours of labor, and he could not "raise the breech" out of the uterus either. Neither was he able to pass his hand around the child (although he tried), "but this the patient could not endure." All of this was done by candlelight, in the midst of a storm, without any meaningful anesthesia. Richmond was desperate. He assumed the fetus was now dead since the afterbirth had been detached for some time, "and considering, at all events, that a childless mother was better than a motherless child," he determined at least to try to save her life. He took a knife and made a transverse incision across the baby's back near the lumbar vertebrae. Once the muscles of the back were divided, he could fold its body into an angle and extract it from the uterus. The placenta followed immediately.

He wiped the blood out of the uterus and cleaned up as best he could, dressing the abdominal wound "with sutures and adhesive straps," but leaving the lower portion of the incision open. The woman fell asleep, and he kept her in bed for four days. He was forced to drain the wound, which had collected a large hematoma, and he irrigated it every day for six days with three pints of water and a little soap until the discharge was clear and the incision closed. His patient was a sturdy woman who "never complained of pain during the whole course of the cure" and was even able to laugh during the irrigations of her wound "because," as she said, "it feels so queer." Miraculously, this pioneer woman recovered and was able to resume work 24 days after the operation; a fortnight later she was able to walk a mile and back on an errand. She survived, later married, but two years later had not gotten pregnant. Her main complaint was that "she suffered great inconvenience on account of the shallowness of the vagina" (it having shrunk to two-thirds the length of a finger in the aftermath of her obstructed labor), but otherwise she was well. Her abdominal incision healed nicely and never gave her any trouble.

In 1830 this ghastly case was a surgical triumph, but it was typical of those rare occasions in which a woman survived Cesarean section. In these early days the risks of this operation were formidable. According to the nineteenth-century Philadelphia obstetrician Robert Harris, who was an indefatigable researcher on operative obstetrics, of the first 100 Cesarean operations performed in Britain, only 16 women survived. The statistics from America were somewhat better, but really nothing to brag about. In his exhaustive 1878 compilation of 71 Cesarean section cases carried out between 1822 and 1877, 34 women lived and 37 died, a mortality of 52 percent. The deaths were due to peritonitis, exhaustion, convulsions, hemorrhage, septicemia, and bowel obstruction. Most of these Cesarean sections were desperate cases like the one encountered by Dr. Richmond, where the pregnant woman had a severely deformed pelvis, sometimes with less than an inch of space between the pubic bone and the sacrum; 16 women were dwarves, one only 3 feet 4 inches tall. "In plain terms," Harris wrote, "there is nothing in surgery, about which the surgeon is so timid, as the Caesarean operation; and nothing in obstetrics, of which the obstetrician stands so much in dread." According to Harris's extensive research, so great was the dread of this operation that prior to 1880 there were only about three Cesarean sections performed in the United States each year; certainly many more women than this had obstructed labor, and many would, potentially, have benefitted from this intervention. Yet unnecessary delay in making the decision to operate led to catastrophic consequences. To pursue "expectant management" in the hopes that "nature would find a way" to deliver the child was fatal. "If left to nature," he said, "the foetus will die and decay in utero, come away piecemeal with a horrid odour, and ultimately the woman will die, a perfect loathing to herself." If she survived, she might develop a fistula, which many regarded as a fate worse than death.

Harris recognized (and demonstrated in paper after paper) that the extremely high mortality from Cesarean section (which he calculated to be 56 percent overall in cases performed in the United States) was largely due to unnecessary delay in performing the operation when it was absolutely indicated. Fatal delay occurred because Cesarean delivery was generally viewed as procedure of last resort, rather than a viable remedy to be undertaken as soon as the need became apparent. When analyzed according to when in the course of labor the operation was undertaken, Harris found the results to be quite different from its overall dismal reputation. "There is a fair prospect," he wrote, "of saving both mother and child by an operation during the first hours of labour, and this hope diminishes as labour advances, until there is a marked falling off; and, finally, the prognosis becomes exceedingly unfavourable, as very few escape." He calculated that 75 percent of women (and children) would survive the operation if performed very early after the onset of labor, but that only one-third of women would survive a Cesarean performed "moderately late," and that only a pitiful 15 percent or so would survive an operation performed very late (from 2 to 15 days after the start of labor).

Harris clearly understood that surgeons get better results if the patients on whom they operate are healthier rather than sicker at the time the operation is performed. In the 1870s, mortality from Cesarean delivery was largely due to infection, which spread throughout the abdomen and pelvis through the incision in the infected uterus, ultimately overwhelming the patient, who likely was exhausted after three or four days in obstructed labor (and who was often in poor health from the very beginning of her pregnancy). Lengthy labors with the amniotic membranes ruptured greatly increased the risk of uterine infection and a fatal outcome. Prolonged labor exhausted the woman, exhausted the uterus (which would gradually lose its contractile power, which was critical for reducing blood loss), and put the surgeon in the unfortunate position of performing a heroic salvage operation on a moribund patient. "To avoid this condition," he thundered, "there is only one remedy, *operate early.*" He pleaded with his obstetrical colleagues to change their ways, writing, "We have, for years past, been making history in the most discreditable way, losing case after case, by operating in extremis as a last resort, under a fear of the abdominal section being almost necessarily fatal, when, in fact, it is chiefly made so by delay and tampering with the patient."

To make his point that a healthy, robust pregnant woman who was operated on early in labor would do much better than those for whom the operation was markedly delayed, Harris compared the results of Cesarean delivery as then practiced in the United States with the results of extraordinary accidents in which pregnant women had been gored by cattle, ripping open their abdomen and uterus. He collected nine such cases of cattle-horn "laparo-hysterotic rips" and found that the cows had better outcomes than the surgeons: five out of the nine cattle-horn cases survived (55 percent) whereas in the seven years previous to his paper only 5 of 27 women undergoing Cesarean delivery in the United States had lived (18.5 percent). "This is a far better showing for the cow-horn than the knife," he wrote glibly, "and has a world of meaning in determining the risks and cause of death under the latter." The main reason, he declared, was that the pregnant women who survived goring by a cow horn were "in the full possession of their usual strength and health" and had not been subjected to the delays of "meddlesome midwifery" that occurred in cases of prolonged obstructed labor in which the operation was used late.

From the standpoint of surgical technique, Cesarean section was not a difficult operation to perform compared with many other surgical procedures, yet the mortality following the operation from infection and hemorrhage was so dreadful that surgeons avoided it at almost any costs. There were still heated debates about how to avoid Cesarean section using high forceps deliveries or destructive operations such as craniotomy as late as the 1870s. As surgeons gained more experience with the operation, Cesarean section started to pull even with or even to surpass these violent techniques for vaginal delivery, but the cost in morbidity and mortality was unacceptably high.

The First Advance: Porro's Cesarean Hysterectomy

A dramatic development in the technique of Cesarean delivery took place on May 21, 1876, in Pavia, Italy. Until that date, no woman there had ever survived Cesarean section. A month earlier, 25-year-old Julia Cavallini was referred to the obstetric clinic of Dr. Eduardo Porro because of her malformed pelvis. Julia was a challenging obstetric case: she was a dwarf (only 148 cm tall) and had suffered with rickets since her childhood. The distance between her pubic bone and her sacrum (the diagonal conjugate of the pelvis) was only 7 centimeters, and the pelvis was severely deformed as well. Porro examined her and presented the case to his colleagues, all of whom agreed that vaginal delivery by any means would be impossible. Julia would have to undergo a Cesarean section.

The operation was carefully planned. Because the risks of infection and bleeding associated with Cesarean delivery were so high, Porro planned to perform a hysterectomy after the baby had been delivered—an operation that also carried an extremely high risk of death. At 4:42 p.m. on May 21, about six hours after her membranes had ruptured, Julia Cavallini was anesthetized with chloroform, and Porro began the operation. She was delivered of a healthy, live-born, 3,300 gram male infant, and the placenta was removed. The surgeons lifted the uterus out of the abdomen for better access, but they were unsuccessful in controlling the bleeding from the uterine incision.

Porro then placed a strong wire snare around the uterus and left ovary just above the point where the cervix joined the body of the uterus. As the wire snare was wound tight, the bleeding stopped. Porro then cut the uterus away above the wire ligature. The stump that was left remained constricted, with no further bleeding. He then passed a curved clamp through the posterior vaginal wall and inserted a 5-millimeter drainage tube into the peritoneal cavity. This would allow infected blood and serum to drain out of the pelvis. The surgical team irrigated the abdomen and pelvis and closed the abdominal wall with four strong sutures of silver wire (an inert metal that resists infection). The wire snare was left around the uterine stump, which was then sewn into the lower angle of the incision so that it drained through the abdominal wall—another procedure to reduce infection. It did leave a pretty hideous-looking surgical wound, however.

Julia's postoperative course was rocky: she developed decubitus ulcers over her sacrum, an infection of her abdominal incision, a urinary tract infection, and also vulvovaginitis—but she survived. The wire snare and the gangrenous portion of the remaining uterus were removed four days after surgery. The silver wire sutures were removed two days later and the vaginal drain was taken out a week after that. The bishop of Padua gave his blessing to the whole procedure; it was justifiable to save the patient's life. Surgeons around the world noted Porro's success. This was an awkward surgical technique, to be sure—but it appeared to work. Better an awkward operation than a dead patient.

Porro's operation of Cesarean hysterectomy was radical but lifesaving. Removing the uterus after delivery of the fetus reduced mortality from both hemorrhage and infection. In cases of long labor where the amniotic membranes had been ruptured for several days, the uterus is inevitably infected. Making an incision through the uterus to deliver the child in a case like this would always mean that infected blood, serum, membranes, and placenta would spill into the abdominopelvic cavity, creating an infection that was usually fatal. Centuries of surgical practice (such as it was) had taught that the uterine incision should be left to close naturally through the mechanism of postdelivery contractions (afterpains)—but in many cases (particularly cases in which labor had been obstructed for several days) the muscle would be weak and would not contract properly to seal off the incised uterine blood vessels, and so hemorrhage would ensue (along with continued spillage of infected matter into the abdomen). By removing the body of the uterus and sewing the remaining stump into the edge of the abdominal incision, Porro greatly reduced both the risk of continued hemorrhage as well as the risk of infection. It wasn't particularly elegant, but it worked.

At roughly this same time, there was a small spasm of enthusiasm for an operation called "gastro-elytrotomy" (sometimes also called "laparo-elytrotomy"). This operation had been tried earlier but was independently rediscovered by American surgeon T. Gaillard Thomas. In this operation, an incision was made from the pubic bone to the right anterior superior iliac spine (much as one might make for a very generous appendectomy). The operator could then bluntly push the tissues apart with a finger down to the side of the cervix and vagina, make an incision in the vaginal wall, and "pull the baby out the side door," as it were, then up through the abdominal incision. This operation had the advantage that it was extraperitoneal; that is, it did not risk spilling infected lochia into the intra-abdominal cavity, but it was not terribly straightforward. The results were similar to other operative techniques: in his history of Cesarean section, Young noted 15 cases of gastro-elytrotomy with a 53 percent maternal mortality and a similar fetal loss. One of the major problems was that there was a high rate of bladder injury (6 of 14 cases) with this operation, and, as Young wrote, "this, together with technical difficulties and fear of haemorrhage, did not make the operation commend itself to the profession." Today it is only a footnote in the history of operative obstetrics.

Sanger's Triumph

In 1882 a young professor of obstetrics named Max Sanger published a book in Leipzig with the typically formidable German title of *Der Kaiserschnitt bei Uterusfibromen, nebst vergleichender Methodik der Sectio Caesarea und der Porro-Operation—Kritiken, Studien und Vorschlage zur Verbesserung des Kaiserschnittes.* In this remarkable volume, Sanger, in a thoroughly Germanic manner, scrutinized the history of the development of Cesarean delivery in detail, meticulously analyzed this past experience, and synthesized everything into a new carefully delineated approach to the operation that revolutionized obstetric practice. It was the single most important step in making Cesarean section part of normal obstetric practice rather than a desperate attempt to salvage the life of a pregnant woman who was at the point of death. Eventually this came to be called the "conservative Cesarean section," so called because, unlike Porro's operation, the Sanger method did not involve hysterectomy, thereby preserving the uterus.

Sanger regarded Porro's operation as a grotesque, cumbersome, mutilating procedure (a point of view with which most objective observers agreed). Surely something better could be devised. He reasoned that the ideal obstetric operation for difficult cases like Porro's patient Julia Cavallini would achieve three goals: it would preserve the life of the child (unlike craniotomy, which killed the child to preserve the mother), preserve the life of the mother, and preserve the uterus and the woman's future fertility. These three goals appeared achievable by Cesarean section if the operation was carried out early in labor (before infection, maternal exhaustion, and other complications set in) and if it was carried out using proper aseptic techniques. Infection was the biggest killer of women delivered by Cesarean section. Was there a way to modify the operation to achieve these goals? (Recall that at this point in time antibiotics did not yet exist.)

Sanger's approach was carefully thought out and planned in detail. Every step in the operation was done for a specific reason, and each step was designed to advance achievement of his overriding goal: a living child born to a healthy mother who kept a healthy uterus afterward.

The conservative "Sanger method" for Cesarean section was as follows. The patient was carefully selected and the decision to operate was made early, before labor had been unduly prolonged and infection had set in (American obstetrician Robert Harris had been arguing for this approach for years; Sanger listened). The bladder was emptied, the external genitalia were shaved, and the abdomen and vagina were carefully disinfected with an antiseptic solution. A vertical incision was made in the skin, and three sutures were passed through the upper portion of the incision (these were to be used to close the incision temporarily after the uterus had been lifted out of the abdominal cavity). The amniotic membranes were then ruptured in the vagina if they were still intact (this would allow the amniotic fluid to drain out through the vagina, thereby reducing the possibility of contaminating the peritoneal cavity). The uterus was lifted out of the patient's belly, and the abdomen was covered with a waterproof sheet soaked in 5 percent carbolic acid, a disinfectant. A vertical incision was made in the anterior wall of uterus and the fetus, placenta, and membranes were removed, after which the uterus was compressed manually to reduce bleeding from the placental site. Specific bleeding points along the incision were clamped with small artery forceps. When the uterus had contracted down, a drainage tube was inserted through the cervix into the vagina, and the uterine cavity was carefully cleaned with a sponge soaked in carbolic acid.

What made all the difference, however, was what followed next. Sanger developed a new method for closing the uterine incision. Previous practice for suturing the uterus (if it was done at all), used only a few sutures that left large gaps between them in the incision, an imperfect closure through which infected lochial fluid could enter the abdomen, typically leading to a fatal infection. Sanger's technique aimed to achieve a watertight closure of the incision. The details of the procedure changed over time, but the basic principle was both sound and simple: multiple sutures of silver wire were used to close the uterine musculature, avoiding the passage of any sutures into the uterine cavity itself. After this, the outer peritoneal surface of the uterus was closed with superficial sutures, so placed as to turn the incision in upon itself, just as the French surgeon Antoine Lembert had described in his method of closing incisions on the intestine. The use of multiple sutures in two layers gave a strong, secure closure of the uterus and prevented the wound from gaping; this in turn prevented infected matter from seeping into the abdomen and setting up a fatal peritonitis.

The remarkable thing about Sanger's operation was that it was entirely (but soundly) theoretical: when he published his book, he had never done the procedure. The first "Sanger operation" was carried out by Sanger's friend and colleague Dr. Christian Gerhard Leopold, with Sanger's assistance, on May 25, 1882. Both the mother and the child survived. The operative technique spread slowly across Europe and to the United States. It had a high rate of success and much lower mortality than Porro's operation, it preserved the uterus, and it was easier to perform.

Cesarean Section Comes of Age

It is difficult for Americans in the twenty-first century to understand how difficult and daunting the operation of Cesarean section was at the end of the nineteenth century. I can remember, as a chief resident in obstetrics at Duke University Medical Center in the late 1980s doing as many as four Cesarean deliveries in a day. The operation was routine, common, and straightforward. Compare my experience with that of Dr. Howard Kelly, professor of gynecology at Johns Hopkins University (whom most would consider to be the founder of modern American gynecologic surgery). Kelly wrote an article in 1891 in the *American Journal of Obstetrics and Diseases of Women and Children* entitled "The Steps of the Cesarean Section—the Dos and the Don'ts." He based this article on the vast experience he had obtained by, he wrote, "having recently completed my fourth successful Cesarean operation in the Johns Hopkins Hospital!" The article is a model of lucidity and common sense, even though it was based on limited personal experience. Kelly thought Sanger's approach was safe and well established, forming the "gold standard" for operative abdominal delivery. He insisted "that my countrymen, in particular, shall cease making useless experiments, unwittingly repeating over and over again the errors of their predecessors." Kelly declaimed, "No man has any longer a right, unless upon the basis of a large experience, to materially modify any details of this operation, if he be unwilling to bear the imputation of unwarrantable trifling with the most sacred trusts committed to his care."

Infection was the unseen killer that lurked behind every obstetric intervention, most especially Cesarean section. Before the discovery of antibiotics (which completely changed the practice of medicine) in the twentieth century, all obstetric practitioners—and especially those contemplating the performance of a Cesarean delivery—had to be absolutely fanatical about cleanliness, or they would risk killing their patients from sepsis. Consider the technique advocated by Egbert Grandin and George Jardin in their 1895 book *Obstetric Surgery* (recalling as well that rubber examination gloves had not yet been introduced into clinical practice—it was the naked hand that came into contact with the patient during surgery at this time):

"In the lying-in [delivery] room," they wrote, "the physician should remove his coat and roll up his shirt-sleeves above the elbow." The hands must be rendered absolutely aseptic since, "aside from instruments, the hands are most likely to septicize the woman from direct contact." If there is any chance of the doctor having been in contact with "any infectious material," the normal routine of washing the hands with soap and water and scrubbing them with a solution of bichloride of mercury was not enough. Under these circumstances the following was required: "The hands and arms are scrubbed for at least ten minutes in hot soap and water, the latter being frequently changed." Special attention must be paid to cleaning the fingernails, which are likely to trap infectious matter. "The hands and arms are next covered with a hot saturated solution of permanganate of potash, and are then immersed in a hot saturated solution of oxalic acid until the stain of the permanganate has entirely disappeared. The oxalic acid is next removed by soaking the hands in hot sterilized water." The authors even recommended scrubbing out the vagina using a toothbrush with soapy water and a solution of bichloride of mercury before proceeding with the operation.

By the turn of the twentieth century, maternal mortality from Cesarean section was largely due to sepsis. Sanger's operative technique, when performed early, before labor was prolonged or before unsuccessful attempts at vaginal delivery had been undertaken, was successful in reducing infectious complications.

According to Amand Routh, in Britain at the turn of the twentieth century, the case fatality rate for Cesarean section (irrespective of the indication for the operation) was 12 percent (155 deaths in 1,282 cases, 1906–1910). Of this series, 602 cases were performed for contracted pelvis with 37 deaths, a mortality of 6.1 percent. Within subgroups, however, the rates were very different, rising rapidly in cases with ruptured membranes or where "meddlesome midwifery" in the form of repeated examinations or attempted delivery had preceded operation. The mortality associated with Cesarean delivery undertaken in cases of contracted pelvis in Britain between 1891 and 1910 is shown in table 3.1. Cases A and B can be considered relatively "clean" cases, with a combined mortality of 2.9 percent, whereas the "suspected infected" cases (C and D) have a mortality of 17.3 percent.

In infected cases, Routh was of the opinion that craniotomy and vaginal removal of the fetus was preferable to Cesarean section, since craniotomy "enables the uterus

Table 3.1. Case fatality of cesarean section for contracted pelvis in Britain, 1891–1910

Patient condition	Number of cases	Number of maternal deaths	Case fatality rate (%)
A. Not in labor	245	9	3.6
B. In labor, membranes intact	224	5	2.2
C. In labor with membranes ruptured	166	18	10.8
D. Frequent examinations or attempts at delivery	64	22	34.3

Source: From Amand Routh, "The Indications for, and Technique of, Caesarean Section and Its Alternatives, in Women with Contracted Pelves, Who Have Been Long in Labour and Exposed to Septic Infection," *Journal of Obstetrics and Gynaecology of the British Empire* 19 (1911): 236–252, table 1.

Table 3.2. Case fatality in contracted pelvis with suspected infection in Britain, 1891–1910.

Condition of patient	Number of cases	Treated by Cesarean section only	Deaths	Treated by supravaginal hysterectomy	Deaths
In labor, membranes ruptured	166	158	18 (11.4%)	8	0
Frequent examinations or attempts at delivery	64	58	22 (37.9%)	6	0
Total	230	216	40 (18.5%)	14	0

Source: From Amand Routh, "The Indications for, and Technique of, Caesarean Section and Its Alternatives, in Women with Contracted Pelves, Who Have Been Long in Labour and Exposed to Septic Infection," *Journal of Obstetrics and Gynaecology of the British Empire* 19 (1911): 236–252, table 2.

to be emptied of its contents with antiseptic precautions, and at the same time the uterine wound of a Caesarean section is obviated and a septic peritonitis is thereby prevented." Furthermore, in craniotomy cases, after the fetus was extracted the uterus could be irrigated with "3 or 4 pints of iodised water," a procedure that could also be performed after delivery of the placenta. This, it was hoped, would further reduce infectious morbidity and mortality. But "if the patient were feverish and ill and the uterus tender, indicating that the infection had probably spread into the uterine tissue or even into the patient's blood . . . hysterectomy should be performed to prevent further infection."

In support of that policy, Routh produced the data given in table 3.2.

In 1925, American obstetrician Joseph Bolivar DeLee noted that Sanger's Cesarean operation, with its emphasis on tight uterine closure combined with rigorous aseptic surgical technique, had freed Cesarean delivery from most of its dangers. Sanger's operation "sprang into favor and soon became standard all over the world. The mortality sank from 65 per cent to 30 per cent, to 20, 10, 5,—indeed series of 100 or more cases without maternal death were published." Unfortunately, however, mortality remained high "in just those cases which were most common and where abnormal delivery was most needed, i.e., the neglected labor with the suspicion of infection." The biggest problem still lay in what to do with women who had labored unsuccessfully for a long time and needed delivery after being subjected to much "meddlesome midwifery," with multiple vaginal examinations, failed attempts at forceps, and other such interventions. In the preantibiotic era, the risk of sepsis in such cases was high, and patients still faced the very real possibility of dying if operated upon. The answer to this problem appeared to lie in some revised form of extraperitoneal operative technique that would further prevent the escape of infected amniotic fluid into the belly. The technique that eventually evolved would become known as the lower-segment Cesarean section.

Although there were numerous early variations (particularly with respect to whether the incision in the uterus should be vertical or transverse), the new technique involved moving the site of incision down into the lower uterine segment, away from the upper uterus or fundus, diminishing the risk of subsequent uterine rupture and also diminishing potential leakage of infected fluids from the uterus into the abdomen. The operator would incise the peritoneum over the uterus, dissect under the bladder (which normally rests on the cervix and lower uterine segment), mobilizing the bladder so that it could be swung anteriorly, away from the operative field. The incision through which the fetus was delivered would then be made in the lower uterine segment. After delivery of the fetus and removal of the placenta, the uterus would be closed à la Sanger, the bladder restored to its normal position over the uterine incision, and the reflected peritoneum was then reclosed to ensure a watertight seal through which infected amniotic fluid and lochia would not be able to enter the abdominal cavity.

As a result of these improvements in technique, mortality following Cesarean delivery started to fall. For example, W. E. Welz reported on all of the Cesarean deliveries that had taken place in Detroit in 1925. He noted that the performance of this "grave obstetric procedure" had increased dramatically over the previous 25 years. Whereas once it was a rarity, it had now become "an everyday occurrence." In 1925 there were 33,480 births in Detroit, of which 10,425 (only 31 percent) took place in hospitals. Of these in-hospital deliveries, there were 154 Cesarean sections, or 1 for every 68 deliveries, the most common indication for the procedure being "contracted pelvis." There were 20 maternal deaths, for a case-fatality rate of 13 percent. He noted that the Cesarean section rate was too high, that the death rate from Cesarean section was far too high, and he noted, in passing, with respect to maternal mortality overall (which was not declining) that overall "one usually thinks of a maternal mortality of 2 per cent"—a statistic that would put Detroit on par with the worst obstetric outcomes prevailing today in the Third World.

But things changed. Five years later, in 1930, Ward F. Seeley again analyzed Cesarean sections in Detroit. At that time 33,988 births took place, with 14,836 in hospital, of which 203 were by Cesarean section, a rate of 1 Cesarean for every 73 hospital deliveries. Of these operations, 73 were done for pelvic contracture, and 34 were repeat operations on women who had had a previous Cesarean. There were nine maternal deaths from all causes among the 203 Cesarean deliveries, a case fatality rate of 4.43 percent. Mortality had dropped by two-thirds in only five years, and among the 87 women who had lower segment operations, there were no deaths.

That same year, Greenhill reported a series of 874 lower segment Cesarean sections from the Chicago Lying-In Hospital, where, in spite of a rising rate of Cesarean delivery (to just over 2 percent), the case fatality rate had dropped to 1.3 percent. The most common indication was still cephalo-pelvic disproportion, but other reasons for Cesarean section were starting to make a more frequent appearance. Surgeons (particularly specialist obstetricians) were gaining proficiency and were perfecting their surgical techniques. Greenhill stated, "I personally have performed 109 consecutive cervical cesarean sections, without a single maternal death." Such a statement would have been unheard of 30 years before. In 1950, Dieckmann and Seski reported 2,871 Cesarean sections from the same hospital performed between 1931 and 1949 with a case fatality rate of 0.42 percent. Thirty years later, in 1980, Frigoletto, Ryan, and Phillippe could report 10,231 Cesarean sections out of 68,645 births at the Boston Hospital for Women with *no* maternal deaths following Cesarean delivery between 1968 and 1978.

The Decline of Maternal Mortality and the End of Obstetric Fistula

Medical historian Irvine Loudon wrote in 1992, "There can be no doubt that the most remarkable feature of childbirth in this century is the profound decline in maternal deaths throughout the Western world." In 1920, maternal mortality throughout Europe, North America, Australia, and New Zealand existed at levels characteristic today of the Third World. Maternal mortality—as measured by the number of maternal deaths per 100,000 births (the maternal mortality ratio)—ranged from a relatively admirable low of 235 deaths per 100,000 births in Denmark in 1920 to an appallingly high 689 deaths per 100,000 births in the United States. Between 1930 and 1960 this situation changed dramatically. In less than 30 years, maternal mortality fell precipitously and consistently throughout the entire Western world so that by 1960 the rates of maternal death were virtually the same in every one of these countries (figure 3.9). Never in human history had maternal mortality been this low, and, with the precipitous fall in maternal deaths, there was a concomitant fall in numbers of women suffering with vesico-vaginal fistulas in these countries. Obstructed labor was no longer a public health problem. How did this happen?

Loudon has convincingly demonstrated that the reason for the appalling maternal mortality throughout Europe and the Western world at the turn of the twentieth century was the terrible organization of maternal health services in those countries.

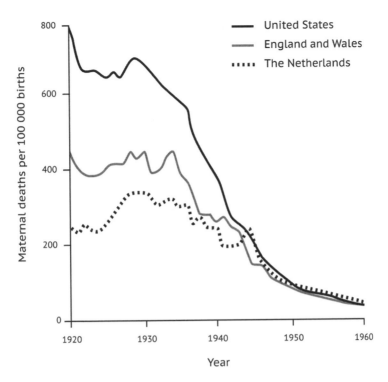

FIGURE 3.9. Annual trends in maternal mortality in western Europe and the United States, 1920–1960, shown as maternal deaths per 100,000 births. *Redrawn from Irvine Loudon, "The Transformation of Maternal Mortality,"* BMJ *305 (1992): 1557.*

Writing in the *BMJ*, Loudon noted, "We find the reasons for maternal mortality in the disparate, ill organised, and often poor standard of maternal care in the first 30 years of this century. The chief culprits were the teaching hospitals, where obstetrics was often a despised specialty. A derisory standard of training instilled bad habits and the low standard of obstetrics in general practice. Moreover, with the exception of a few individuals . . . leadership from the top was timorous and indecisive, and funding was through local authorities, who spent as little as possible on maternal and child health." As we shall see, this is still the case in those Third World countries with high levels of maternal death and large numbers of vesico-vaginal fistulas.

The precipitous drop in maternal death was *not* due to increasing economic prosperity throughout the region: these were the years of the Great Depression, the Second World War, and the postwar reconstruction of Europe. Rather, the decline in maternal mortality was due to dramatic improvements in standards of obstetric care, reorganization of health services, and the introduction of numerous lifesaving technologies that addressed specific causes of maternal death: hemorrhage, infection, hypertensive disorders of pregnancy, and obstructed labor. For example, the first antibiotics (the sulfonamides) were introduced into clinical use in 1937, followed by penicillin in the 1940s. Ergometrine (a uterine contractant) became available during this period, due to the work of J. Chassar Moir. Blood transfusion also became practical on a broad scale on the basis of wartime experience. Most important, however, was the development of obstetrics as a vigorous medical discipline. For example, the Royal College of Obstetricians and Gynaecologists in Britain was founded in 1929, and the American College of Obstetricians and Gynecologists followed in 1950. It was largely the diffusion of specialist expertise in the management of difficult labor and delivery, along with refined skills in performing Cesarean section, that dropped maternal mortality to levels previously unachieved in world history.

The End of Obstetric Fistula as a Public Health Problem in the West

The persistent and dramatic fall of vesico-vaginal fistulas in the twentieth century can best be documented by the career of Dr. John Chassar Moir, Nuffield Professor of Obstetrics and Gynaecology at Oxford University, described in his 1977 obituary in the *BMJ* as "one of the most distinguished and best-loved men in obstetrics and gynaecology in Britain in the twentieth century." Moir graduated from the University of Edinburgh, served for a time in general practice, and then began a distinguished research career (discovering and developing the drug ergometrine, widely used to make the uterus contract after delivery, which saved thousands of women from postpartum hemorrhage). He was appointed to his professorial position in Oxford in 1937, where he remained until he retired in 1967. His career thus very nicely parallels the developments outlined by Irvine Loudon that led to the dramatic fall in maternal mortality that took place in Britain between 1935 and 1950.

Moir developed an interest in vesico-vaginal fistula early in his career and soon acquired a reputation as the best fistula surgeon in the British Isles. His obituary noted, "In this, as in everything that he did, he was a perfectionist: it was not unknown for him, at the end of a three-hour operation on a fistula, to look at the result and decide to take out every stitch and begin again. His results were so good that other men's failures were increasingly referred to him, and even after his retirement from the chair at Oxford he was in such demand that he returned to Hammersmith as visiting professor to continue this work."

As a result of his well-deserved reputation, Moir found himself at the apex the "referral pyramid" in Britain for women with fistulas: if you were British and had a fistula, Chassar Moir was the surgeon you wanted to do your case. In 1973, Moir published an overview of his fistula experience, reviewing 431 fistula cases that he had seen in Britain (cases on which he operated in Africa, India, and elsewhere were not included). "In Britain," he wrote, "vesico-vaginal fistula is rare, and usually results from surgical misadventure and not from obstetrical neglect." By 1973, 80 percent of the vesico-vaginal fistulas referred to him were due to injury occurring during gynecological surgery, most commonly during hysterectomy. In fact, he reported that, of the last 100 cases that he had seen, 93 were related to surgery, and only 7 were of obstetrical origin; and actually "some of the obstetrical cases were in fact 'surgical,' having been caused by injury to the bladder or ureter at Caesarean section or other operative intervention."

Vesico-vaginal fistulas resulting from hysterectomy are completely different from those arising from obstructed labor. In obstructed labor the fistula develops in a central area of necrosis produced by prolonged pressure of the fetal head on the vulnerable tissues of the vesico-vaginal septum. These tissues slough away, creating the fistula, but the tissues around the fistulous opening are also severely (though not lethally) injured. As these badly injured tissues heal, profound scarring and retraction often develop, creating a very difficult environment for future surgical repair. In the posthysterectomy case, however, the mechanism of fistula formation is different, with a consequentially more favorable prognosis. Here the fistula develops as the result of an unrecognized injury to an otherwise healthy bladder. Urine leaks from the injured bladder and begins to pool over the portion of the vagina that has been sutured together after removing the cervix. The pooled urine interferes with healing of the edges of the vaginal incision. Because the edges do not heal, the pooled urine drains through the incision into the vagina and a fistula forms. This process typically results in the formation of a small fistula at the top of the vagina that is located in a field of normal surrounding tissue—an injury that has a far better prognosis than the fistula from prolonged obstructed labor.

Earlier in his career, Moir saw a greater proportion of obstetric fistulas: as he reported in 1954, roughly 36 percent of his first 100 fistula cases were of obstetric origin. Some of these were catastrophes from outlying areas involving women who had suffered unbelievable obstetrical neglect. One case involved a woman from Ireland who "had been left unattended for twenty-four hours" during a breech delivery. Because the head is the largest part of the fetus, breech deliveries in which the baby presents hindermost-fore are feared because the cervix may not be dilated enough to allow the head to pass at the end of the second stage of labor. If the head becomes entrapped within the cervix, this is an obstetrical emergency: first because the umbilical cord can be compressed between the cervix and the fetal head, resulting in the death of the fetus from asphyxiation within a matter of minutes, and second because the physical circumstances of an entrapped fetal head expose the mother to considerable danger from hemorrhage, infection, and damage to surrounding tissues during frantic obstetric manipulations. For a woman to be left like this for an entire day is unbelievable, and the injuries she sustained were reflective of that fact: "The whole anterior vaginal wall had sloughed," and so much bladder had been lost that the pubic bones themselves were widely exposed within the fistula.

Reflecting on his experience with obstetric injuries as a cause of vesico-vaginal fistula, Moir remarked (in a paper on bladder injuries presented to the New York Obstetrical Society in 1959, subsequently published in the *American Journal of Obstetrics and Gynecology* in 1961), "Almost all the cases which have been referred to me have been caused by the failure of the attending doctor to detect [cephalo-pelvic] disproportion—pelvic contraction, hydrocephalus, and the like—with the result that he attempts to deliver the baby with forceps when vaginal delivery is impossible. It is a deplorable fact that so many doctors, having applied the forceps blades, feel themselves irrevocably committed to deliver the baby, and will not give up the effort even when it becomes obvious that only be brute force can the baby be extracted." Such injuries were the last remnants of the nineteenth-century reluctance to embrace Cesarean delivery. As safe, effective Cesarean section became widely available, the devastating consequences of prolonged, obstructed labor dissipated, and the obstetric vesico-vaginal fistula became a rarity in the Western world.

In 1888, when obstetric fistulas were common occurrences, Francis Champneys, obstetric physician to St. George's Hospital in London, could devote an entire meeting of the Obstetrical Society of London to a detailed case presentation of a single Cesarean section performed for contracted pelvis and generate a vigorous discussion among the membership. Today, when Cesarean section has become the most common major surgical operation performed in the United States, a meeting devoted to this routine operation would be hard to imagine, but a fistula resulting from obstructed labor is now worthy of a case report. How the world has changed.

The development of effective techniques to alleviate obstructed labor led to a rapid decline in the number of fistula cases. But, as Francis Henry Ramsbotham noted earlier in the nineteenth century, the woman who developed a sloughing of the vagina after obstructed labor and developed a fistula was in serious trouble: "Little can be done by medicine under this unfortunate condition." The quest to develop a successful method for repair of a vesico-vaginal fistula was an equally challenging chapter in the history of surgery.

CHAPTER 4

Dr. Sims Finds a Cure

Until the middle of the nineteenth century, the history of surgical attempts to close an obstetric fistula was one of continuous failure. Sir James Young Simpson, one of the leading obstetrician-gynecologists of the Victorian age, quoted French surgeon Auguste Vidal as saying, "I do not believe that there exists in the science of surgery a well-authenticated complete cure of vesico-vaginal fistula." Alfred Velpeau, another famous French surgeon, declared in his 1847 book *New Elements of Operative Surgery* that none of the cases in which someone had reportedly managed to cure a fistula were "entirely free from contestation." Joseph Pancoast, professor of surgery at the Jefferson Medical College in Philadelphia, said that of all the surgical operations that had ever been developed, those devised for the cure of vesico-vaginal fistula had produced the least satisfactory results. Indeed, many medical authors referred to vesico-vaginal fistula as "the opprobrium of surgery." The intractable failure of surgeons to cure vesico-vaginal fistula was a shame, a disgrace, a humiliation, an embarrassment, a dishonor to the profession.

The Plight of the Fistula Patient

But they tried, and often tried mightily. No surgeon could fail to be moved by the suffering of the fistula patient. Dr. Peter Kollock referred to "the sad and disgusting picture which is presented by the victims of this fearful malady." Robert Liston, the leading London surgeon of the first half of the nineteenth century stated, "I have been consulted in some dreadful cases, incurable and loathsome . . . the bladder, without any part of its posterior fundus has been rent so as to admit the fingers; the rectum also torn extensively—in some, merely a shred of the sphincter remaining; feces and urine constantly mixing in one vast offensive cavity." Pancoast sadly called the vesico-vaginal fistula "one of the most afflicting and disgusting maladies to which the female can be subjected." New Orleans surgeon Mortiz Schuppert, reflecting philosophically upon one patient, wrote how her unhappy condition "impressed on me still more forcibly the amount of suffering and pain that human flesh is heir to."

The extent of the injuries that some women sustained from obstructed labor was simply stunning. Schuppert reported one case that he saw in New Orleans in February 1860. The patient was named Betsey, a 16-year-old slave girl from rural Louisiana, who had become pregnant when she was 14 years old. She was in labor for a week. In fact, she had been in labor for four days before anyone even sent for medical help, and, unfortunately, the doctor who attended to her during her last three days in labor was not a skilled obstetrician. Betsey finally delivered on her own, without the use of surgical instruments, probably because the baby had died and had softened enough from putrefaction to finally slip through her pelvis. When Schuppert saw her she had been living in misery for nearly two years, constantly leaking urine.

He was dumbfounded by what he saw. "Upon examination," he wrote, "the whole vesico-vaginal septum, including the neck of the bladder, was found destroyed." Only a single centimeter of the urethra remained; the rest had vanished. Her vulva and buttocks were encrusted with urinary salts and covered with ulcers. The fistula was so large that the bladder had turned completely inside out, the dome had prolapsed through the opening of the fistula and was now resting completely outside the vagina. You could see the whole bladder lining, red and inflamed. Even the ureters—the small muscular tubes that carry urine from the kidneys down to the bladder—were exposed, shooting out small streams of urine from their openings every 10 to 12 seconds. The rest of the vagina was completely obliterated from the crush injury she had sustained during labor. Schuppert couldn't even find her cervix. All he could see was a narrow crevasse in a cul-de-sac of scar tissue, through which menstrual blood would flow during her periods.

The Irish surgeon, Maurice Collis, who had extensive experience with fistula patients, wrote, "The unhappy lot of those females who are the subjects of vaginal fistula are proverbial. Shut off from society, if they are rich; and in constant pain and anguish, if they are poor; subjects often of loathing to their friends and to themselves—I know of no beings so much to be pitied." Even more poignantly, he said, "it is not the old and decrepid, those whose race is well nigh run, but the young, and often the beautiful, that are thus afflicted"; his heart broke for them.

Faced with such suffering, surgeons tried their best to provide relief. The problem was clear enough: there was a hole in the bladder. The solution was also clear enough: the hole needed to be closed. Unfortunately, neither the surgical skill nor the technology of the times was suited to the task.

Early Attempts at Cure

Writing in 1847, the German surgeon J. M. Chelius, professor at the University of Heidelberg, summed up the treatments available for patients with a vesico-vaginal fistula. "The prognosis in vesico-vaginal fistula is always unfavorable inasmuch as the continual wetting of the fistulous edges with urine prevent it from closing; this, however, must always be attempted, especially when the opening depends on considerable loss of substance." He admitted that therapy was rarely successful, but the absence of reliable palliative measures to reduce the suffering of the patients also meant there were few alternatives to attempted surgical closure. He enumerated five methods by which a surgeon might seek a cure.

The first method involved drawing off the urine with some kind of drainage device. This, in theory, would allow the bladder to collapse, causing the edges of the fistula to fall together where they would (he hoped) heal spontaneously and close the hole. The trouble was that urinary catheters were not technologically satisfactory; keeping them in the bladder was difficult. They usually fell out. If this therapy was to work, it had to provide continuous, around-the-clock bladder drainage; otherwise, the bladder would fill partially and pull the edges of the fistula apart. Most of the time the catheters had to be harnessed to a truss that the patient wore around her abdomen. In conjunction with this, the surgeon would pack the vagina with linen "stuffed with lint and smeared over with resin or wax," to try to bring the edges of the fistula together. Such catheter-holding devices were incredibly cumbersome to wear and the course of treatment was onerous in the extreme: "During this treatment," Chelius wrote, "the patient must avoid lying on her back"—which meant that she would have to lie on her belly with the catheter falling through a hole in the bed into a receptacle below—and "the cure is rarely effected before six or twelve months."

When this treatment failed (as it almost certainly would), the next recourse was cauterization of the fistula. The idea here was to close the fistula by traumatizing its edges, after which the raw edges would stick together and gradually heal. After cauterizing the fistula, surgeons often placed small hooks through the tissues at its edges to try to pull them more closely together. The hope was that the traction from the hooks would help the fistulous opening contract as the scar tissue formed, and eventually the hole in the bladder would be closed completely. This treatment usually lasted five to eight days—shorter than a year with a catheter—but the initial therapy was rather daunting. Cauterization was achieved either chemically or thermally. In the first instance, a substance such as "lunar caustic" (known to us as silver nitrate) was applied to the edges of the fistula. In the second instance, cautery was a red-hot iron applied directly to the fistula edges.

It takes little imagination to conjure up what this would have been like for the patient, lying on her back, her legs apart, her most private parts boldly exposed so the surgeon could try to get access to the fistula. The fistula, of course, was up inside the vagina, a troublesome organ whose walls naturally fall together, constantly collapsing to obscure the surgeon's view. At this time there were no electric lights to shine into such dark spaces; everything would have to be done by light of day, perhaps with sunlight reflected from a mirror, or, as Chelius suggested, "the position of the fistula may be illuminated by a candle held before it." It would take great fortitude (born of immense suffering) to submit to therapy of this kind: an open flame immediately in front of her genitals, the surgeon struggling to see the fistula with the aid of a crude speculum, cautiously advancing a hot iron poker up into the vagina in hopes that he could sear the edges of her injury enough to produce a healing inflammation.

Assuming the external genitalia could be navigated successfully, application of the cautery itself was quick and relatively painless. Dr. William Keith of Aberdeen, Scotland, described the process: "The speculum was introduced, and the edge of the false passage [fistula] touched with a button-headed cautery, at a white heat. The operation did not occupy three seconds: a smoke and a singed smell were created, but not the slightest pain was felt." Chelius admitted that cauterization often had to be repeated multiple times. He further believed that it was worth the attempt only if the fistula was small and indurated. Keith reported two fistula cases cured by the cautery; such reports of occasional successes were enough to keep hope alive and to persuade some women that the chance of cure was worth the ordeal.

When cautery failed (as it usually did), the next step was an attempt to sew the fistula closed after first having "refreshed" its edges (again, to produce a healing inflammation). It was widely reported that a suturing operation had been successfully performed by the Dutch surgeon Hendrik van Roonhuysen in 1663. Roonhuysen's procedure involved denuding the vaginal wall around the fistula to create a field for the formation of scar tissue, stitching the fistula edges together using pins made from the stiff quills of swan's feathers, finally plastering over the repair with wicks soaked in warm oil, after which the vagina was packed with moistened sponges. The packing had to be removed and replaced every time the patient needed to void, and she was required to remain quietly in bed until she healed—an arduous regimen, like all the others.

Most surgeons were skeptical of Roonhuysen's claimed success; nevertheless, there were intermittent, sporadic, irregular, and almost always irreproducible reports of successful cures of fistulas from time to time. The medical community regarded them skeptically. By the beginning of the nineteenth century, a few successful cases had been reported, but the prognosis for a patient with fistula was always regarded as grim. Success, when it was achieved, came only after heroic perseverance by both the surgeon and the patient. In a lecture on vesico-vaginal fistula given in 1829, British surgeon Henry Earle remarked, "It must be confessed that under the most favourable circumstances, these cases present the greatest obstacles, and are certainly the most difficult that occur in surgery. I do not mention this to discourage you from making attempts to relieve patients suffering under this great calamity; on the contrary, I would strongly urge you not to abandon them, and not to be deterred by many failures. I have succeeded in perfectly restoring three such cases [out of 21 seen]; in one of which I performed upwards of thirty operations before success crowned my efforts." He conceded, however, that "in the majority of cases, little can be done to obtain a cure."

Medical research (such as it was) was poorly designed, imperfectly controlled, incompletely observed, and sporadically reported in the early nineteenth century. Communication was bad, access to medical journals was difficult, and doctors had to try to solve clinical problems with what they had at hand. Serendipity played a major role in discoveries when they did occur, but discoveries were often lost or neglected because nobody heard of them.

A flicker of light appeared in in 1834, when Montague Gosset of London reported the successful repair of a fistula in "Mrs. H," a 45-year-old woman who had lived with her injury for 11 and a half years following the birth of a child. Her main complaint (aside from the constant loss of urine) was the unceasing pain and "bearing down" sensation produced by a large stone in her bladder above the fistula. Gosset introduced a sound into the bladder, dilated the fistula enough to insert a forceps inside, then crushed the stone and extracted it in pieces, after which he flushed her bladder with injections of warm water for several days to remove the residual "sand" created by this process. He wisely waited four months for her to recover from this operation and to let the inflammation subside, after which he proceeded to attempt the closure of her fistula.

His operation was straightforward. He "seized the upper part of the thickened edge of the bladder" around the fistula with a hook and, using a "spear-shaped knife," he excised the "whole of the callous lip surrounding the fistula." Following this, he closed the fistula using three gilt-wire sutures on "needles very much curved." The ends of the wires were twisted to hold them in place and to bring the incised edges of the fistula together. The patient was put to bed, face-down, with a gum-elastic catheter in her bladder, held in place by series of tapes. And there she lay, for three weeks.

Unlike silk, the gilt-wire produced little inflammation, thereby promoting wound healing. He removed one suture 9 days after surgery, the second at 12 days, and the last three weeks after the operation. The patient was cured. "She had not the slightest discharge of urine through the vagina after the operation," he wrote, "which has completely succeeded in restoring the healthy function of the parts."

But this was only one case, briefly reported, of a technique that was not pursued by others. The flicker of hope that had appeared briefly winked out.

Surgeons faced three main technical challenges in the course of this long and generally dismal history of attempts to cure vesico-vaginal fistulas: (1) How could you expose the fistula so that you could repair it? (Not only was seeing the fistula up inside the vagina a problem, but visualization was often further obscured by extensive scar tissue from the trauma of obstructed labor.) (2) What sort of suture material should be used to close it? (A chronic problem was finding a material that did not create inflammation at the surgical site and therefore cause the suture line to break down.) (3) How could you drain the bladder reliably so that it would not fill up, stretch the suture line during healing, and cause the repair to split open? Together, these three problems seemed insoluble.

In their desperation to find something—anything—that would work, many different surgical procedures for fistula closure were devised, most rather desperate and unlikely to succeed. On several occasions the French surgeon Jobert de Lamballe tried to close a vesico-vaginal fistula by transplanting skin flaps from the external genitalia over the opening. Although these first attempts to use flaps in reconstructive vaginal surgery were impressive in concept, in practice they were failures. Other surgeons tried to close fistulas using ingenious systems of hooks along their edges, making "relaxing incisions" in the surrounding tissues that would allow the edges to fall together more easily. These didn't work either. Velpeau described how others, such as Vidal, decided that the only hope for fistula patients was to close off the vagina entirely, trying to sew it shut so that it could become an "auxiliary bladder." The hope was that the vagina itself would then fill up and retain the urine. These operations always failed, but even had they had succeeded, the problem of how to empty the vagina of the accumulated urine (not to mention how menstruation would be dealt with) would have been an insuperable problem.

It is no wonder that some patients came up with their own solutions, which were at least as good as these surgical innovations. The ingenious Janet Shirress of Aberdeen, who became a fistula victim during her first delivery in 1831, decided to plug her fistula with a cork taken from a pint bottle. This worked for many months, until the cork slipped into her bladder, where it became the nidus around which a large and exquisitely painful bladder stone formed. The irritation from the stone caused great pain and unremitting bladder contractions, which produced in poor Janet "an unceasing desire to make water" and led to continual incontinence. She was seen by Dr. William Keith, who managed to crush the stone with a lithotrite, broke it (and the cork around which it had formed) into pieces, and removed it, eventually giving her relief by application of the cautery.

In 1839, Boston surgeon George Hayward published the first report of a successful cure of a vesico-vaginal fistula in North America in the *American Journal of the Medical Sciences*. The patient was a 34-year-old married woman who had had a fistula for 15 years, ever since the stillbirth of her first child. She had been in labor for three days and not urinated at all for the whole time of her travail. The child was finally removed, dead, with instruments, and 10 days later her bladder sloughed to form the fistula. She had had 11 pregnancies since the first, all miscarriages, and had previously sought relief from her fistula. She wore a catheter "for a considerable length of time" and had had the edges of the fistula touched "with caustic" as described, but to no benefit. Hayward said, "She regarded her case as almost hopeless."

When he examined her, however, he was cautiously optimistic. The fistula was not large (it admitted only the end of his forefinger), and it was favorably located in the mid-vagina. "I told her that an operation for the difficulty had been several times successful," he said, but "that it had more frequently failed, and that in a few instances it had been followed by very serious consequences" (by which he meant, of course, that she could die). She consented to treatment, and the operation proceeded on May 10, 1839.

The operation was performed without anesthesia, which had not yet been discovered. Hayward was assisted by Drs. Channing, Putnam, and Jackson. He inserted a sound into the urethra, depressing the bladder base toward the vagina to expose the fistula. While his assistants held the sound and comforted the patient, he made a rapid incision around the fistula with a scalpel and removed the external edge. He then dissected the vagina away from the bladder, and, without penetrating the bladder but only suturing the vagina, he passed three sutures from side to side and tied them tightly. He did not want to injure the bladder with the needles and, he reasoned, having freed the bladder from the underlying vagina, tying down the vaginal sutures would pull the edges of the fistula together in the bladder, where they would heal.

The patient was put to bed and laid on her right side with a short silver catheter in her bladder. She had two or three hours of pain (which she described as "smarting"), after which she was comfortable. She was placed on a minimalist diet of arrow root, milk, water, and "a solution of gum Arabic." The catheter was removed and cleaned every few hours so that it would not become obstructed. The sutures held.

Five days later, Hayward examined the patient, and the wound appeared to be healed. He removed the sutures but left a catheter in place to drain the bladder. He then removed the catheter but had her insert it herself every three hours or so to make sure the bladder was draining. Seventeen days after the operation, she was cured. Hayward was quite surprised. "Everything connected with this case proved more favorable than I had anticipated," he wrote. "The operation was not difficult, nor very painful; it was followed by no bad consequences and afforded complete relief." Was this the way forward, or had Hayward simply been lucky? It was, after all, only one case.

For the vast majority of patients, none of the interventions outlined here provided durable or substantial relief. Many, if not most, patients were reduced to the pitiful state eloquently described by Dr. Peter Kollock in his address to the Georgia State Medical Society in 1857. Following the "tedious labour" of obstructed childbirth when the vagina sloughs away and a fistula forms, Kollock said:

> The poor woman is now reduced to a condition of the most piteous description, compared with which, most of the other physical evils of life sink into utter insignificance. The urine passing into the vagina as soon as it is secreted, inflames and excoriates its mucous lining, covering it with calcareous depositions, and causing great suffering. It trickles constantly down her thighs, irritates the integument with its acrid qualities, keeps her

clothing constantly soaked, and exhales without cessation its peculiar odour, insupportable to herself and those all around her. In cases where the sloughing has been extensive, and the loss of substance of the tissues great, and where neither palliative nor curable means have availed for the relief of the sufferer, she has been compelled to sit constantly on a chair, or stool, with a hole in the seat, through which the urine descends into a vessel beneath.

Truly, American surgeon Samuel D. Gross would write, "a female affected with a vesico-vaginal fistula must necessarily be an object of deepest commiseration."

J. Marion Sims

A more unlikely candidate for solving the surgical conundrum of vesico-vaginal fistula closure could hardly have been found than J. Marion Sims. He was not a distinguished clinician at the acme of his career when he made his contribution to surgery, nor was he a renowned professor at one of the world's great medical institutions. Rather, he was simply a hardworking, incredibly persistent, country practitioner in the backwater town of Montgomery, Alabama, deep in the slaveholding American South.

Sims came from a humble, but respectable, background. He was born (as he wrote in his autobiography) "in Lancaster, South Carolina the 25th of January, 1813, about 10 miles south of the village of Lancaster, and a mile or more west of the old wagon-road from Lancaster to Camden." His parents were John Sims and Mahala Mackey Sims. His father's family was English and had arrived in America in 1740. His red-headed mother was of Scots-Irish ancestry. They were respectable but not wealthy people. His father, after military service in the War of 1812, was known as "Colonel Jack" Sims, and later he was elected high sheriff of Lancaster County. Acutely aware of his own educational shortcomings, Jack Sims was determined to educate his eight children. Young Marion was sent to the local schools where he appears to have been a clever but indifferent student. In 1825 a secondary school opened in the area, named Franklin Academy, in honor of the American polymath and patriot, Benjamin Franklin. Sims told his father that, as the family was so poor, he would prefer to drop out of school, abandon his seemingly pointless classical education, and go to work in a local business, but the colonel would have none of it. Sims would have preferred to take up a position in Mr. Stringfellow's store at the then-handsome salary of $300 per year, but his father insisted upon his further education. In 1830 he was admitted to Columbia College in Columbia, South Carolina, well enough prepared to be admitted as a junior. Colonel Sims saw his son as a future lawyer; his mother, Mahala, expected him to become a Presbyterian minister. Sims was interested in neither occupation and wrote, candidly, "I knew I should disappoint both of them."

He graduated from Columbia College in December 1832 and summed up his experience by saying, "I never was remarkable for anything while I was in college, except good behavior. Nobody ever expected anything of me, and I never expected anything of myself." He returned home to Lancaster at 20 years of age, in love with his childhood sweetheart, Theresa Jones, but too poor and undistinguished to wed a girl of her social class and growing ever more aware that his parents were likely to be disappointed in him. He was especially worried about his father, who still entertained hopes that young Marion would take up the study of law. (His mother died unexpectedly two months before he finished college; though tragic, he was off the hook with respect to her expectations.)

Colonel Jack wanted to know his son's plans. As a college graduate, Marion could not now enter a "trade" (which saddened him, because he could now be making the princely salary of $500 per year at Stringfellow's store); he was expected to follow a profession. The only options were law, the ministry, or medicine. Marion Sims had a terrible aversion to writing and speaking publicly, which ruled out the law. He had no desire to enter the ministry. That left only medicine.

His father was highly displeased. He bitterly told his son, "If I had known this I certainly should not have sent you to college." Marion retorted that he was none too pleased about the situation himself. His father responded, "Well, I suppose that I can not control you; but it is a profession for which I have the utmost contempt. There is no science in it. There is no honor to be achieved in it; no reputation to be made, and to think that my son should be going around from house to house through this country, with a box of pills in one hand and a squirt in the other, to ameliorate human suffering, is a thought I never supposed I should have to contemplate."

Colonel Sims's opinion seems bizarre to twenty-first-century American readers. In our experience, physicians come from the very top ranks of college graduates. In a Harris Interactive Poll conducted in September 2014, doctors topped the list of professions deemed to have "prestige or great prestige," being admired by 88 percent of the population. Admission to medical school today is highly competitive. The medical curriculum is intellectually rigorous and exceptionally demanding—both mentally and physically. It involves a preliminary college degree, followed by two years of intensive study of sciences basic of medicine (biochemistry, pathology, physiology, anatomy, histology, genetics, microbiology, etc.), followed by two years of carefully supervised clinical training. After this the fledgling physician enters a residency for three to five years of tightly mentored training in the hands-on business of caring for ill patients in fields ranging from internal medicine to obstetrics and gynecology to surgery. Still further opportunities for subspecialty clinical training or scientific research can be pursued thereafter. Only the best and brightest are up to the challenges, which is why half of the incoming freshmen at my own university declare they want to become physicians.

But in his day, Colonel Jack Sims was perfectly justified in the low opinion he had of the practice of medicine. The medical realities of the 1830s were far different from the high-technology, science-driven practice of the twenty-first century. The entire medical infrastructure with which we are now familiar is a product of only the past 100 years. Medicine became "modern" in the scientific sense of being grounded in a detailed understanding of human biology and pathophysiology only toward the end of the nineteenth century. In 1833 when Marion Sims reluctantly determined to become a doctor, medicine was an unregulated, slapdash affair. It was almost impossible to separate the quacks from the "regular" physicians if for no other reason than the quacks were just about as successful in clinical practice as were the regulars. Medical education was neither standardized nor regulated. Any doctor could set up a "medical school" and enroll students. Many doctors trained under an apprenticeship system, "reading" medicine with some country practitioner for a few months before setting up their own practices. There were no residencies or fellowships, and clinical appointments at major hospitals were few and far between.

A twenty-first century physician who picks up a medical textbook from 1830 will find herself incomprehensibly lost almost immediately. The physiology and disease states described in these textbooks were still based on causal assumptions about disease derived from ancient Greek humoral theories in which illness was believed to result from an imbalance of blood, phlegm, yellow bile, and black bile, brought on by too much heat or cold, too much moisture or excessive dryness. The mainstays of the pharmacopeia were brandy and other "cordials" for use as stimulants, quinine for intermittent and relapsing fevers (malaria not yet having been recognized as a parasitic infection), and opium for almost everything else. Aggressive medical treatment employed bloodletting, leeches, blisters and plasters, purgatives to make you vomit or develop copious diarrhea to force the evil humors out and restore bodily balance, or sialagogues designed to purge you through copious salivation (generally involving ingestion of potentially toxic doses of mercury). There were no antibiotics, no anesthetics, no blood transfusions, no intravenous fluids, no conception of sterile (or even antiseptic) technique. Medical practice was based on the dispensing of a hodgepodge of traditional mixtures and concoctions, often harmful rather than beneficial, so much so that the famed Dr. Oliver Wendell Holmes could state even as late as 1860 that "I firmly believe that if the whole materia medica, as now used, could be sunk to the bottom of the sea, it would be all the better for mankind,—and all the worse for the fishes." As a doctor training in the 1830s, Sims would not have much to work with.

Surgical practice was equally bad, but at least surgery was based on a meticulous understanding of anatomy. In 1830 the repertoire of surgery was limited almost exclusively to the drainage of abscesses, the removal of tumors located close to the surface of the body, and the amputation of limbs, since entry into any one of the three major cavities of the body (the skull, the chest, or the abdomen) was a virtual death sentence for the patient due to inevitable infectious complications. The physical and emotional trauma from undergoing an operation was also substantial, since effective anesthesia remained unknown. These factors meant that surgical operations were undertaken only when justified by overwhelmingly clear indications. The benefits had to be substantial to compensate for the enormous risks. Robert Liston, perhaps the greatest surgeon of the first half of the nineteenth century, wrote that operations could be justified on a patient only when the disease was "of such a nature as to render the part in which it is situated unserviceable, or of such severity as evidently to be wearing out his constitution by violent and continued suffering, or destroying his health and threatening his existence by excessive and wasting discharges." No wonder Colonel Sims was disappointed in Marion's proposed choice of profession.

Sims started his medical training by reading medicine with Dr. Churchill Jones in his hometown of Lancaster, South Carolina. "Church" Jones was the brother of the town's most distinguished citizen, Dr. Bartlett Jones (with whose daughter, Theresa, Marion Sims was desperately in love). Sims said Church Jones was regarded as "a man of great ability" and "a very great surgeon," but these qualities were offset by the fact that he was a drunkard whose addiction to alcohol often made him unfit to practice. In addition, Jones had no facilities for medical instruction, and he was by no means a great reader himself. His medical library was almost nonexistent, and Sims was forced to scrounge around to find the minimal resources needed to start his studies. Unsurprisingly, he made very little progress toward becoming a doctor.

In November 1833, Sims left Lancaster to enroll at the Charleston Medical School, recently opened with a small faculty. With far better resources at his disposal than he had found with Church Jones, Sims threw himself into his studies and worked diligently, "earnestly taking notes" of what he saw and heard and working "in the deadhouse with interest" on his studies of anatomy—but the course of instruction in Charleston was only 14 weeks, hardly enough to even scratch the surface of human disease and medical practice.

Sims was smart enough to recognize this. In company with his friend Ben Robinson of North Carolina, he resolved to pursue further medical studies in Philadelphia at the Jefferson Medical College, which had been established in 1825. He spent the spring and summer back in Lancaster again reading with Church Jones and set off for Pennsylvania in September 1834. Philadelphia was a great improvement over either Lancaster or Charleston. The leading light of the Jefferson Medical College was Dr. George McClellan, a surgeon (and also the father of a little boy named George Brinton McClellan, who would eventually become the commander of the Union Army of the Potomac during the Civil War). It was Dr. McClellan who really aroused Sims's interest in surgical practice, frequently calling upon Sims to assist him in his surgical operations.

William Hunter, the great eighteenth-century obstetrician-anatomist, said that the study of anatomy "informs the head, gives dexterity to the hand, and familiarizes the heart with a sort of necessary inhumanity, the use of cutting instruments upon our fellow creatures." Learning this "necessary inhumanity"—the ability to unflinchingly inflict pain on a fellow human being—quickly, adroitly, and skillfully—in service of a greater good was one of the most important characteristics that surgeons needed in the preanesthetic age.

Sims recounted one operation in particular (a surgical triumph at the time) in which McClellan operated on a man to excise a portion of a necrosed rib (without anesthesia) and did so without entering or injuring the underlying pleural membrane (which likely would have been fatal). Sims wrote, "He talked to the patient all the time of his operation, for it was before the days of anesthesia, and when it required great nerve to be a good surgeon. He would gouge and chisel and work away, and say to the man 'Courage, my brave fellow, courage; we wound but to heal. It will soon be over.' Then he would work away again, and again he would cheer up the patient, saying 'Courage, my good fellow; be brave, for we wound but to heal; it will soon be over. Courage, my dear fellow, it will soon be over.' " The fortitude of both patient and surgeon made a great impression on Sims. Those who dithered from lack of will, deficiency of skill, or wont of understanding of the local anatomy, caused grievous suffering to those upon whom they operated. Such fortitude was not easily learned, but it was an absolute necessity if one were to become a good surgeon.

Sims graduated from the Jefferson Medical College on March 1, 1835. He had less than two years of formal medical education and a few months of nearly worthless reading with the alcoholic Church Jones. No wonder, then, that he joined together with 30 or 40 of his classmates to pay for an additional month of private lectures given by Professor Patterson on regional and surgical anatomy before setting out for home.

He arrived back in South Carolina around the middle of May 1835, ready to set up practice. "I had," he wrote, "no clinical advantages, no hospital experience, and had seen nothing at all of sickness. I had been able to buy a full set of instruments for surgical operations, and I laid in a full stock of medicines in Philadelphia. My father rented me an office on Main Street. I had a sign painted on tin, that would reach one third of the way across the end of my office." He moved in and waited for patients.

They were slow in coming. And the results were disastrous.

His first two patients were infants with chronic diarrhea. Today, as in South Carolina in the 1830s, diarrhea is the great killer of children in poor countries, where they rapidly succumb to infection and loss of fluids. Sims was just out of his training and had no experience in treating pediatric problems. He tried mightily to come up with solutions, but to no avail. Both children died.

Sims was distraught beyond consolation. He went home, took down the shingle from his office front, tossed it down an old well in the back of his house, and resolved to leave South Carolina for some place out in the west. Maybe his luck would change in Alabama.

With his father along for companionship and emotional support, Marion Sims set out for Mount Meigs in Montgomery County, Alabama. The trip took about three weeks. There were two doctors in Mount Meigs: Dr. Lucas and Dr. Childers. Dr. Lucas was a wealthy bachelor plantation owner who was deeply involved in Alabama politics and was frequently absent from Mount Meigs on business. Dr. Childers was afflicted with wanderlust. He never stayed in one place longer than two years, and when Marion Sims arrived Childers sold him his practice—books, medicines, and all—for a promissory note for $200 and an agreement that he would recommend Sims to his patients.

It took some time for Sims to develop a practice, but gradually he began to prosper. He was finally able to return to Lancaster, South Carolina, to marry his childhood sweetheart, Theresa Jones, in spite of the protestations of her mother that Sims was not a suitable husband for a genteel girl like her. Sims was determined to prove his mother-in-law wrong, and he did. Marion and Theresa were deeply in love with one another: 50 years later Sims could still show visitors the rosebud that his future wife gave him the day she agreed to marry him.

Eventually they moved to Montgomery. He was popular, well liked, and respected in the city. He started practice with the free Negroes of Montgomery as his primary clientele, but within two years he was becoming a physician to the richest members of society. He was embraced by Montgomery's Jewish community as their doctor, and he wrote, "At the end of five years, I had established a reputation as a judicious practitioner and as a skilful surgeon, and was getting as much as I could do."

His surgical practice in particular boomed. He was practically minded, deft with his hands, and had a good bedside manner. He seems to have been one of those men with a gift for surgical practice, and, as he acknowledged candidly (but less than humbly), he "performed all sorts of beautiful and brilliant operations." People came to see him from 40 and more miles away when they were in need of an operation—and Alabamans of the 1840s did not seek out surgery for trivial reasons. He developed an interest in medical politics and became well known throughout the state. He was proud of his reputation.

Reconstructive Surgery in the 1840s

Surgical operations fall roughly into two categories: extirpative procedures, in which a diseased body part is removed, and reconstructive or restorative procedures, where the goal is to put something back together again so that it works properly. It is almost always easier to take something out than it is to repair a damaged structure. Sims was skilled at both. He undertook complex operations for cancers of the head and neck—fearful procedures in the 1840s that he had seen his old mentor George McClellan perform back in Philadelphia in his student days—but he took a special interest in reconstructive operations and understood their life-transforming power.

For example, in late 1844, Dr. Sims was visited by a young woman from Lowndes County. She was about 30 years old, and when she came to see him, her entire face was covered by a blue, double-thick veil. She had been born with a large double harelip and felt unable to show herself in public. When she raised her veil to show him her face, "the sight was horrible," he admitted. "I had never seen such a bad case of hare-lip before. It was sickening. Out from the end of her nose was a little bone—a snout—and from the tip end of her nose there was a small piece of skin, about three fourths of an inch long, looking like a shriveled-up gobbler's snout. She had no teeth, and I could look clear down her throat." In the surgical article that he later wrote about this case, Sims described her situation this way: "Her voice is nasal and very unintelligible to one unaccustomed to it. She swallows fluids with great difficulty, as they regurgitate by the fissures in the lip and superior maxillae. This mortifying deformity has excluded her altogether from society. Modest, diffident and sensitive, she avoids the presence of every one, except her own brothers and sisters. Life has no charms for her; and her only solace here is her hope of a blessed immortality hereafter." He took on her case.

He operated on her twice over the course of one month. The surgical procedure was relatively straightforward, complicated mainly by the fact that, "in spite of every entreaty she persisted in talking most vehemently, during the whole cutting pro-cess." Since this was done on the sensitive tissue of the lip and mouth before anesthe-sia existed, this would have been a pretty formidable undertaking. At the end of Sims's two operations, she was completely cured and had "a very presentable mouth, and Dr. Belanges, who was the leading dentist of the town, took a cast of the roof of her mouth, and made her a set of four handsome teeth. When he had finished his part of the work, she was a very presentable person indeed, and really a pretty woman. Her life, of course, was enlivened and revolutionized."

It may seem a long way from harelip to vesico-vaginal fistula, but the operation to repair a harelip was actually very important for reconstructive surgeons. It combined a number of principles that seemed applicable to the repair of a vesico-vaginal fistula: permanent closure of a defect, technical skill in manipulating delicate and sensitive structures, and the ability to enlist the full cooperation of the patient during the op-eration. Sims's subsequent attempts to repair vesico-vaginal fistula took place against this background: poorly developed techniques of reconstructive surgery, no anesthe-sia, precious few drugs of any benefit, patients hardened by difficult life experiences and used to dealing with pain, and a persevering surgical practitioner. The fistula operations would never have happened but for a coincidence: a fall off a pony by a short, fat neighbor lady that coincided with Sims's first encounter with a vesico-vaginal fistula.

Sims Encounters a Vesico-Vaginal Fistula

By this time Sims had been in practice for about 10 years, and he was doing well. He confined his work to surgery and general family practice. He had nothing to do with midwifery or obstetrics except when called in occasionally for consultation by another doctor. He did not practice gynecology and referred any such cases to his local colleagues, Dr. Henry or Dr. McWhorter.

In June 1845, Dr. Henry asked Sims to accompany him to the Westcott place a mile outside of town to see a slave woman who had been in labor for three days but still had not delivered. The slave, named Anarcha, was about 17 years old and had been in labor for 72 hours with the fetal head impacted in the pelvis. After seeing her, they both agreed that she needed to be delivered immediately; she was exhausted, and her uterine contractions had almost ceased. Waiting any longer would only increase the risk of complications and the likelihood that she would die. Sims had a pair of obstetrical forceps among his instruments and used them to deliver the (stillborn) baby without difficulty.

Anarcha seemed to rally from her ordeal and was improving. Five days later Dr. Henry stopped by Sims's office to give him an update. Anarcha's vagina had sloughed away from the prolonged pressure of her labor, leaving her with both a vesico-vaginal and a recto-vaginal fistula. "Aside from death," Sims remarked, "this was about the worst accident that could have happened to the poor young girl. I went to see her, and found an enormous slough, spreading from the posterior wall of the vagina, and another thrown off from the anterior wall. The case was hopelessly incurable." Never having encountered a case like this before, Sims went home and looked through all of the medical literature he could find on obstetric fistulas. It was totally discouraging. The medical consensus was that nothing could be done. Anarcha was doomed to be an outcast because of her injuries.

The following day, Sims ran into Mr. Westcott, Anarcha's owner, and told him, "Mr. Westcott, Anarcha has an affection that unfits her for the duties required of a servant. She will not die, but will never get well, and all you have to do is to take good care of her so long as she lives." Westcott, whom Sims called "a kind-hearted man," promised he would take care of her.

For Sims, Anarcha's case was only an unfortunate surgical curiosity, and he put it out of his mind. He wasn't particularly interested in gynecology generally or obstetric fistulas specifically. Then, a month later Dr. Harris from Lowndes County stopped by to see Sims and told him that one of his married slaves, Betsey, who was 17 or 18 years old, had had a baby a month ago, and since that time she had been completely incontinent. This was the second fistula.

Sims told Harris that there was nothing to be done. He knew about these cases, in fact he had just seen one. He had researched the subject and had to tell him that Betsey was incurable. Harris would not be denied. He insisted that his slave overseer send the girl to Sims for an examination. The following day, when Sims saw Betsey, he found the base of her bladder had also been destroyed. He kept her in Montgomery for a day or two, then sent her home with a note to Harris explaining that she was incurable, as he had already told him. "I supposed," he later wrote, "that I should never see another case of vesico-vaginal fistula."

But clinicians say that bizarre cases come in sets of three. Only a month later he was visited by Tom Zimmerman from Macon County. Tom had been one of Sims's patients when he lived out on Cubahatchee Creek in rural Alabama, but they had not seen one another for four or five years. Zimmerman told Sims that one of his slaves, Lucy, had given birth to child about two months previously after a difficult labor, and ever since she had "been unable to hold any water." This was the third fistula in less than three months.

Decades later Sims still recalled his conversation with Zimmerman. "Tom," he said:

> I know all about this case, and there is no doctor in this town or country who can afford any relief. I have just been reading up the subject; I have consulted all the authorities I can find in every doctor's library in this city. She has fistula in the bladder—a hole in it. It may be no larger than a pipe-stem, or it may be as large as two or three inches in diameter; but, whether big or little, the urine runs all the time; it makes no odds what position she is in, whether asleep or awake, walking or standing, sitting or lying down. The case is absolutely incurable. I don't want to see her or the case. You need not send her to town. I have just seen two cases, one in this town, and another that was sent to me from Lowndes County, and I have sent the last one back because there is no hope for it.

Zimmerman was undeterred—and pretty caustic—in his reply. He told Sims that having moved to Montgomery he was now "putting on airs" as a big-city doctor. Back in the day, he said (or words to this effect), when you were a simple country doctor in Cubahatchee, you would never have refused to see a member of my family or one of my slaves. Now that you are a fancy-pants doctor in Montgomery, you think you can pick and choose your patients. But you can't. I'm sending Lucy to see you tomorrow morning on the first train, whether you like it or not. You had better be ready to see her. And he left.

Sims took care of a lot of slaves. In fact, he had built a little eight-bed hospital on the grounds of his house for slaves who needed surgery or a medical consultation, and when Lucy arrived he gave her a bed. He examined her and told her, frankly, that he had nothing to offer her. She was incurable; that was the consensus of the established medical authorities. He would send her home the next day. "She was," he wrote, "very much disappointed, for her condition was loathsome, and she was in hopes that she could be cured."

Lucy's case now disposed of (so he thought), he set off to make rounds. He had a busy schedule of house calls, usually seeing 18 or 20 patients in the morning. Just as he was setting off, a little black boy came running up to tell him that Mrs. Merrill had been thrown off her pony and was badly hurt. He had to come see her right away. Not knowing whether it was a fractured skull, a broken bone, or something else, Sims hurried off.

Mrs. Merrill lived about three-quarters of a mile away. She was an old woman married to a "dissipated old man." In spite of her disreputable spouse, Mrs. Merrill was a hardworking, upright woman who lived by taking in laundry and sewing. She was in her mid-40s, "stout and fat," weighing some 200 pounds (large for then, not so much now). She had been riding her pony only a few yards from her house, when a hog had darted out into the road, spooking the pony, which threw her off. She landed hard on her pelvis. Although she had no broken bones, she was confined to bed, "complaining of great pain in her back, and a sense of tenesmus in both the bladder and rectum, the bearing down making her condition miserable." This was exactly the kind of case Sims hated.

"If there was anything I hated," he later wrote, "it was investigating the organs of the female pelvis. But this poor woman was in such a condition that I was obliged to find out what was the matter with her." He performed a digital examination and discovered that her uterus was retroverted—flipped backward—and apparently trapped up against the sacrum. The entrapped, impacted uterus was causing these feelings of unbearable, unrelievable pressure. The diagnosis seemed straightforward; the question, though, was what to do about it?

The voice of old Dr. Prioleau from his days at the Charleston Medical College suddenly came to Sims's mind: "Gentlemen, if any of you are ever called to a case of sudden version of the uterus backward, you must place the patient on the knees and elbows"—the so-called knee-chest position—"and the introduce one finger into the rectum and another into the vagina, and push up and pull down; and, if you don't get the uterus in position by this means, you will hardly effect it by any other."

Sims placed her in the appropriate position (discreetly covered by a large bedsheet) and started to work. He placed his fingers into her vagina (avoiding the rectum out of a combination of discretion and reluctance to stick a naked finger—rubber exam gloves not having yet been invented—into that particular orifice), found the uterus, and began pushing first upward and then downward, as hard as he could. Suddenly, he couldn't feel the uterus at all. He wondered where in the world it had gone, when Mrs. Merrill exclaimed, "Why, doctor, I am relieved." Sims still didn't understand what had happened but told her she could relax.

Mrs. Merrill, exhausted from her ordeal, fell over on her side. As she did so, a loud sound like a tremendous fart exploded into the room. The poor woman was mortified. She immediately began to apologize for the indiscretion of breaking wind in such an unladylike manner, but Sims suddenly realized what had happened. The noise was not the escape of gas from her rectum; rather, it was air that had rushed into the vagina and had expanded it while Sims was performing his therapeutic maneuvers. It was the inrush of air at atmospheric pressure, combined with her knee-chest position and his intravaginal manipulations, that had restored her uterus to its normal position.

It all clicked. "If I can place the patient in that position," he thought to himself, "and distend the vagina by the pressure of air, so as to produce such a wonderful result as this, why can I not take the incurable case of vesico-vaginal fistula, which seems now to be so incomprehensible, and put the girl in this position and see exactly what are the relations of the surrounding tissues?" If he could clearly see the location and nature of the injury, it would be the first step in figuring out whether a vesico-vaginal fistula could actually be cured.

Fired with this sudden insight, Sims forgot about the rest of his rounds and hurriedly headed home, stopping only to buy a pewter spoon at the store of Messrs. Hall, Mores, and Roberts. He ran to his office, grabbing two medical students who were working with him, and rushed off to the little hospital behind his house, hoping that Lucy had not yet left for home. To his relief, she was still there. He told her that he wanted to examine her again, to see whether anything could be done for her. She willingly consented.

They got a small table about three feet long and draped it with a coverlet. Lucy mounted the table, kneeling, and placed her head on the palms of her hands. The medical students were on each side to steady her and help expose the anatomy. Sims had planned to use the bent spoon handle as a speculum to examine the vagina, but as soon at Lucy assumed the knee-chest position with the help of the medical students, "the air rushed in with a puffing noise, dilating the vagina to its fullest extent." Sims gently introduced the bent spoon handle and, as he later wrote, "I saw everything, as no man had ever seen before. The fistula was as plain as the nose on a man's face. The edges were clear and well-defined, and distinct, and the opening could be measured as accurately as if it had been cut out of a piece of plain paper. The walls of the vagina could be seen closing in every direction; the neck of the uterus was distinct and well-defined, and even the secretions from the neck could be seen as a tear glistening in the eye, clear even and distinct, and as plain as could be."

Sims had solved the first great challenge of fistula surgery, which was how to get adequate exposure of the operative field. The vagina is a space deep in the pelvis. The walls of the vagina collapse together unless they are somehow held apart. If the vaginal walls are not somehow held apart effectively, any surgeon attempting to close a fistula would have to operate blindly, by touch—a formidable undertaking (and one of the main reasons why fistula repair had been such a failure up to this time). Sims had stumbled, quite by accident, upon a position for the patient that would allow easy visualization of her injury. Modified later from knee-chest to a more comfortable position in which the patient lies on her left side with her lower leg out straight and her upper right leg flexed, this "Sims position" became the preferred position for patients during vaginal surgery (see figure 4.1 below). It is still used extensively in gynecology today, being (for example) the preferred position for pelvic examinations in the British Isles. The "Sims speculum"—a later, more sophisticated version of his original bent pewter spoon—is still a valuable gynecological instrument used daily in clinics around the world.

The other two challenges would prove to be more formidable for Sims, although he didn't realize it at the time. These challenges would be closing the fistula with a suture material that would allow its edges to heal without suppuration and finding a way to drain the bladder effectively after surgery so that it did not become distended and split the line along which the edges of the fistula had been sewn together.

Before the development of the germ theory of disease toward the end of the nineteenth century and the concurrent development of "Listerism" (antiseptic, then aseptic, surgical technique), wound infection was a persistent and daunting challenge for surgeons. This was a particularly vexing problem in fistula surgery, since the edges of infected wounds do not heal properly and will not close. The critical part of fistula repair is getting the edges of the fistula to heal together; otherwise, they will not seal, the bladder will not be watertight, and thus the fistula will continue to leak. This had been the most important reason that fistula repairs had failed so often in the past: the wound would heal only partially after surgery because of infection. The fistula would generally shrink in size, but there would still be a residual defect that did not close. If there was a residual defect of any size in the bladder, urine loss would continue, and the patient would remain wet and miserable. Fistula surgeons using unsterile silk, horsehair, or various threads made from animal gut were continually plagued by wound infections that caused the repair to fail.

The third challenge, related to the second, was finding a way to drain the bladder continually as it healed. The bladder is a distensible organ, perhaps best likened to a balloon. A fundamental principle of surgery is that wounds should be closed without tension on the suture line, tension always tending to pull the repair apart. Urine is produced continuously by the kidneys, and therefore spurts of urine are always entering the bladder through the ureters (the tubes that connect the former to the latter). Unless it is drained, the bladder will start to fill. As it fills, it stretches. As it stretches, it places tension on the suture line, which pulls the repair apart. A distended bladder combined with a dirty, infected suture line was implicated in virtually every failed fistula repair that had ever been attempted.

In the flush of his discovery, however, Sims had yet to learn these lessons. With the optimism of inexperience, he exclaimed, "Why can not these things be cured? It seems to me that there is nothing to do but pare the edges of the fistula and bring it together nicely, introduce a catheter in the neck of the bladder and drain the urine off continually, and the case will be cured." Bursting with excitement, he finally managed to complete his morning rounds, but as soon as he had finished them he went to work inventing the instruments he would need to repair Lucy's fistula. "I felt sure that I was on the eve of one of the greatest discoveries of the day," he recalled. "The more I thought of it, the more I was convinced of it."

Sims Attempts to Cure a Fistula

He wrote Tom Zimmerman to tell him that he had changed his mind. He would be keeping Lucy in Montgomery after all. He told him to come down for a visit. He saw Mr. Westcott, Anarcha's owner, to tell him that there was a good chance he could do something for her after all. He also wrote to Dr. Harris and told him that he had changed his mind about Betsey. "I ransacked the country for cases," he wrote, and "told the doctors what had happened and what I had done, and it ended in my finding six or seven cases of vesico-vaginal fistula that had been hidden away for years in the country because they had been pronounced incurable." He needed more beds for the patients and those looking after them, so he added another story to his little hospital. He was confident and enthusiastic. Optimistically, he expected to cure all of these women of their horrible affliction within six months.

He told the slave owners that he would perform no experiment or operation on the women that would endanger their lives, that he would keep them at his own expense and would not charge for his services, but that the owners would have to be responsible for any taxes owed and to pay for the slaves' clothing. "I never dreamed of failure," he said, "and could only see how accurately and how nicely the operation could be performed." It took him three months to have his specialized instruments made, to collect all the patients, and to make the necessary preparations for his great surgical experiment.

The first patient whose fistula Sims tried to cure was Lucy. He described her case as "a very bad one. The whole base of the bladder was gone and destroyed, and a piece had fallen out, leaving an opening between the vagina and the bladder, at least two inches in diameter or more." The operation lasted about an hour and "the poor girl, on her knees, bore the operation with great heroism and bravery." Anesthesia had not yet been discovered, so none was used. The operation could not have been done without the full cooperation of the patient, who had everything to gain from success—restoration of urinary control and the dignity which that would bring—and very little to lose.

Sims had a crowd of doctors present to observe the operation, which he described as "tedious and difficult." His newly crafted instruments were serviceable but needed further modifications. Overall, he thought it was "very good work." The operation concluded, he put Lucy to bed. In retrospect, he wrote, "it does seem to me now, since things were so simple and clear, that I was exceedingly stupid at the beginning."

The fistula closed (at least for the moment), Sims needed a reliable way to drain the bladder. This was one of the most challenging aspects of fistula surgery at that time. All surgeons were hampered by the inadequate medical technology that existed in the middle of the nineteenth century. Plastic tubing and modern materials processing did not exist. The reliable and now-familiar latex Foley catheter that could be inserted simply into the bladder and kept comfortably in place with an inflatable balloon housed in the tubing was not invented until 1935. Sims recalled that the German surgeon Wurtzer, unable to find a way of retaining a catheter successfully in the bladder of his fistula patients, finally resorted to poking a hole in the bladder through the abdomen just above the pubic bone, inserting a tube into the bladder, which in turn was then affixed by screws to a large "belly harness" worn by the patient, after which she was placed flat on her abdomen on leather cushions in a special bed, so the tube could drain freely into a receptacle placed below. Sims was looking for something much simpler, but his initial selection of a method for bladder drainage was a huge mistake.

Sims decided to try to drain Lucy's bladder using a sponge wick with a silk thread running through it. The idea was that the little piece of sponge would act like a capillary tube, wicking the urine out of the bladder. It appeared to work like a charm. "As soon as it was applied," he wrote, "the urine came dripping through, just as fast as it was secreted in the bladder, and so it continued during all the time it was worn." But things did not go well. Five days after surgery, Lucy became very ill. She was obviously infected and starting to develop urosepsis, although, as Sims noted, "We did not know what to call it at that day and time." She had a high fever with a racing pulse and was dangerously ill. Sims was smart enough to know that he had to take everything out if Lucy was going to be cured, so he cut his sutures loose, got rid of the "peculiar mechanical contrivance" that he had used to hold the sutures in place in the vagina, and started to pull out the sponge wick that was resting in the bladder. To his horror, it did not budge. It had become encrusted with uric acid salts and adhered to the bladder like a stone. It had to be pulled away by "main force," causing great agony to his patient. Lucy "was much prostrated, and I thought she was going to die," he wrote. "But by irrigating the parts of the bladder she recovered with great rapidity, and in the course of a week or 10 days she was as well as ever"—except, of course, for the fact that she still had a fistula.

When she was well enough, Sims reexamined her. To his surprise, "the appearance of the parts was changed entirely. The enormous fistula had disappeared, and two little openings in the line of union, across the vagina, were all that remained. One was the size of a knitting-needle, and the other was the size of a goose quill." She was not cured, but her "enormous fistula" had been markedly reduced in size. If he could find a better way of draining the bladder, he thought, maybe he could cure these women after all.

Perseverance

Sims tinkered with his instruments, catheters, and suture while Lucy recovered from her surgery. By December 1845, he had made enough alterations that he felt confident about trying again. This time he operated on Betsey, whose fistula "occupied the base of the bladder, and was very large, being quite two inches in diameter." He repeated the operation exactly as he had attempted it on Lucy, but by this time he had developed a self-retaining catheter for draining the bladder. After anxiously waiting for a week, he reexamined Betsey. Her postoperative course was unremarkable, without chills, fever, sepsis, or other complications. He was hopeful of a cure. However, "To my great astonishment and disappointment, the operation was a failure. Still, the opening had been changed entirely in character, and, instead of being two inches in diameter, it was united across entirely, with the exception of three little openings, one in the middle, and one at each end of the line of union."

After further tinkering and revisions, Sims tried again. This time Anarcha was the patient. She was the first fistula patient Sims had ever seen, and she was one of the most challenging. She had a double fistula. Not only did she have an enormous fistula in the base of her bladder, she also had suffered extensive damage to the posterior vagina as well. Both the rectum and the bladder were involved, and her suffering, as Sims described it, was intense. Anarcha

> had the very worst form of vesico-vaginal fistula. The urine was running day and night, saturating the bedding and clothing, and producing an inflammation of the external parts wherever it came in contact with the person, almost similar to confluent small-pox, with constant pain and burning. The odor from this saturation permeated everything, and every corner of the room; and, of course, her life was one of suffering and disgust. Death would have been preferable. But patients of this kind never die; they must live and suffer. Anarcha had added to the fistula an opening which extended into the rectum, by which gas—intestinal gas—escaped involuntarily, and was passing off constantly, so that her person was not only loathsome and disgusting to herself, but to every one who came near her.

Sims made some more modifications to his equipment and then operated on Anarcha's vesico-vaginal fistula. Once again, "like the others, she was only partially cured." The large fistula was partially closed and greatly reduced in size, leaving only two or three small holes along the suture line. But, as Sims readily declared, "The size of the fistula makes no difference in the involuntary loss of urine. It will escape as readily and as rapidly through an opening the size of a goose-quill as it will when the whole base of the bladder is destroyed." He was discouraged.

Sims had attempted only three fistula operations, but already the entire history of attempted fistula repair had opened before him in all its frustration. The words of the great German surgeon Johannes Dieffenbach would have resonated with Sims's now-chronic disappointment. Dieffenbach had summarized his experience as a fistula surgeon in these eloquent yet melancholy words:

> The cure of vesico-vaginal fistula is one of the most difficult operations in surgery. With grief do we look at the imperfection of our art, accusing it and good mother Nature for their insufficient assistance. For centuries researches have been made for new and sure

methods, because the old ones have proved to be worthless; and with shame have we to acknowledge that the progress we have made is but small. The cure of vesico-vaginal fistula is still of a rare occurrence, at least more rare than its failure. Over sanguine in seeing once a fistula of great extent successfully obliterated by eight sutures, I was full of hope now to be able to defeat the grim enemy forever; but then I saw a small needle-hole remaining after an otherwise successful operation, or a fistula not larger than the point of a probe, defying all efforts to close it; I saw a fistulous opening of the size of a small pea, after cutting, sewing, cauterising, attain the extent of a large pea, a hole of 5 mm diameter, getting as large as one centimetre to two centimetres; then I stopped. I have operated on a woman eighteen times, and discharged her unrelieved. I have gathered together large rooms full of these unhappy women from all parts of the country, and I have exhausted all resorts and have cured only a few.

Sims was in exactly the same position as Dieffenbach, but he was remarkably resilient and perseverant. He wrote, "It would be tiresome for me to repeat in detail all the stages of improvement in the operation that were necessary before it was made perfect." He continued to collect patients with this soul-destroying malady. "Besides these three cases, I got three or four more to experiment on, and there was never a time that I could not, at any day, have had a subject for operation. But my operations all failed." He kept trying for two, three, even four years. He was obsessed with curing the vesico-vaginal fistula. His practice suffered. The costs of keeping a hospital full of slaves with fistulas was substantial. Although he had plenty of doctors eager to help him when he started, the continued failure of his efforts depleted their enthusiasm, and before long he had no assistants. His brother-in-law, Dr. Rush Jones, tried to persuade him to give it up, but Sims was resolute: "I am going on with this series of experiments to the end. It matters not what it costs, if it costs me my life," he declared stubbornly. "But, notwithstanding the repeated failures, I had succeeded in inspiring my patients with confidence that they would be cured eventually. They would not have felt that confidence if I had not felt confident too; and at last I performed operations only with the assistance of the patients themselves."

On reflection, Sims's surgical team was one of the most extraordinary groups ever assembled in the history of medicine. Operating without anesthesia, Sims repeatedly tried to close the defects between the bladder and the vagina to stop the maddening, debilitating, offensive stream of urine that ruled these patients' lives. The patients themselves, working as his surgical assistants, could see him inching closer to success. They could see the size of the holes being reduced almost to the point of closure, but not quite. Having experienced the misery of a fistula themselves, they were extraordinarily sympathetic to their fellow sufferers. Having experienced the challenges of attempted fistula repair themselves, they were constantly supportive of one another when they were patients on the table. They truly formed a "sisterhood of suffering," united in their desire to conquer the fistula problem. This phenomenon is well known in sub-Saharan Africa today. In many fistula centers the most devoted nurses, the most passionate patient advocates, and sometimes the most skilled surgeons are former fistula patients themselves.

Sims got more and more skilled as he performed more operations. They now took only 20, perhaps 30, minutes to perform, but he could not get the defect completely closed. The Sims position and the Sims speculum gave him exquisite exposure of the operative field. He had developed a technique of holding the sutures in place with little beads of lead shot that he crimped along the end of the suture, obviating the need to tie stitches high inside the vagina where it was difficult to reach. He had developed a remarkable S-shaped silver catheter with slits and holes along the side that drained the bladder magnificently. Once inserted into the bladder, one end rested up behind the pubic bone, while the other dangled outside the urethra. His catheter was easy to remove and clean, and comfortable for patients. He had honed his surgical technique to maximum efficiency, but he still could not succeed.

The Key to Success

To this point, however, he had been using silk thread as his suture material, as most surgeons still did at that time. He said to himself, "There must be a cause for this. I have improved the operations till the mechanism seems to be as perfect as possible, and yet they fail. I wonder if it is in the kind of suture that is used? Can I get a substitute for silk thread?" As he was pondering these thoughts one day, walking from his house to his office, he stopped to pick up a little bit of fine brass wire that was lying in his yard, the sort of thing that was "used as springs in suspenders before the days of India-rubber." An idea came to him as he pondered this piece of trash. He took the wire to a local jeweler, Mr. Swan, and asked him whether he could make a similarly fine pure silver wire for him. Mr. Swan obliged, and the spark first struck by Montague Gosset in London more than a decade previously had been rekindled in Montgomery, Alabama.

Anarcha, the first fistula patient that Sims had ever seen, was the first person on whom Sims used his silver wire sutures. In spite of all her operations, she still had a fistula in the base of the bladder that would accept the end of his little finger. (He had cured her other fistula.) The edges of the fistula were denuded and then brought together with four fine silver wires. The wires were passed through small strips of lead on each side of the fistula. The wires were held in place against the lead strip by small perforated pieces of lead shot threaded along the wires, which were then crimped with a pair of forceps. It was Anarcha's thirtieth vesico-vaginal fistula repair operation.

Sims put her to bed, introduced a catheter into her bladder and waited for the healing to occur. He noted that "the next day the urine came from the bladder as clear and as limpid as spring water," a hopeful sign. Cystitis had always occurred postoperatively when silk sutures were used, but that did not occur this time. Something was different.

A week after surgery, Sims examined Anarcha. "With a palpating heart and an anxious mind I turned her on her side, introduced the speculum, and there lay the suture apparatus just exactly as I had placed it. There was no inflammation, there was no tumefaction, nothing unnatural, and a very perfect union of the little fistula."

He had succeeded. Silver wire made all the difference. It was late in the spring of 1849. He had been struggling with this problem for nearly four years.

Over the next two weeks, he operated on both Lucy and Betsey, with the same results. They "were both cured by the same means, without any sort of disturbance or discomfort." For the first time in history, a surgeon had developed a consistent, repeatable method for closing a vesico-vaginal fistula. It was a huge achievement.

What was Sims's operation? How had he succeeded, where so many others before him had failed? The operation was simple and straightforward (although many of the fistula cases were not). He "pared" the edges of the fistula by saucerization, removing a thin strip of vaginal tissue but avoiding all but the edge of the bladder itself. (He described this as "the most tedious and difficult part of the operation.") The operative field was kept clear by the use of sponges (surgical suction did not yet exist). With the fistula exposed and its edges thus "scarified," Sims placed several silk sutures along the edges of the fistula using a needle, the precise number depending on the size of the fistula. The suture was placed into the vagina about half an inch from the edge of the fistula without going through its full thickness. The thread was then brought out just at the edge of the bladder lining, carried across the mouth of the fistula to the other side, where it was again inserted just at the edge of the bladder, then carried through the vaginal wall, exiting half an inch on the other side. Silver wire sutures were then fixed to the silk threads, which were used to pull the silver wire through to the other side. The silk sutures were then discarded, the silver wires were inserted through small openings in a small lead or silver bar (in the manner of a traditional "quill" suture). A small perforated lead shot was then threaded over the silver suture and crimped at the edge of the bar, holding each suture in place. Another bar was then placed on the other side and the silver wires similarly threaded into place, at which point the sutures could be tensioned to close the fistula completely, after which perforated lead shot was placed at that end of each wire and crimped to complete the closure and hold the sutures in place.

"The operation," he wrote in 1852, "which may have lasted some twenty or thirty minutes, or, under any circumstances, not more than an hour, is now over; and our patient is ready for bed, complaining only of fatigue from the constrained position."

His silver catheter was then placed to allow the bladder to drain continuously while healing took place. The catheter could be removed periodically, cleaned and rinsed, and reinserted. Constant vigilance to make sure the catheter was draining was important, for if it became blocked, the bladder could distend, ripping the healing suture

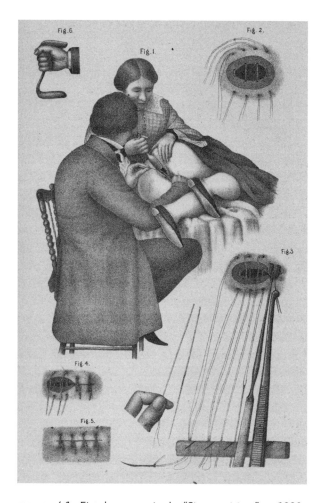

FIGURE 4.1. Fistula surgery in the "Sims position," ca. 1880. This is a recognizable modification of Sims's original operation. Lucy, Anarcha, and Betsey would have been on their hands and knees during the operation, a position that proved to be exhausting to the first patients. Sims subsequently discovered that having the patient lie on her left side with the operative field exposed with a retractor in the fashion shown here, was much more comfortable for the patients. *From Henry Savage,* The Surgery, Surgical Pathology and Surgical Anatomy of the Female Pelvic Organs, *3rd ed. (New York: William Wood, 1880), plate 24.*

line apart. "I have seen a failure result from a neglect of this precaution," he warned. Patients were given opium twice a day for pain relief and as a sedative and constipating agent. "It calms the nerves, inspires hope, relieves the scalding of the urine, prevents a craving for food, produces constipation, subdues inflammatory action, and assists the patient, doomed to a fortnight's horizontal position" due to the need for continuous catheter drainage, "to pass the time with pleasant dreams, and delightful sensations, instead of painful forebodings, and intolerable sufferings." The vulvar area was rinsed with tepid water several times a day for cleanliness and comfort.

He carried out an examination of the suture apparatus every few days to make sure nothing was amiss. He removed the clamps and the sutures around postoperative day 9 or 10, but he kept the patients in bed for another few days, with the catheter in place "to prevent any strain or traction on the delicate new cicatrix."

A new day in surgery appeared to be dawning, and Sims, thoroughly familiar with the struggles faced by previous surgeons, "realized the fact that, at last, my efforts had been blessed with success, and that I had made, perhaps, one of the most important discoveries of the age for the relief of suffering humanity."

These years of struggle had been difficult. The run-up to success was particularly trying because in October 1848, his three-year-old son had died of chronic diarrhea (the same illness that had killed his first two patients in Lancaster, South Carolina, many years previously). Six weeks after successfully closing Anarcha's fistula, Sims himself came down with severe dysentery. This affliction was "a chronic disease of the climate," endemic throughout the Mississippi River valley and undoubtedly due to infectious causes, considering the poor sanitary conditions prevalent in the South at that time. (It may have been an amoebic infection.) His health deteriorated rapidly. He became so weak and emaciated that he could not work. He feared that he was going to die. He struggled with gravely poor health for three years, with only intermittent relief from his gastrointestinal disorder. His weight dropped to 90 pounds. Finally, he sold all of his possessions (including several slaves) and moved permanently to New York City with his family in hopes of recovery.

He settled in a house at 89 Madison Avenue but struggled (as a Southerner transplanted to the North) to find a professional foothold in New York. His health gradually improved. Little by little he made the acquaintance of surgeons in New York and helped some of them with their operations. As a country practitioner from the South, he was an outsider, but many people had read his paper on the treatment of vesicovaginal fistulas in the *American Journal of the Medical Sciences*, and soon they were bringing cases to him, asking his assistance. But, he noted sadly, "As soon as the doctors learned what they wanted of me, they dropped me. As soon as they had learned how to perform these operations successfully in the New York Hospital and elsewhere, they had no use further use for me. My thunder had been stolen, and I was left without any resources whatever." Without a hospital in which to operate, Sims's career was doomed. The medical fraternity of New York City was largely opposed to helping him gain a position in practice.

Through a series of fortunate events—coupled with dogged persistence—Sims advanced a proposal to develop and open a hospital dedicated exclusively to women, particularly women who had obstetric fistulas. He managed to get the ear of several prominent, wealthy women, who backed him in this venture, and on May 1, 1855, the Woman's Hospital of New York was opened at 83 Madison Avenue. "The hospital was full from the day it opened," he noted. "We had about thirty beds. It was a charity; there were no 'pay-patients' admitted." He worked hard, still not fully up to health. Patients started coming from long distances and in larger numbers than could be accommodated in the facility. Within six months, he had to have an assistant—but whom should he choose?

The Contributions of Thomas Addis Emmet

Thomas Addis Emmet was a Virginian who, like Sims, had inadvertently fallen into a medical career for lack of a better idea. He had also attended the Jefferson Medical College in Philadelphia. After graduation, he took up a position as resident physician to the Emigrant Refuge Hospital in New York City, which had been established on Ward's Island, largely to accommodate Irish refugees fleeing the famine in their home country. The health problems of these people were formidable; many of them were suffering from typhus, and Emmet had to see roughly 100 men and 150 women and children each day, twice a day, in his position at the hospital. He sometimes was responsible for 3,000 or 4,000 patients at one time. He was regarded as an outstanding doctor who acquired extensive clinical experience working at the Refuge Hospital. There were 5 to 10 obstetrical deliveries a day in addition to the other clinical problems. He worked extra time in the hospital pharmacy, and he carried out more than 1,000 postmortem examinations of those who had died over the course of three years in this capacity. He was one of the hardest-working physicians in the history of American medicine.

One night, in the spring of 1855, Emmet was hard at work in his home tallying up each typhus-fever case that he had treated on Ward's Island. It was a cold day. It had been snowing, and he found the resulting quiet conducive to his work. While concentrating on his casebooks, there was suddenly a loud rap on his window. He opened the door, and there was J. Marion Sims, standing out in the cold. Sims told him the streetcar in which he had been riding had gone off the tracks just outside Emmet's house, and, as it was a cold night and he saw a light burning in the window, he wondered whether he could come inside to warm himself up. Emmet obliged. They started talking, and, before he knew it, Emmet was appointed to be Sims's assistant at the Woman's Hospital.

Aside from his wife, Theresa, Dr. Emmet was the best thing that ever happened to J. Marion Sims. Sims was an "idea man," full of new conceptions and brilliant ideas, but he was not by nature a "detail man" who would look after the practical considerations of bringing his ideas to fruition. Emmet was the perfect foil for Sims. Emmet was used to backbreaking hospital work after his stint at the Emigrant Refuge Hospital. It was easy for him to extract the pertinent clinical details from a case history, make drawings in medical records to illustrate problems, and tend to the details of medical administration. Before long he was doing two-thirds of the surgical cases at the Woman's Hospital, while Sims occupied himself with other matters, and after a few years (to be perfectly honest) the student surpassed the master as a fistula surgeon.

In his autobiography, *Incidents of My Life*, published in 1911, Emmet remarked concerning vesico-vaginal fistula, "I did not realize that it was to be part of my life's mission to render this loathsome and almost incurable injury not only curable, but that I was to be the means of restoring to perfect health nearly six hundred women thus afflicted, and finally to discover the cause and thereby revolutionize the obstetrical practice of the world, so that now the occurrence of this injury is almost unknown."

With the outbreak of the American Civil War, Sims was torn between his loyalties to his native South and to the national government of the United States. He decided to immigrate to Europe for the duration of the conflict, leaving Emmet in charge of the Woman's Hospital. In Europe, Sims was a fabulous success. He became one of the leading gynecologists in the world, personal physician to the nobility of France, and a sought-after writer and consultant. His book, *Clinical Notes on Uterine Surgery, with Special Reference to the Management of the Sterile Condition*, based on a series of articles he wrote for the British medical journal, the *Lancet*, was published in 1868. It was an international hit. This book, combined with his extensive surgical experience in treating gynecological disorders such as vesico-vaginal fistula, laid the foundations for much of modern gynecological practice.

During Sims's absence, Emmet continued the fistula work at the Woman's Hospital of New York, and his dogged perseverance and hard work paid off. He did several cases nearly every week and had done 270 fistula repairs up until October 1867. Of these he cured 200, had 5 complete failures, and the rest were improved or in various stages of preparation for final surgery. In 1868, the same year that Sims published his pioneering book on uterine surgery, Emmet published his own book on obstetric fistula, *Vesico-Vaginal Fistula from Parturition and Other Causes: With Cases of Rectovaginal Fistula*, a landmark text in the history of pelvic surgery, which was dedicated by Emmet, "To J. Marion Sims, M.D., my instructor."

Emmet's book clearly described how far fistula surgery had come since Sims began his preliminary efforts to close these defects in 1845. With a state-of-the-art institution in which to work, Emmet had perfected the protocol for the care of women with fistulas as much as possible within the limits of the surgical technology of the times.

He believed that the understanding of these injuries had progressed to the point where their treatment should be within the skill set of any competent, dedicated surgeon. He wrote, "No more training or tact is needed in the execution of this than in many other operations of surgery which have long since become familiar to the many." Done properly, the odds of success in a fistula repair operation were now high; what an enormous change from the situation 50 years before! However, achieving success required meticulous attention to detail, patience, and the understanding that several preparatory operations might be needed before the fistula could finally be closed. The operating surgeon often had to deal with extensive vaginal scarring, shrinkage, and distorted anatomy before the fistula could be repaired. Considerable thought and ingenuity was required to overcome these challenges.

Proper hygiene for the fistula patient was always a challenge, but getting the tissues into a healthy condition was the first—and most important—prerequisite for successful fistula repair. As Emmet wrote, "Unless the greatest care has been given to cleanliness, the sufferer, in a few weeks after receiving the injury, becomes a most loathsome object." The constant irritation of urine excoriated the vulva and made it swell. Ulcers on the labia were very common; occasionally they turned into abscesses. The injured vagina became coated with an "offensive phosphate deposit from the urine." If the fistula was large, it was common to find that "the inverted posterior wall of the bladder protrudes in a semi-strangulated condition, more or less incrusted with the same deposit, and bleeding readily." As a result he often found that "the sufferer becomes unable to walk or even to stand upright, without the greatest agony."

Care of the patient started with good hygiene to promote proper healing. Operating on inflamed, unhealthy tissues increased the risk of failure. The encrusted deposits had to be removed by cleaning with a soft sponge, after which the raw surface was covered with a weak solution of silver nitrate. Warm sitz baths were then instituted, which were greatly comforting to the patient. The vagina had to be irrigated regularly with large volumes of warm water to keep it clean and to reduce inflammation. Thereafter, the vaginal outlet and surrounding tissues were covered "with any simple ointment," which acted as a barrier to protect the skin. Urine was (partially) contained by the use of external menstrual pads or napkins, which had to be washed frequently when they became saturated. The expedient adopted by some patients to simply let the urine-soaked pads dry out and use them again was not acceptable. It would only irritate the tissues and prevent their healing. Emmet's regiment required "judicious attention to such details."

Every fifth day the excoriated surfaces were covered with silver nitrate solution—a course of treatment that could last weeks as the tissues healed. It was important to wait until the extent of the injuries revealed themselves and the tissues were in "a perfectly healthy condition." Only then could the attempt be made to close the defect. "This is the secret of success," he wrote, "but the necessity is rarely appreciated; without it, the most skilfully performed operation is almost certain to fail."

Each case was unique: the extent of the injuries, the location of the fistula, the presence and specific distribution of scar tissue all posed unique challenges that had to be overcome. The surgeon had to plan carefully, think topographically, and adapt his technique to the arrangement of the injuries before him. "The operator," he wrote, "like an engineer, must fully appreciate the peculiarities of the situation, and make each point available in his defense, and his success will be in proportion to his ingenuity in turning to the best account the peculiar features of each case." This approach often required considerable time and multiple operations to prepare the surgical field for final closure of the fistula. "The soft parts," he noted, "are susceptible of such great modification that it is often impossible for the surgeon to fully anticipate from the first what may be the result of his labors. It is only step by step, as the parts are relieved of tension, that they become moulded to their new condition. A full conception of what may be accomplished can only be formed with the gradual disappearance of the cicatricial [scar] tissue, and after a more healthy condition has been brought about by proper treatment." Some patients, being from poor circumstances, were unable to spend the time away from home that was necessary for a full and complete cure. As a consequence, some lost faith in the face of "the many progressive operations so often requisite" to achieve the final goal. But perseverance was usually crowned by success. His book contained numerous case studies that showed how, by patience, careful dissection, and proper preparation and aftercare, remarkable success could be attained.

An example was case 37, "Mrs. R.," a 40-year-old Irishwoman who had previously given birth to four children, all stillborn. In her last pregnancy (the "index pregnancy" that resulted in her fistula), she was in labor for nearly five days, only to deliver a very large stillborn baby with the aid of forceps. The urine began to run away almost immediately, and three weeks later a large slough of tissue was expelled through the vagina.

Emmet saw the patient at the request of the delivering physician and immediately admitted her to the Woman's Hospital for rehabilitation. "She was very much prostrated," Emmet noted. In fact, she spent almost five months as an inpatient recovering her strength and actually went home without having an operation. She was later readmitted for surgery.

At her readmission, Emmet found that she was missing the entire base of the bladder "from the neck of the uterus to the neck of the bladder," a horrific injury. Even the pubic bone was denuded and exposed. Furthermore, the bladder was turned inside out, protruding through the gigantic fistula, but the remaining vaginal tissues appeared to be relatively uninjured. Where would one even start to tackle pathology this extensive?

Emmet decided first simply to try to reduce the size of the fistula, since it was "impossible to bring the edges together in any continuous line." He freed what remained of the bladder from the pubic bone, mobilizing it enough so that he could draw it into the middle of the vagina. There he pulled its edges together using 13 sutures. This pulled the uterus down into the pelvis nearly an inch closer to the bladder and "half-closed" the fistula, but an opening still remained "in the shape of a right-angled triangle." At that point, he stopped. The fistula was not closed, but it was dramatically modified. A catheter was left in place and routine care was instituted. When the catheter was removed 12 days later, the edges that he had pulled together had all united, and the bladder no longer prolapsed through the opening that remained. This was good progress, but the patient was still totally incontinent from loss of urine through the defect that remained.

A little more than a month later, "Mrs. R" underwent a second operation. The remaining edges of the triangle-shaped fistula that still remained were "scarified," and the edges were joined by seven sutures, which succeeded in converting the triangular opening into a small circle. The fistula had been reduced from its enormous size down to one only about half an inch in diameter.

About six weeks after the second operation, Emmet performed a third surgery. This time he freed up the edges of the fistula, created lateral tissue flaps, and drew these flaps together with an additional 10 sutures. "The sutures were removed on the eleventh day," he wrote, "and the union was found perfect, except a small opening caused by the cutting out of a suture. This, however, closed in a few days, and the case was discharged, cured, shortly afterward." This was a triumph of patient, meticulous surgical care that would not even have been dreamed possible a few decades earlier.

The Legacy of Sims and Emmet

By the twentieth century the obstetric fistula was no longer the public health problem it had been a century earlier. Obstetric care was improving, and, as Cesarean section for obstructed labor became safer and more widely available, the number of fistula cases declined. The fistula hospital moved several times over the course of its life, and in 1900 Emmet carried out his last operation in the old facilities before a new ward was opened at 110th Street and Amsterdam Avenue as part of St. Luke's Hospital. The Woman's Hospital had been a proving ground for gynecological surgery. Sims—and especially Emmet—developed creative approaches to reconstructive surgery there, expanding their skills to encompass the operative treatment of many other gynecologic disorders. Howard Kelly, the first professor of gynecology at the new Johns Hopkins Medical School in Baltimore, poetically acknowledged the landmark work of Sims and Emmet in the *Dictionary of American Medical Biography* in 1928, writing of the two men that "in the history of gynecology, they abide serene like Castor and Pollux in the starry firmament of the midnight sky, well-known and welcome beacon lights destined to shine long after thousands of lesser luminaries have palled into oblivion."

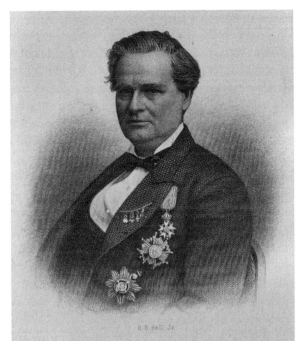

FIGURE 4.2. J. Marion Sims, at the end of his life, in full regalia, wearing some of his many medals and honors. *J. Marion Sims,* The Story of My Life *(New York: D. Appleton, 1888), frontispiece.*

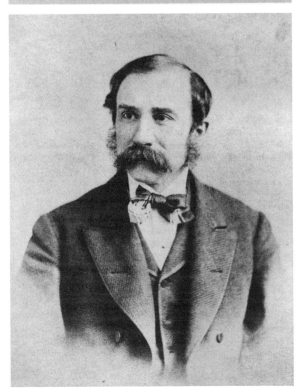

FIGURE 4.3. Thomas Addis Emmet in 1854, about the time he started his association with J. Marion Sims. *From Thomas Addis Emmet,* Incidents of My Life *(New York: G. P. Putnam's Sons, 1911), 162.*

Obstetric fistula surgery today is vastly different from what it was in the days of Sims and Emmet. There have been huge technical advances in instruments, sutures, drugs, fluid management, catheter drainage, anesthesia, and pre- and postoperative care that are beyond anything that Sims and Emmet could have envisioned in their time. Lessons from battlefield and trauma surgery have expanded the use of flaps and grafts and led to the development of extraordinary operative techniques that can be used to reconstruct the entire genito-urinary tract. New bladders, new ureters, and even new vaginas can be created out of segments of intestine, and current research has even successfully grown new bladders in the laboratory. Within the realm of fistula repair itself, however, the basic principles of fistula closure remain unchanged from those developed by Sims and Emmet: (1) mobilization of the fistula from the surrounding tissues so that the defect can be closed without tension on the suture line, (2) watertight closure of the fistula, and (3) prolonged catheter drainage after surgery so that the incision heals without being stretched. Today the most common causes of vesico-vaginal fistula in industrialized countries are surgical injuries during another operation (such as a hysterectomy or removal of a urinary stone) or complications of radiation therapy. These injuries are very different from the devastating crush injuries caused by prolonged obstructed labor.

Emmet noted that most of the fistula patients he saw were poor and from rural areas. This is still true today, although the epidemiological distribution of these injuries has shifted. Globalization and the spread of modern medical technologies has eliminated childbirth injuries from obstructed labor as a public health problem throughout the industrialized world. These injuries now occur only sporadically and under unusual circumstances in high-income countries. Obstetric fistulas persist in large numbers only in the poor and rural areas of the globe, especially in sub-Saharan Africa. Today the obstetric fistula problem affects mainly poor women in the "bottom billion" of the world's population. To understand why this preventable, treatable, obstetric malady persists in such large numbers, we need to dive deeper into the social circumstances in which such women live. I do this by examining the position of women in the Hausa culture in West Africa to see how their social circumstances affect their reproductive lives.

CHAPTER 5

Structural Violence and Obstetric Fistula among the Hausa

The labor of any pregnant woman can become obstructed, but the incidence and prevalence of fistulas are not evenly distributed throughout the population of reproductive-age females around the world. In a completely just society, the incidence and prevalence of injuries and ill health would be spread relatively evenly across all age groups and socioeconomic classes (after adjusting for inherent biological variables). But the world is not just; extraordinary inequalities exist everywhere. Fistula is one such inequality that is suffered by the world's poorest women.

In this chapter I examine the Hausa people of West Africa, among whom obstetric fistulas are common. I will show how this form of obstetric injury is linked to the social institutions and value structure of Hausa society. I have chosen the Hausa because I know them well, having lived among them intimately as an anthropologist and having visited this region many times over the past 40 years both as a researcher and as a clinician. Hausaland covers the northern half of Nigeria and the southern edge of Niger, but the Hausa language is spoken over a much greater area. Hausa is the most widely spoken indigenous language in West Africa, and it may well be spoken over a broader geographical range than any other African language.

The best way to enter the domain of obstetric injury in Hausaland is by explaining a song that I encountered on a visit to northern Nigeria several years ago. The Hausa title of the song is "Fitsari 'Dan Duniya," which may be loosely translated as "Urine, the Oppressor of the World." The song was composed by a young woman named Fatu, herself a victim of obstetric fistula. The song was enthusiastically performed by a large group of incontinent women, all of whom had developed obstetric fistulas from prolonged obstructed labor. These women lived together in a special hostel for fistula patients on the grounds of Evangel Hospital in the city of Jos, Plateau State, in north-central Nigeria. The hostel had been constructed with the assistance of the

Worldwide Fistula Fund, the oldest US charity supporting fistula work, and I was there on its behalf. The women of the Evangel Fistula Hostel had adopted "Fitsari 'Dan Duniya" as their anthem. Performing it helped them develop the sense of community and group solidarity that was critical for their rehabilitation, and it aided the psychosocial healing that is so important for the fistula patient. African praise songs usually follow a stylized pattern, a verse being called out by the lead singer with a chorus responding to the call. Through this cycle of call and response, vocalization and repetition, accompanied all the while by vigorous drumming, this community of patient-victims found its common voice and struggled to establish both its identity and its dignity.

Here is the Hausa text, along with an English translation.

"Fitsari 'Dan Duniya"
(Urine, the Oppressor of the World)

Fitsari 'dan duniya. Fitsari 'dan Dandi.
(Urine, the Oppressor of the world. Urine, who has forced me from my home.)

Muna neman lafiya; sun ce mu tafi Dandi.
(We went out looking to be healed, but they said we were all whores.)

Ciwo ya same ni tun ina yarinya ta.
(This sickness "caught me" when I was only a young girl.)

Ina zauna a gida na ji labari mai kyau.
(I sat confined at home until I heard the good news.)

Na ce: Wayyo, iya! Sai ki ba ni ku'di.
(I said, "My word, mother! Give me the money!")

Zan je Jos Jankwano zan sauka zan ga sabbin Turawa.
(I will go to Jankwano in Jos! I will go down there and see the new Europeans.)

Kamman gobe haka tiata zan sauka.
(By this time tomorrow I will have arrived in the operating theater.)

Can wurin Karshima zaune.
(I will remain there at Dr. Karshima's place.)

Dakta Karshima sai godiya muke Allah saka mar.
(Doctor Karshima I thank you! May God bless you!)

Ya dinken mata masu ciwon gana yoyo.
(You have sewn up the leaking women.)

Maigida ya yarda ni domin ina ciwon yoyo.
(My husband threw me out because I was leaking.)

Ciwo ya same ka sai su kai ka su yarda kai.

(If this sickness "catches you" they'll carry you out and throw you away too.)

It takes more than a literal translation to unpack the meaning of this song. *Fitsari 'dan duniya* literally means "urine, son of the world." The Hausa word *'dan* means "son of," but it is commonly used in a broad metaphoric sense to express an intimate relationship between objects. For example, a policeman is often called *'dan sanda*, which literally means "son of a cudgel," a reference to the intimate relationship between a policeman and his baton or nightstick. The Hausa word *duniya* literally means "the world," but in Hausa thought *duniya* (this world) is often contrasted unfavorably with *lahira* (the next world, or the afterlife). As C. H. Robinson glossed the word in his *Dictionary of the Hausa Language* in 1925, "'Duniya is often used to denote the evil principle which characterizes the world, so *'dan duniya* (lit. 'son of the world') a bad man." In this sense, then, *fitsari 'dan duniya* means something like "urine, the evil oppressor" or "urine that puts the weight of the world upon us." For a woman who experiences total, unremitting urinary incontinence from a vesico-vaginal fistula, this is an apt description.

The expression *fitsari 'dan dandi* or "urine, son of Dandi" likewise requires explication. *Dandi* is a generic Hausa expression for places south of the city of Zaria, which lies on the southern fringes of Hausaland between the Hausa heartland and Nigeria's "middle belt," in which the city of Jos is located. To call someone a *'dan Dandi* ("son of dandi") or *'yar dandi* ("daughter of *Dandi*") is to characterize her as a person who migrates out of her own "proper" sphere into a state of marginality. The implication is usually that she is leaving home to lead a morally dissolute life, in which case *Dandi* becomes not so much a physical location as it is a state of abnormal being. *Fitsari 'dan Dandi* thus refers to the urinary incontinence that forces these women with fistulas to leave their homes, their social positions, their normalcy and to take up a despised, liminal existence on the fringes of society. Many women with a vesico-vaginal fistula, especially those who have suffered with this condition for years, have lived as "fistula pilgrims," continually wandering in search of a cure. As a result, they have often been divorced by their husbands and sometimes abandoned by their families as incurable outcasts. They have become "children of *dandi*" in literal as well as figurative terms.

This is why the next line of the song goes, "We went out looking to be healed," referring to their quest for medical help for this terrible affliction, "but they [their families and neighbors] said we were all whores," out to lead dissolute lives. In traditional Hausa society, proper married women are secluded at home within the family compound and cannot go out without their husband's express permission. The Hausa word *karuwa*, which is generally translated as "prostitute," actually refers to a woman who is not under proper male control. Hausa culture imputes to women an inherent tendency to promiscuity; thus, a mature woman who is out by herself in the world without male supervision is regarded as a prostitute by definition, irrespective of her actual behavior. Although the vast majority of fistula women have developed their affliction because of an unforeseen and unavoidable complication of labor—which means that they themselves are morally innocent—they may be stigmatized by the community as having contracted a horrible venereal disease through promiscuity or having developed their fistula as a consequence of (or punishment for) adultery. This stigma, along with a common lack of understanding on the part of these women as to what has really happened to them and why they have developed their affliction, adds to the psychological burden that they carry.

The third line of the song goes, "This sickness 'caught me' when I was only a young girl." The age of marriage for girls is young in Hausa society, and many are married before they are physiologically prepared for childbearing. Growth in height or stature stops before full growth of the pelvic bones has been reached, so girls who marry young and become pregnant early are at increased risk of obstetric complications. Although obstructed labor can occur in any pregnancy, the two groups most at risk are young girls in their first pregnancy and older women who are in their fourth or greater pregnancy (because fetal weight tends to increase with subsequent pregnancies, this increases the risk for cephalo-pelvic disproportion).

The line "I sat confined at home until I heard the good news" again explicates the isolation experienced by the fistula patient, sitting alone in her room. These women are cut off from wider society. Their hygienic needs are overwhelming and if neglected even for a short time, they may end up smelling of urine, and sometimes of stool as well. They are reluctant to socialize, and their sense of loneliness can be profound. The "good news," of course, is word carried through the amazing African grapevine of a place where help is available for fistula victims.

The girl exclaims, "Wayyo [Wow!], mother! Give me the money!" (for traveling expenses). She is destitute, dependent upon charity for everything that comes her way. Hausa fistula victims are generally young, illiterate, unskilled women in a culture that values them slightly, and they are afflicted with a socially disgusting condition that often renders them incapable of fulfilling their socially mandated roles as wives and mothers. Thus, she needs help and begs for it from the listener (calling, at the same time, upon the Muslim tradition of almsgiving, which makes "begging" a ubiquitous part of life in West Africa). It is also highly significant that she begs her mother for help. A girl's mother is her last, best hope for solace when all else fails. In a patriarchal society like that of the Hausa, there may not be much sympathy from a male for a woman with a female complaint, but a mother will always understand and try to help. The fistula patients most to be pitied are those whose mothers have died, for they are truly destitute and at the mercy of the world.

The place she seeks is the hospital in Jos, located in the neighborhood of Jankwano. The "new Europeans" there are non-African doctors—usually white European or American missionaries, but the same term is also applied to American blacks who, despite their skin color are recognized as European culturally. The presence of Europeans is significant because there is generally little interest in the welfare of fistula victims in Nigeria. They are "charity" cases in every sense of the word. Almost every fistula hospital anywhere in the world needs an "external lifeline" if it is to function, because local resources are inadequate for the clinical challenges they face.

"By this time tomorrow I will have arrived in the [operating] theater." This expresses the poignant hope for surgical cure—and it is one that is quite realistic. The vast majority of vesico-vaginal fistulas can be closed successfully, sometimes in as little as 20 or 30 minutes of operating time, if conditions are favorable. The transformation in an afflicted woman's life created by a successful repair is staggering, and there is no more overwhelmingly grateful patient in gynecology than a woman who has been cured of a vesico-vaginal fistula.

Thus, the song says, "I will remain there at Dr. Karshima's place." Dr. Jonathan Karshima is an old friend of mine, a dedicated clinician and expert fistula surgeon, who was the medical director of the fistula unit at Evangel Hospital when this song was composed. Having found an environment in which they are welcomed—after all of the suffering they have endured—it is no small wonder that these women do not wish to leave. Although the hostel is designed to house patients for a brief period before and after surgery, many of these women stay for months, having no place else to go, a fact that raises ongoing administrative problems of its own. "Doctor Karshima I thank you! May God bless you!" "You have sewn up the leaking women."

Many African songs of this type end with a moral exhortation or a caution. The words say, "My husband threw me out because I was leaking. If this sickness 'catches you' they'll carry you out and throw you away too." In Hausa, as in many other African languages, one does not "catch" an illness; rather, the illness "catches" you. The world is seen as a dangerous place, where malevolent forces lurk and to which you may fall victim if you are not careful.

Structural Violence and Obstetric Fistula

Structural violence is a concept used by anthropologists and other social scientists to help explain the skewed distribution of injuries and ill health among particular social groupings. Structural violence is indirect, rather than direct, violence. Direct violence is the kind of violence that occurs when someone is beaten and robbed. Structural violence is more subtle than this but often is just as lethal. James Gilligan defined structural violence as "the increased rates of death and disability suffered by those who occupy the bottom rungs of society, as contrasted with the relatively lower death rates experienced by those who are above them. Those excess deaths (or at least a demonstrably large proportion of them) are a function of class structure; and that structure itself is a product of society's collective human choices, concerning how to distribute the collective wealth of society." An alternate way of explaining this concept with respect to obstetric fistulas is to say that structural violence reflects the way in which healthcare resources are allocated within a particular society. Obstetric fistulas are manifestations of the unequal, unjust, and inadequate distribution of healthcare resources to childbearing women. Obstetric fistulas are a violent reflection of the way in which a society fails to value its reproducing women and how it neglects to manage the complications of human reproduction.

Obstetric fistulas result from the interaction of individual physiological violence (obstructed labor) and the social violence produced by badly managed, poorly resourced, inefficient maternal healthcare systems. The physiological violence that afflicts any individual woman in obstructed labor takes place within a particular infrastructure of obstetric care that is in turn determined by the social, political, and economic priorities of each nation. Obstetric fistula is the outcome of two types of structural constraints that come together in devastating ways: the constraints of social structure (beliefs, attitudes, conceptual categories, family relations, economic relationships, political power) and the constraints produced by the quality and distribution of resources devoted to health (doctors, nurses, midwives, clinics, hospitals, ambulances, surgical instruments, medications, ultrasound machines, etc.).

The first set of constraints produces social-structural violence by shaping the social norms that dictate appropriate behavior for pregnant women. The second set of constraints produces infrastructural violence by determining the nature and distribution of healthcare institutions that provide emergency obstetric care. Where crumbling healthcare facilities, bad roads, poor communication, erratic power and water supplies, incompetent management, and indifferent or incompetent doctors, nurses, and technicians are found, there will be high rates of maternal death and disability. Maternal mortality and severe obstetric morbidity (such as obstetric fistulas) are the visible manifestations of social-structural and infrastructural violence.

An overview of how various types of determinants affect the outcome of obstructed labor is provided in figure 5.1. The pregnancy of any individual woman takes place

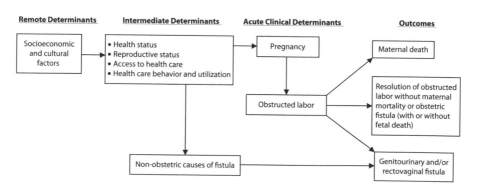

FIGURE 5.1. A framework for analyzing the determinants of obstetric fistula formation. This chart shows how socioeconomic, geographic, and clinical circumstances interact to create the "perfect storm" that creates an obstetric fistula or maternal death. © Worldwide Fistula Fund, used by permission.

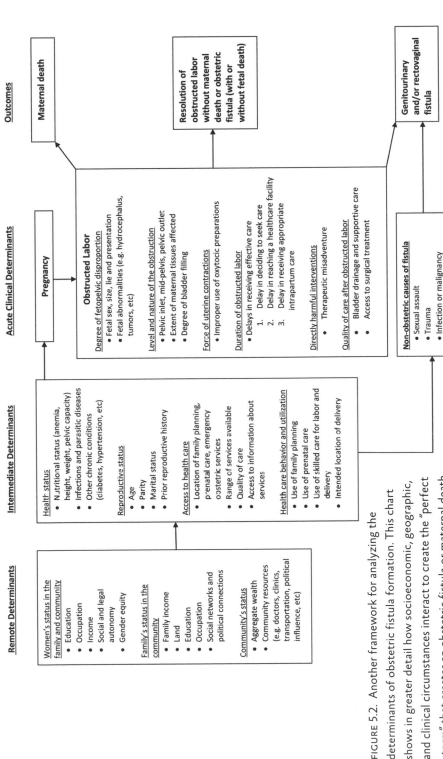

FIGURE 5.2. Another framework for analyzing the determinants of obstetric fistula formation. This chart shows in greater detail how socioeconomic, geographic, and clinical circumstances interact to create the "perfect storm" that creates an obstetric fistula or maternal death.

© *Worldwide Fistula Fund, used by permission.*

within a particular social and economic setting. The immediate determinants of her situation will be defined by her health and reproductive status, her access to care, and the way healthcare is utilized. The outcome of acute problems in pregnancy, such as the outcome of a particular case of obstructed labor, will be determined by specific clinical developments occurring within this larger framework (figure 5.2).

Most maternal deaths and childbirth injuries are avoidable. The skills and technologies needed to prevent these dreadful outcomes are straightforward and have been widely known throughout the international medical community for more than 75 years. The reason that maternal death and maternal childbirth injury have not been addressed more forcefully around the world is because of societies' views concerning women and human reproduction. The Hausa people of northern Nigeria and southern Niger are a paradigmatic case of how a culture's views about women are reflected in the incidence and prevalence of reproductive morbidity and mortality. Recent data gathered by H. M. Salihu and colleagues demonstrate that nearly 35 percent of women who deliver a baby in northern Nigeria will have a significant obstetric complication. Maternal mortality ratios here are among the highest in the world. It is no surprise that obstetric fistulas are extremely common in this part of the world. These statistics reflect the social position of women in Hausa culture.

Obstetrician Kelsey Harrison, whose study of childbirth outcomes at Ahmadu Bello University Teaching Hospital in northern Nigeria launched the international Safe Motherhood movement in the 1980s, agrees with this view. He wrote, "A striking feature of Hausa life is the extremely low status it accords women." When the biological reality that women bear the totality of risk associated with childbearing is combined with a degraded social position and a healthcare infrastructure that devalues women, the result is an enormous gender inequity demonstrated by exceptionally high rates of female death and disability. The Hausa are a dramatic case study of how the prevalence of obstetric fistula reflects its social milieu.

The Political Background of Hausaland

The Hausa people have been prodigious traders and commercial entrepreneurs throughout their history, traveling widely to pursue economic opportunities wherever they can find them. As a result, there are Hausa-speaking communities scattered from Senegal on the westernmost coast of Africa, to Tunisia along the Mediterranean, across the Sudan to the Red Sea in the east, and as far south as the Congo basin. The Hausa heartland in northern Nigeria consists of rolling savanna broken by outcroppings of rocks and scattered acacia trees, arid most of the year but fertile enough to support relatively dense human settlement, particularly around the commercial center of Kano.

This dense population anchored the southern end of the trans-Saharan caravan routes and allowed the Hausa to develop a sophisticated social and political system early in their history. The political consolidation of territories led to the creation of a number of kingdoms, each centered on a large walled capital city and controlled by a hierarchy of chieftains who owed allegiance to the king (*sarki*) in his fortified palace. These independent kingdoms were often at war with one another, with boundaries that expanded and contracted as the fortunes of the various city-states ebbed and flowed.

Although the traditional Hausa kingdoms became nominally Muslim in the sixteenth century, they were relatively tolerant and easygoing. Their "live and let live" attitude resulted in a heterogeneous intermingling of traditional customs covered with a thin veneer of Islam. At the beginning of the nineteenth century, this situation changed dramatically. A revivalist Muslim cleric of Fulani ethnicity named Shehu Usman 'Dan Fodio, preached an Islamic holy war against the Hausa kings, whom he regarded as "pagans" because of their relaxed approach to Islam. 'Dan Fodio's Islamic revivalism sparked a political uprising that grew exponentially. Within a few years, the Hausa kingdoms were overthrown, and the ruling Hausa elite were replaced by Hausa-speaking Fulani overlords, who established an Islamic caliphate in the northwestern Nigerian city of Sokoto.

When the British conquered northern Nigeria at the turn of the twentieth century, to their surprise they found a sophisticated governmental apparatus already established, with its own system of laws, tax collection, and administration. Rather than replace this indigenous system with an entirely new administrative arrangement, the British elected to govern northern Nigeria through the political hierarchy that was already in place (the "policy of indirect rule"). This provided administrative continuity, but it also served to entrench the existing Hausa-Fulani leadership in power (who were not always as powerful, as popular, or as stable as the British thought). The legacy of these colonial policies continues to haunt Nigerian national politics to this day.

Their long tradition of territorially based political hierarchy means that Hausa social organization has not been dominated by lineage and clanship obligations to the same extent as have other African societies. The fundamental unit of Hausa social structure is the household compound (*gida*), headed by a senior male owner of the compound (*maigida*), who is the resident authority within the home. The compound is also often occupied by the householder's adult sons, who may be married but are not yet wealthy enough to form their own compounds.

A typical Hausa compound is constructed with high mud-brick walls and is entered from the street through a small entry hut (*zaure*) where the compound head greets visitors. The number of individuals living in a compound—as well as their relationships to one another—is fluid. Inside the compound there are storehouses for grain, a cooking area, a latrine, possibly a well, and separate huts for each of the wives. Because this is a Muslim society, a man with enough wealth and can marry up to four women if he so desires. Unrelated males do not enter another man's household without permission.

Hausa Women in Their Social Setting

One of the most striking things for an outsider who arrives in a Hausa village is the almost complete absence of adult women in public, except for the very old and, perhaps, the very poor. Goats, sheep, men, boys, and preadolescent girls are everywhere, but women are nowhere to be seen. This is because the Muslim Hausa have adopted a relatively strict form of purdah, or "wife seclusion." In Hausa this is known as *auren 'kulle*, or "locked-in marriage." This spatial configuration of Hausa living arrangements has immensely important implications for Hausa women. As Renee Pittin has written, "No single aspect of Hausa culture gives men such ascendancy over women as this God-given system of unrelenting spatial constraint, often beginning even before a woman is married, and continuing until she is well into middle-age." With rare exceptions, Hausa women have limited personal autonomy and are subject to male social control in almost every area of Hausa life. These arrangements directly impact the health of Hausa women.

Of the Hausa household, anthropologist Barbara Callaway wrote:

To the casual observer, life behind the mud wall of the compound appears secure and peaceful, but time spent there brings hundreds of sad stories. Women complain of heavy labor, of marriages of young daughters against their wills, of child brides brought into the household, of forced sexual cohabitation at puberty regardless of mental or emotional development, of early motherhood and infant death. There is no sewage system, running water is unreliable, and animals roam freely. Illness, needless death, and especially female and infant mortality are commonplace. Said a mother of a twelve-year-old on her wedding day, "may the day be cursed when she was born a woman.

The life cycle of Hausa women revolves around their reproductive capacity, and a fundamental principle of Hausa social organization is that female reproductive capacity must be controlled by appropriate males. Hausa men are quite blunt in stating that the purpose of women is to produce children, which they regard as the "profit" obtained in return for the exchange of goods in marriage arrangements. Women are seen as "fields" to be "tilled" by men, and children are the "crop" that results. The same word (*riba*) is used for the profit that comes from children in a marriage as well as for the profit that comes from selling cotton or groundnuts. Hausa women are not regarded as fully adult until they have produced a child, preferably a male. In the event of divorce, even though a woman may (and should) return to the compound of her father or a brother, her children (especially male children) remain the property of her former husband.

Hausa females move through a series of life stages, each with its own appropriate behavior and social controls, but the most important organizing principle of female social status is reproductive status. Hausa girls and women are readily organized according to pre-reproductive, reproductive, and post-reproductive categories. The young Hausa girl from toddler to preadolescent has great personal freedom, just as do young

Hausa boys. Brothers and sisters of the same mother commonly sleep with one another in their mother's hut inside the family compound, and they may play together throughout the village. As they grow older, the separation of the sexes becomes more pronounced: girls spend more time with the women of the compound, boys with the men. Girls are given increasing responsibilities for household chores, particularly those involving the itinerant sale of snacks and foodstuffs throughout a village, since the seclusion of adult women limits their economic activities.

Nonetheless, the preadolescent Hausa girl (bera) has great freedom of movement and may engage in open joking and friendly banter with men and women throughout the village. This is an important form of social interchange as she sells foodstuffs and runs errands for the secluded female members of her compound. The adolescent Hausa girl is called a budurwa, a word that signals the onset of puberty, marked most conspicuously by the formation of breast buds. A budurwa has many of the same social freedoms as her younger sisters but is expected to assume the more modest demeanor appropriate for one starting to approach womanhood. In this period of her life there may even be innocent (or sometimes perhaps not so innocent) sex play with males, but intercourse is strictly forbidden by social custom, and illegitimate pregnancy remains a rare, but heinous, offense against community standards.

To ensure proper control and to prevent potential sexual misconduct, marriage usually occurs quite early for Hausa girls, frequently before their first menstrual period. It is not uncommon for girls to get married between the ages of 12 and 14, and even sometimes as early as 9 or 10. This practice stems largely from the social requirement that female reproductive capacity should be under strictly acknowledged and well-defined male control. These social arrangements are often implicated in the obstetric catastrophes that are so common in this part of Africa.

When marriage occurs, the social transformation from carefree girl to married woman is instantaneous, abrupt, and emotionally jarring. The Hausa word for "woman" and the word for "wife" are one and the same: mace. These roles are synonymous in Hausa thought. Whereas the day before she had the freedom to roam the village, talk to men and boys, visit with friends, and to enter other households whenever she pleased, the day after marriage she is confined to her husband's compound, cut off from her family, and often subjected to abuse by her new relatives, particularly if she is the second wife of a man whose senior wife feels threatened by displacement by a younger rival. In such circumstances the new bride may be treated as little more than an unworthy servant by the older women of the household. The psychological impact of these changes can be profound, and the sudden and complete disappearance of previously outgoing, friendly young women upon their marriage is one of the more striking aspects of life noticed by a long-term resident of a Hausa village.

Throughout their lives, Hausa females are continually told that they are inferior to males. This viewpoint is codified in Islamic law, according to which women do not receive an equal share of an inheritance, nor is their legal testimony given the same weight as that of a man. Women are often excluded from communal Islamic religious activities because they are seen as recurrently unclean because of menstruation and childbirth. Women of reproductive age rarely participate in communal prayers at the village mosque, undertaking their devotions (when they do so) in the privacy of their homes. Only older, postmenopausal women who have lost their reproductive potential and who no longer pose a threat to society are likely to be seen at the mosque, relegated to a separate area behind and away from the men.

In the eyes of Hausa men, female sexuality is dangerous and disruptive. Hausa men see women as inherently licentious and potentially troublesome, a theme that is abundantly elaborated in Hausa folktales. The control of female sexuality is a constant worry in Hausa culture. One Hausa proverb goes so far as to say, "Matar mutum kabarinsa" (A man's wife is his grave). Women are depicted as unreliable, devious, and unpredictable. A cynical Hausa proverb ridicules men who "fall in love": "Maso mace wawa; bai san za ta ki shi ba" (He who loves a woman is a fool, for he never knows if she hates him or not).

Women can (partially) compensate for their flawed natures by acquiring *kunya*: "modesty," "shame," or "deference." In Hausa eyes, *kunya* is the supreme virtue for a woman. One proverb expresses it well: "Matar na tuba ba ta rasa miji" (A submissive woman won't lack for a husband). In a society where the only respectable role open to a woman is that of wife and mother, getting a husband is vital. The virtuous woman is deferential, submissive, and (ideally) secluded within the family compound away from the view of other men. Numerous Hausa proverbs echo these sentiments: "Matar shige ba ta da daraja" (A woman who "goes out" is without honor). "Kyakkyawar 'kwarya tana ragaya da faifanta a rufe" (The very best gourd calabash stays hung up at home with a lid on top). Not only should a "calabash" stay at home, but it remains closed—sealed up—to be used only by its proper owner, her husband.

Jean Trevor, who taught in a girls' school in Sokoto in the early 1950s, went back 20 years later to find out what had happened to her former pupils, who by that time had all married and started families. As she remembered, "I asked a traditional religious leader to describe the ideal woman, and he described 'M,' a girl I had taught, very intelligent, tactful, and charming who after school devoted herself to Koranic studies and was content to stay in purdah organising the domestic arrangements of a big compound and teaching women and children the Koran, and helping the children with their homework. Unfortunately she preferred traditional maternity care to that of the modern hospital: she died in childbirth. She had been quiet, obedient, emotionally controlled and had not struggled against her fate." This girl was, in many ways, the perfect reflection of Hausa female virtue as well as an all too common example of the reality in which such girls live—and die.

Hannah Papanek has analyzed the institution of wife seclusion through the interaction of two principles, which she calls "separate worlds" and "symbolic shelter": the rigid sexual division of labor that separates men from women and the concomitant moral obligation that men have to provide for their womenfolk. Richard Longhurst has enumerated the obligations a Hausa husband has toward his wives and family as the provision of food, water, firewood, housekeeping money, and shelter, as well as gifts of cloth and perfume at the major festivals. The Hausa wife, in turn, is obligated to provide labor for the preparation of food, childcare, and general domestic chores. In the system of wife seclusion, she is not expected to work in the fields or to fetch water. If the husband cannot provide food from his own farm, he must purchase it on the open market for the family. Wife seclusion is therefore a major determinant in the sexual division of labor, and this in turn results in an economic imbalance between the sexes. Men maintain the household for the benefit of the family unit; women should acknowledge the "shelter" they receive by appropriately modest behavior, including deference to males and covering their heads (and sometimes their faces) in the presence of men. When greeting a social superior, the inferior person crouches submissively: women always crouch when greeting men.

Within these separate worlds, men and women are free to pursue their own economic activities as long as the obligations mentioned above are met, and nearly all Hausa adults—both male and female—vigorously pursue such activities. Men engage in contract labor, farm cash crops such as cotton or groundnuts, sell cloth, kola nuts, or other items in the market, or start small businesses of various kinds. Women engage mainly in local trade carried out among the compounds of the village. Economist Polly Hill has called this the "honeycomb trade" in Hausaland, an economic network composed of many busy but separate and segregated little "cells" of sheltered women interacting together in a widespread (but relatively hidden) network of trading relationships. The economics, however, are markedly unequal: Longhurst calculated that the social constraints imposed on her activities meant that a rural woman could earn only about a quarter of what a man could earn. Thus, the economic game is rigged against women, a fact that makes it almost impossible for them to survive on their own income alone. They remain economically subservient, as well as socially subservient, to men, especially in the rural economy.

Since women should be wives and mothers, secluded within their family compounds, it is not surprising that little value is placed on educating girls or women. Although Islam holds that it is important for females to have an understanding of the Koran and the basic tenets of the religion, in practice (if girls get any schooling at all), their formal education usually consists of only a brief stay at a local religious school where they memorize a few Koranic verses under the guidance of a neighbor who has a reputation for piety. Even in the religious sphere, females get far less education than males. In the late 1970s, Nigeria instituted a program of "universal primary education," but its impact on rural Hausa girls appears to have been minimal even 40 years after the policy was put in place. The rural population does not see the need for secular education, which is, in any case, often perceived as having "corrupting influences" on females.

The name of the Islamic terrorist group Boko Haram, which became firmly entrenched in northeastern Nigeria in the early twenty-first century means "books (Western education) are prohibited (anathema)." Boys are much more likely than girls to receive an education, since the Hausa have lower expectations for females than for males.

While a woman still has reproductive potential, her life should revolve around kitchen, home, and family, ideally separated and secluded from the outside world. After menopause, when a woman has "dried up" and can no longer reproduce, the issue of male control is not as important because there is no reproductive potential to worry about (and old women are not regarded as sexually attractive in any case). As a consequence, when women reach their postreproductive years, they are allowed greater freedom. If they are clever, ambitious, and industrious, postmenopausal women may become more active in the wider economy and occasionally can amass significant wealth.

Women may fall out of their normal social position as wives through divorce or widowhood. One Hausa proverb bluntly states, "Zamanka kai kadai ya fi zama da mugunyar mace" (Living by yourself is better than living with an evil woman). While a man could never live alone and retain any status in Hausa society, the social contempt that exists for an "evil woman" is reflected in the ease with which a man can divorce a woman. Divorce is quite common in Hausaland. It is not unusual for a woman to be married three or more times in the course of her life. If the marriage is childless, the husband may demand the return of a portion of the bridal payments that were transferred to his wife's father at the time of their marriage. But if children have been born, the transaction is complete: the husband has received his "profit" from the marriage in the form of offspring. Understandably, then, divorces are more common in childless marriages, where there is less to bind husband and wife together. Because children remain the property of their father, women are often reluctant to risk losing their offspring through divorce.

Although it is more difficult, women may also obtain a divorce. A woman who is dissatisfied with her marriage may move out of her husband's compound and return to her father's household, an act that is poetically called *yaji* (literally "hot pepper") in Hausa. The embarrassment caused to the husband by such a defiant act on the part of his wife may be enough to force his hand in their dispute and lead to an acceptable resolution, but it may also be the precipitating factor that causes an enraged husband to divorce his unruly wife.

The Hausa word *bazawara* refers to a woman who is no longer married. She may be a divorcée or a widow. To be a *bazawara* is socially acceptable and respectable (as long as the accompanying behaviors are appropriate), but in the ideal world this should be only a temporary state. A *bazawara* is expected to return to the household of a male relative (either her father or a brother) until she remarries, at which time she is given over to the control of her new husband. In Hausaland the duration of this status is regulated by Maliki Islamic law. Divorcées and widows are forbidden to remarry until several months have passed, a practice based on reproductive concerns about paternity in any pregnancy that occurs toward the end of a marriage that has dissolved. A period of enforced celibacy (theoretically) ensures that if a child is born during this liminal period, the father is clearly identifiable. Women are expected to remarry within a reasonably short time unless they are old and are therefore "undesirable." Should a woman not remarry, she can maintain her respectability only by remaining in the household of an appropriate male family member. To behave otherwise is to risk becoming a "prostitute" (karuwa) in the eyes of the community.

The Hausa word karuwa is generally translated into English as "prostitute" or "courtesan." In English, such words designate a woman who earns her livelihood by selling sexual favors for money, often having multiple partners in a single day. While there is no question that a Hausa karuwa may engage in sexual intercourse for financial gain, the term "prostitute" is not really an accurate translation as karuwa does not require the exchange of sex for money. In fact, a karuwa may be celibate. More precisely, the term karuwa refers to a woman who is no longer under the control of a socially appropriate male. She is a woman who has lost her modesty (kunya) and who has moved beyond the bounds of social respectability. This may be the only option for some women to escape an intolerable living situation. In the context of rural village life it generally means escaping from relatives and starting a precarious and unrespectable life on the edges of urban society.

The interrelated concepts of dangerous female sexuality, the need for women to be controlled and supervised by men in a secluded social environment, and the cultural definition of a virtuous woman as one who is modest, deferential, and submissive (as well as fertile), have important consequences for Hausa women's health. Added together, these factors have a tremendous impact on pregnancy and childbirth.

Childbirth in Hausaland

A Hausa girl, even a bride, is not really considered a woman until she has given birth. Rehan accurately described Hausa society in 1984 as "pronatalist." Attitudes have not changed since then. Children are regarded as a gift from God, the desired and prescribed outcome of marriage, and the greatest fulfillment of being a woman. Hausa proverbs express the importance of childbirth in maintaining the continuity of life, stressing the social role of childbearing women: "Haifuwa maganin mutuwa" (Birth is the medicine for death). Rehan's 1984 study from Katsina reported that the average desired family size for Hausa women is seven children, with only 12 percent of women desiring fewer than five. Producing many children brings respect and honor to the family and to the mother who bears them. Even today, few women have any knowledge of birth control, and most consider family planning the moral equivalent of murder. Only an unbeliever would even contemplate abortion (at least openly). Such attitudes are generally shared by Hausa men and women alike.

Because marriage occurs at an early age in Hausaland, sometimes even before a girl's first menstrual period, it is not surprising that early teenage pregnancy is common. Rahan and Sani found that over 32 percent of obstetric patients in Katsina were under the age of 20, as compared to only 18.5 percent of a similar population in Nairobi, Kenya. Pregnancy in young teenage girls places an enormous strain on their bodies. Since these mothers are still growing themselves, they actually compete with their fetuses for nutrition. The extent of this problem among the Hausa is clearly seen from the work of Kelsey Harrison and colleagues, who gave young pregnant teenagers iron and folic acid supplements during pregnancy and documented a huge difference in growth between the supplemented and unsupplemented groups. These studies also found significant correlations between lack of antenatal care, lack of iron-folate supplementation, and the need for operative delivery due to cephalo-pelvic disproportion at the time of delivery.

Kunya, or "shame," is supremely important during childbirth, especially during a woman's first pregnancy. Social convention dictates that the newly pregnant girl should avoid drawing attention to her gravid state. She should avoid all mention of the pregnancy in conversation and behavior. Older women stand ready to scold her should she deviate from this norm. The social pressure to "remain modest" may well prevent her from asking questions about pregnancy and childbirth, even in the face of a pressing clinical problem. This creates an enormous barrier to providing and obtaining prenatal care, to delivery in a hospital or at a community health center, or in accessing emergency obstetrical services when problems arise.

In spite of the increased demands placed on her body by pregnancy, the pregnant adolescent is still expected to carry her full share of household work without receiving any special consideration. Overall there seems to be a general tendency to ignore pregnancy in Hausa culture, particularly as a girl begins the transition to full womanhood during her first pregnancy. So great is this sense of shame surrounding the first pregnancy that traditionally a woman's firstborn child was often given to another relative to raise, and a culturally sanctioned avoidance relationship is often present between parents and their firstborn child.

As term approaches, the first-time pregnant bride is usually sent back to her parents' home for delivery. In this setting she probably receives more compassionate treatment than she would if she stayed in her husband's family compound. Her mother, other relatives, and a local midwife usually stay with her during labor, but her fear and her sense of shame may be so great that she says nothing to them until labor is well advanced.

Women labor in several positions, but typically they deliver kneeling or squatting, often with another woman supporting her. The Hausa recognize both how difficult childbirth is and how important is its outcome. The proverb says "Azabar uwa ta sami 'da" (A mother's agony gets her a son). Nonetheless, there is great social pressure on a pregnant woman to remain modest during labor and to avoid crying out or showing any evidence of pain. To labor quietly and patiently is a sign of courage and great character, and it shows proper modesty. A proverb also says "Haifuwa 'daya horon gutsu ne" (The first birth "breaks" the bottom). Just as a horse is broken to become docile, domesticated, and useful, so too a Hausa woman is domesticated to a life of patient childbearing. The expectation is that after the woman is "broken," many more births will follow. In subsequent deliveries, women are often left to labor by themselves and to deliver alone, away from the prying eyes of jealous cowives and busybodies.

Lorna Trevitt's observations here are particularly interesting. After investigating Hausa childbirth practices, she wrote:

> It is unusual for a girl to deliver alone the first time. Her mother or another older relative stays with her. If there is nobody immediately available, however, it is unlikely that the girl will send for someone, for quite apart from the fact that she may not realise that she is going into labour, *kunya* will prevent her from saying anything. One woman thought that even in later deliveries, anyone who was over-anxious to have people around her was a coward, and she made explicit what others had implied, that it is a source of pride after the first child to deliver alone. Others suggested in addition that this was the only way to prevent exaggerated gossip afterwards.

Only an older woman who has borne children herself can become a Hausa midwife (*ungozoma*). These women usually have little education of any kind and do not receive any formal training in midwifery. They acquire their skills through family tradition, trial and error, and perhaps by assisting other midwives in the community (although there may also be considerable competition and personal jealousy between them). Hausa midwives also typically provide traditional remedies for medical conditions other than pregnancy (especially treatments for infertility and pediatric problems), and they dispense wisdom to their clients as liberally as they give out herbal medications.

Although they are often respected within their communities and may hold high status among local women, as a group, Hausa midwives do not possess any particular manual skills for dealing with complicated deliveries. The astoundingly high maternal mortality in Hausaland, along with the prevalence of fistulas, confirms this. The *ungozoma* is a ritual officiant for pregnancy and childbirth rather than a technical expert in obstetric emergencies. The Hausa midwife serves a social role in maintaining and promoting normative community values. This role is far more prominent than any technical contribution she might make to the process of childbirth. In fact, Hausa midwives are largely responsible for overseeing two traditional practices that are directly harmful to childbearing women: the mandatory hot ritual baths taken after childbirth and *gishiri* cutting in obstructed labor.

The balance between hot and cold is an important concept in the traditional Hausa medical beliefs. Either too much heat or too much cold is thought to produce serious adverse effects on the body, particularly on the blood. If the body is "open," cold can come in and cause illness. Because of their recent deliveries, postpartum women are considered to be particularly "open" and thus vulnerable to the deleterious effects of cold. To ward off illness due to the pernicious effects of cold (*sanyi*), newly delivered Hausa women are kept hot. There are several methods by which this is achieved. For example, they may rest on a clay bed built with a small fireplace underneath to allow them to be "roasted." This small furnace is stoked with hot coals around the clock and can dramatically drive up the temperature of the room, especially during the hot season.

In addition to such "roasting," recently delivered women (particularly women who have delivered their first child) are expected to undergo a series of hot ritual baths for at least 40, and sometimes as long as 90, days after delivery. These baths (called *wankan jego* or *wankan biki*) serve both ritual (purifying) and medicinal purposes. They are undertaken with a pot of very hot water into which various herbal ingredients with purported medicinal power have been added. The recently delivered woman (or her attendant) then uses a bundle of small leafy branches from a tree to slap herself with steaming hot water, beating herself with the leaves to drive the heat into her body. This is not a trivial procedure: Lorna Trevitt actually measured a water temperature of 82° Celsius (148°F) just prior to the start of one such ritual bath.

The practices of "roasting" puerperal women over a bed of hot coals and "steaming" them with hot water has a number of serious health consequences. Many Hausa women are admitted to hospital each year with serious burns they have sustained by being immersed in scalding water or falling onto beds of glowing coals during these ritual baths. These customs also result in large number of burn injuries to children and newborns, who are often innocent but injured bystanders of these ritual practices.

In addition to producing direct thermal trauma, the prolonged ritual heating of puerperal women contributes to the significant clinical problem of peripartum cardiac failure in northern Nigeria. Peripartum cardiomyopathy is a somewhat obscure form of heart failure that occurs during pregnancy or after delivery in previously healthy women. The condition is relatively rare, with an incidence ranging between 1 in 1,300 to 1 in 15,000 pregnancies. In the United States peripartum cardiomyopathy occurs approximately once in every 3,780 pregnancies, but it is the single most common cardiac disease seen in Zaria, Nigeria, at the Ahmadu Bello University Teaching Hospital, where it complicates approximately 1 percent of all Hausa deliveries—an astonishingly high rate. The condition is uncommon among other Nigerian ethnic groups and appears to be confined almost exclusively to Hausa women.

In addition to the hot baths and traditional "roasting" that a Hausa woman undergoes after delivery, she is fed large quantities of a special gruel ostensibly to increase her strength and to increase the flow of her breast milk. This gruel contains a large amount of a local lake salt called *kangwa*, which contains large amounts of sodium carbonate. *Kangwa* is a common ingredient in Hausa traditional medicines and is used for a variety of gastrointestinal and other complaints. E. H. O. Parry and coworkers reported that newly delivered women ingested as much as 30 grams of this salt per day. High salt ingestion and excessive heat appear to combine with a number of other common conditions (hypertension, seasonal temperature rises, anemia, splenomegaly, low serum albumin, and perhaps a genetic predisposition) to increase extracellular fluid and plasma volumes, to increase cardiac work, and ultimately to produce an extraordinarily high incidence of peripartum cardiac failure. Many women who develop this condition never recover, either dying or becoming permanently disabled by cardiac disease.

Although the problem of peripartum heart failure is extremely disturbing, it is probably overshadowed by another ethnomedical condition, called *gishiri* among the Hausa. *Gishiri* is the Hausa word for "salt." It is used particularly to refer to the salt encrustation that forms on the bottom exterior of an earthen waterpot as its contents slowly seep through and evaporate. This word is also used to describe a medical condition that many Hausa believe affects women, particularly pregnant women. The proper balance among bodily fluids is an important concept in Hausa traditional medicine. This is thought to be especially important during pregnancy, when imbalances of body fluids or substances are thought to be harmful to the mother and her developing child. Such imbalances are also thought to contribute to gynecological problems, particularly sexual dysfunction and difficult delivery. One such belief is that if a woman ingests too much sugar or salt, it may seep through the vagina, "encrusting" it (as it would the bottom of a waterpot) and leading to a vaginal constriction that causes menstrual difficulties, pain with intercourse, or obstructed labor.

Traditional Hausa midwives do not cut episiotomies to open the perineum in order to expedite delivery. This unpopular practice is one of the common reasons Hausa women give for avoiding hospital deliveries (along with an aversion to losing *kunya* by exposing their genitals to strangers—possibly men—during delivery). If labor is prolonged, a diagnosis of obstructed labor due to *gishiri* is often made, and a village midwife or barber may be called in to perform an operation called *yankan gishiri* (salt cutting). In an attempt to alleviate the obstruction, the midwife or barber takes a sharp object such as a knife, razor blade, piece of glass, or other available instrument, inserts it into the woman's vagina, and makes a series of random cuts. Since the Hausa do not possess any detailed knowledge of human anatomy (most of what they know is based upon analogies derived from the casual study of animals during butchering), *gishiri* cutting is not done with any knowledge of the anatomic structures involved or of the actual pathophysiology of obstructed labor. As a result, *gishiri* cutting often leads to serious hemorrhage, infection, and injury to the urethra, bladder, rectum, or vagina. In most series of fistulas reported from northern Nigeria, *gishiri* cutting is responsible for up to 15 percent of cases. Most *gishiri* cuts are associated with the treatment of obstructed labor, but they may also be made to treat other "gynecological" conditions, such as attempting to enlarge the vagina of an 11-year-old bride who is "too small" to permit her new husband to have intercourse with her.

Hausa women are defined by low social status, poor education, economic inequality in a context of general poverty, restricted social mobility, spatial confinement, high fertility, low personal agency, and a general cultural expectation that virtue requires modesty, subservience, and compliance if they are to avoid bringing shame upon themselves or their families. Each of these factors reinforces and compounds the effects of the others. When obstetric complications are added to this mix, the results are frequently fatal.

Maternal Mortality in Hausaland

A maternal death is traditionally defined as the death of a woman while pregnant or within six weeks of the termination of pregnancy, from causes related to pregnancy or worsened by the pregnant state. Within this six-week window the most common causes of death for pregnant or recently pregnant women are hemorrhage, infection, hypertensive disorders of pregnancy (preeclampsia and eclampsia), complications of unsafe abortion, and obstructed labor (which also causes fistula). The most common measurement of the incidence of maternal death is the maternal mortality *ratio*: the number of maternal deaths per 100,000 live births. To put this discussion in context, consider that the maternal mortality ratio in the United States in 2015 was 14 maternal deaths per 100,000 live births. Other industrialized countries have similar (and usually better) maternal mortality ratios, for example, Canada (7), Great Britain (9), Germany (6), France (8), Australia (6), Sweden (4).

According to estimates for 2015 developed by the World Health Organization, approximately 201,000 women die in sub-Saharan Africa each year from pregnancy-related causes. Africa accounts for more than half of the world's maternal deaths, even though it produces less than a quarter of the world's births. Sub-Saharan Africa has the highest maternal mortality ratio in the world: 546 maternal deaths per 100,000 live births. Nigeria has more maternal deaths (40,000 per year) than any African country, and a Nigerian woman has a 1 in 22 lifetime risk of dying from a pregnancy-related cause (compared to 1 in 3,800 in the United States or 1 in 12,900 in Sweden). These numbers are worse in northern Nigeria than in the rest of the country, and equally poor if not worse in the poverty-stricken country of Niger directly to the north.

While maternal death is tragic (and almost always preventable, at least in theory), maternal mortality measures only fatal outcomes. Nonfatal maternal birth injuries (such as obstetric fistula) have consequences that may be even more devastating than death itself. Whereas a tragic death in childbirth brings release from suffering, the woman who is seriously injured while delivering a stillborn child may live a life of unremitting misery for decades afterward. The term "severe obstetric morbidity" is used to refer to serious nonfatal obstetric events or "near misses" in which the pregnant woman is gravely ill or seriously injured but survives. Severe obstetric morbidity is always much higher than maternal mortality, and it may be a better indicator of obstetric practice than the maternal mortality ratio. For example, a study by Mark Waterstone and colleagues from the UK analyzed 48,865 deliveries from all 19 maternity units and six hospitals in the South East Thames region of England over a one-year period and found a maternal mortality ratio of 10.2 maternal deaths per 100,000 live births but a severe obstetric morbidity ratio of 1,200 severe morbidities per 100,000 births, a hundredfold increase in the "burden of disease" compared to maternal death. But circumstances in resource-poor countries are much, much worse. Alain Prual and colleagues performed a similar study in Niamey, Niger, and found severe obstetric morbidity to be an astonishing 6,450 cases per 100,000 deliveries—and these statistics included only the most severe complications. Recall as well that these statistics refer only to a single pregnancy; women who have many pregnancies face similar risks in *each* pregnancy, raising the lifetime risk of death or injury to astoundingly high levels.

Where rates of maternal death are high, rates of nonfatal obstetric injury will be sky high, and fistulas will be prominent where obstructed labor is a common contributor to maternal death. In Prual's study, obstructed labor occurred at a rate of 3,614 cases per 100,000 deliveries. It is no wonder that maternal mortality is only the "tip of the iceberg" with respect to African women's health problems.

Comprehensive statistics on maternal mortality are not available for the whole of Hausaland, but numerous studies over 40 years have accumulated enough data to paint an extraordinarily dismal picture of maternal health in this part of West Africa. The most important maternal health study in northern Nigeria was conducted by the Department of Obstetrics and Gynaecology at Ahmadu Bello University in Zaria, Kaduna State. Professor Kelsey Harrison, himself a Nigerian, supervised the analysis of 22,774 consecutive deliveries at Ahmadu Bello University Teaching Hospital over a two-and-a-half-year period between January 1, 1976, and June 30, 1979. During the study period, there were 238 maternal deaths among 22,774 deliveries, for a crude maternal mortality ratio of 1,050 maternal deaths per 100,000 births. This represents the death of slightly more than 1 percent of all women in childbirth.

The most common causes of maternal death in Harrison's study were bacterial infection, anemia, hemorrhage, pregnancy-induced hypertension, and obstructed labor. An old medical adage says, "People don't die from complications—they die from the complications of complications"; that is to say, the situation most often turns deadly when several confounding factors interact. Two or more confounding factors were often present in the maternal deaths that Harrison reported. A later study (also in Zaria) by Kisekka and colleagues confirmed this and noted that obstructed labor was often a precipitating factor in the cascade of complications that lead to maternal death. Although the most common reasons for death were sepsis, hemorrhage (complicated by preexisting anemia), and eclampsia, these often occurred in the setting of obstructed labor. "For instance," they wrote, "among the patients whose deaths were associated with haemorrhage, the antecedent event was obstructed labour in 58.3% of the cases. Haemorrhage occurred as the result of ruptured uterus, difficult caesarian section or uterine atony [a noncontractile uterus] from prolonged obstructed labour. Similarly, in those dying from eclampsia and sepsis, obstructed labour was the underlying cause in 46% and 63% respectively."

One of the most striking facts in Harrison's study was the extremely high proportion of maternal deaths (92 percent) that occurred in women who had no prenatal care (219 of 238 maternal deaths). Most of these women presented for treatment gravely ill and very late in their clinical course, already knocking at death's door when they reached the hospital. None of these unfortunate women had any formal schooling, and none had registered for antenatal care. They were typical of childbearing women among the rural Hausa.

Looking more closely at Harrison's statistics, we find that among women without prenatal care ("unbooked deliveries") there was a maternal mortality ratio of 2,860 per 100,000 births, as compared to a maternal mortality ratio of 130 per 100,000 births in the "booked" group that had received prenatal care. (Compare this to the US statistic of 14 deaths per 100,000 births). Unbooked women in their first pregnancy—one of the highest risk groups—had a maternal mortality ratio of 3,320 deaths per 100,000 births, unbooked patients who had several previous pregnancies (multiparous women) had a maternal mortality ratio of 2,600 deaths per 100,000 births, and unbooked women who had had five or more pregnancies (grand multiparas) had a maternal mortality ratio of 3,480 deaths per 100,000 births. Among booked patients who had received prenatal care, the comparable maternal mortality ratios were 110, 130, and 140 maternal deaths respectively per 100,000 births—still high by the standards of the industrialized world, but good for sub-Saharan Africa. More detailed analysis of the data revealed staggering numbers of maternal deaths in certain subsets of this population, with maternal mortality ratios as high as 7,360 maternal deaths per 100,000 births among 15-year-olds in their first pregnancies who received no prenatal care and 4,530 maternal deaths per 100,000 births among women 30 years of age or older who had had five or more pregnancies but no prenatal care. These statistics can only be described as obstetric carnage.

Unfortunately, the situation in northern Nigeria has not improved since Harrison's day; in fact, there are indications it is actually getting worse. Since Harrison's pioneering work in the late 1970s, additional studies on maternal mortality have been carried out at medical centers throughout northern Nigeria. All of these studies have documented large numbers of maternal deaths and tremendously high maternal mortality ratios. The data are summarized in table 5.1.

The studies from Zaria, Jos, Kaduna, Sokoto, Birnin Kudu, and Nguru were all undertaken at hospitals and therefore are subject to potential institutional biases due to the nature of the case mix at those institutions (sicker patients are generally found in hospitals), whereas the study from Kano State is a population-based study and the study

Table 5.1. *Maternal mortality in northern Nigeria (Hausaland)*

Location	Lead author	Dates of study	Number of maternal deaths	Number of deliveries	Maternal mortality ratio (maternal deaths per 100,000 deliveries)
Zaria	Harrison	1976–1979	238	22,774	1,050
Sokoto	Shehu	1984–1987	405	14,179	2,856
Jos	Ujah	1985–2001	267	38,768	740
Kaduna	Onwuhafua	1990–1997	69	10,572	652
Sokoto	Audu	1990–1999	197	9,158	2,151
Sokoto	Airede	1990–1999	46	946	4,863*
Kano State	Adamu	1990–1999	4,154	171,621	2,420
Sokoto	Nwobodo	2000–2009	165	3,047	5,415*
Birnin Kudu	Tukur	2002 2005	51	2,233	2,284
Nguru	Kullima	2003–2007	112	3,931	2,849
Zamfara	Doctor	2011	584	n/a	1,732**

Source: Full citations to the source papers of these data are in the bibliographical essay.
*These were maternal deaths in pregnant adolescents, 12–19 years of age.
**Maternal mortality ratio calculated on the basis of demographic surveys using the "sisterhood method" of maternal mortality estimation.

from Zamfara is a demographic study based on a sampling technique called the "sisterhood method," in which individuals are questioned about the obstetric experiences of their adult sisters. The results of these studies are shocking but consistent with one another. The maternal mortality ratio of 2,420 maternal deaths per 100,000 live births from Kano State is one of the worst maternal mortality ratios documented anywhere in the world using a large population base. What is consistent among all studies is the staggering rate of maternal death and childbirth injury across northern Nigeria.

As with Kelsey Harrison's original work from Zaria, these subsequent studies have all shown dramatically increased rates of maternal death among pregnant women who do not receive prenatal care, among adolescents (who really should not be pregnant in the first place), among women in their first pregnancies, among "grand multiparas" who have had at least five previous deliveries, and among illiterate, uneducated women. Each of these findings is a concrete example of the way structural violence affects women. The increased mortality found in each of these groups of pregnant women is a direct reflection of a value system that restricts women's freedoms, constrains their social lives, limits their personal agency, and refuses to allocate adequate resources to meeting critical female-specific healthcare problems. In the study from Sokoto, for example, 84 percent of maternal deaths occurred among women who had received no prenatal care, and 95 percent of the maternal deaths occurred among women with no education who were secluded at home, dependent solely on their husbands for support. In the study from Jos, pregnant women aged less than 15 years or more than 40 years accounted for only 1.8 percent and 1.0 percent of total pregnancies, respectively, but these two groups had maternal mortality ratios of 573 and 2,325 maternal deaths per 100,000 live births. There was also a twentyfold increase in risk of death among pregnant women who did not receive prenatal care.

As noted before, the Hausa have traditionally advocated early marriage to ensure that female reproductive capacity is under clearly defined, socially sanctioned male control, but because girls become fertile before their pelvic growth is complete, early marriage sets the stage for adolescent pregnancy, with higher rates of obstructed labor and potentially devastating health consequences. Several studies from Sokoto, Nigeria, clearly demonstrate this. In Sokoto, over 90 percent of unschooled women are married by the age of 16, and, unsurprisingly, this is associated with high rates of adolescent pregnancy. A retrospective analysis of 337 young adolescents aged 16 years who had given birth in Sokoto (7.9 percent of all deliveries) found poor attendance at prenatal clinics among this group (probably indicative of the effects of *kunya* on a young pregnant adolescent), with nearly 80 percent of these girls receiving no antenatal care. When compared to other pregnant women, these young adolescents had longer labors and a much higher rate of instrumental vaginal delivery (forceps or vacuum extraction), higher risk of Cesarean section, and more destructive obstetric operations undertaken in order to attempt to preserve maternal life and health. These are all direct indicators of high rates of cephalo-pelvic disproportion and obstructed labor brought on by childbearing before pelvic growth is complete. Anemia, postpartum hemorrhage, preeclampsia/eclampsia and maternal deaths were more common in this subgroup than in the general obstetric population. These 337 16-year-old girls had an astonishing overall obstetric complication rate of 58 percent. There were 194 serious obstetric complications, including 69 cases of anemia, 27 cases of hemorrhage after delivery, 31 cases of obstructed labor, 31 cases of preeclampsia or eclampsia, 26 maternal deaths, and four vesico-vaginal fistulas. Among older adolescents aged 17–19 years (528 cases), there were 150 serious obstetric complications, a rate of 28 percent. Among this group there were 42 cases of obstructed labor, and two women who developed fistulas.

In another study from Sokoto by Airede and Ekele that evaluated maternal deaths at Usumanu Danfodiyo University Teaching Hospital in the 1990s, 10.3 percent of deliveries were to adolescent females aged 10–19 years, but 23.4 percent of maternal deaths occurred among females aged 12–19. The mean age of adolescent girls who died was only 17 years. All of the deaths occurred in young married women who were full-time housewives; 87 percent had no formal education, and 85 percent had no prenatal care. Prolonged labor was common. Of the 40 young women who died during or after delivery, labor lasted more than 24 hours in 24 girls and more than 72 hours in 9. The most common causes of death were eclampsia (21 cases, 46 percent) and prolonged obstructed labor (14 cases, 30 percent). Three girls died from a ruptured uterus (7 percent), and in many cases several complications were present simultaneously.

The authors of this study eloquently summed up their bleak findings: "The general picture of adolescent maternal deaths . . . is one of poverty, powerlessness and neglect." These young women were married and living respectable lives as housewives but were cut off from the wider world by traditional Hausa social practices. They were excluded from decision making in their households and were not empowered to act by themselves even when in personally desperate circumstances. They were dependent for others for financial support, access to supplies, and medical services. Over 85 percent had no education and no prenatal care, either of which might have saved their lives. Unable to access quality obstetric care, they ended up dead, often after considerable suffering. "In most instances they were brought to hospital only as a last resort after some complication was deemed to have occurred. As a result, 60% of them were in labour for over 24 hours and in nine of these labour lasted for over 3 days." By the time they finally reached the hospital, "a chain of events had already been set into motion placing them far down 'the maternal death road.'" Even though each woman managed to cross the threshold of a healthcare facility, adequate supplies and timely treatment was not available. Having struggled for medical care as a last, desperate act, they ended as victims who were blamed themselves: "In some instances the situation was compounded further by delays in the health facility due to inability or unwillingness of the girls' relatives to purchase drugs and materials required for intervention." The notion that prompt, competent care is the responsibility of healthcare institutions is sadly lacking in Hausaland.

Obstetric Fistulas in Hausaland

A Hausa proverb proclaims, "Duniya mace da ciki ce" (The world is a pregnant woman), meaning that life, like pregnancy, is uncertain: life, like the pregnant belly, is full of momentous portents, but no one knows what will happen or how things will turn out. In a region where maternal death is common and catastrophic pregnancy complications occur with horrific regularity, the proverb is both accurate and ominous.

The worst pregnancy outcome is an obstetric fistula. Death, although tragic, ends suffering, but fistula is a nonhealing wound, relentlessly gnawing at a woman's physical and psychosocial well-being. Several days after she has passed her (invariably) stillborn infant, exhausted from the ordeal of prolonged obstructed labor, and grief stricken by the death of her child, the injured woman now must face the sudden, constant, and uncontrollable loss of urine (and possibly stool). These developments are tremendously frightening and not easily explained or understood. Those afflicted often lie motionless in bed for days or even weeks, hoping that if they stay quiet and do not get up, perhaps the flow of urine somehow will stop. When it becomes sadly obvious that the leakage will not resolve by itself, more troubling questions begin to arise. Many of these girls and women feel guilty. Are they being punished for some unknown transgression? Excretory control is a hallmark of adulthood; to lose that control is to regress to an infantile state. This is tremendously embarrassing and women strive mightily to conceal their leakage because the consequences of exposure can be shattering. Sometimes, with great effort, the outward manifestations of urine loss can be hidden successfully, but often they are not. When the leakage is obvious, their situation worsens. Because they have a genital injury, there is speculation as to how and why it occurred. Gossip about one's genitals is rarely favorable (or polite), and if the injured woman is the second, third, or fourth wife in the compound, her rivals are rarely kind. The Hausa word for cowife is *kishiya*, from *kishi*, the Hausa word for "jealousy." The "jealous ones" are likely to smirk and gloat and talk behind her back; compassion is unlikely to be the predominant response, particularly when it becomes obvious that the injury is not going to heal on its own.

Most obstetric fistulas among the Hausa result from pressure necrosis from prolonged obstructed labor, sometimes in conjunction with a *gishiri* cut. But, as we saw in chapter 2, obstructed labor also often produces concurrent injuries in other parts of the pelvis, such as foot drop. Not only must the afflicted woman struggle to control excretory control, injuries like foot drop may worsen her social circumstances in other ways, creating further suffering. Foot drop and pelvic injuries may make normal women's work impossible. In a culture where a woman at best can expect to produce only one-quarter as much income as a man, this is an economic disaster for her, especially if she has no children to help. Obstetric fistula most commonly occurs during a young woman's first pregnancy, but a large number of women who develop a fistula do so after five or more pregnancies. When this happens, their injuries may make it impossible for them to care for their surviving children, a social "ripple effect" that often goes unnoticed. Since fetal mortality is high (usually 90 percent or more) in cases of obstructed labor where a fistula develops, many women have no further children after their fistula occurs, and many fistula victims have no living children at all. In the study of obstetric fistula cases from Jos, Nigeria, by Wall and colleagues, the 899 women involved had had 2,729 pregnancies but only 819 living children—a childhood mortality of 70 percent. The widespread problems of menstrual irregularity or menstrual cessation, injuries to the cervix, vaginal scarring, and subsequent pelvic inflammatory disease mean that many women never have another chance at childbirth: a devastating blow in a family-oriented continent like Africa.

Since fistulas rarely heal without surgical intervention, these injuries are generally chronic and highly stigmatizing once their presence becomes known. Concealment becomes key, and if that is not possible, the constant obvious presence of urine means that women with a fistula are often segregated from the rest of the family, sleeping and eating by themselves, since they are prohibited from cooking for others. Because personal cleanliness is a prerequisite for worship in Islam, and because fistula patients are obviously unclean, they are also excluded from participation in religious activities. This may diminish their sense of self-worth even further, removing even the prospect of spiritual solace for their affliction.

What to do? Immediately after the index pregnancy in which a fistula develops, women may be treated sympathetically by their husband, remaining in his compound. If the woman has children from previous births, there is more invested in the marriage, and the bonds between husband and wife are likely to be stronger, but even these relations can be strained over time. This is no different from the marital strains experienced by people in our society who are dealing with chronic, long-term health issues. As sociologist Margaret Murphy noted in her pioneering study of Hausa women with fistulas, "With prolongation of the illness, support for the fistula patient falls sharply." As the length of time with leakage increases and the injury reveals itself as chronic, the afflicted woman typically moves back home with her parents and may spend much of her time traveling from place to place looking for a cure. An incurable, stigmatizing condition coupled with prolonged absence from the home in the quest for therapy has devastating consequences for marriage. In the Jos study referred to above, only 26 percent of women with fistula were still married and living with their husbands; 49 percent were divorced, and 22 percent were separated. These findings are similar to those in Murphy's earlier work. She found that while only 14 percent of new fistula patients were divorced and 42 percent were still living with their husbands, by the time their condition had become chronic, only 11 percent were still living with their husbands, and over 77 percent had been separated for more than two years.

The shocking level of maternal mortality in northern Nigeria reflects the general lack of access to emergency obstetric care. The result is large numbers of maternal deaths, extremely high levels of near-miss events, widespread morbidity, and large numbers of women with obstetric fistulas. As noted previously, obstructed labor is common in this part of Africa. In Kelsey Harrison's pathbreaking maternal health study from Zaria, there were 203 cases of uterine rupture and 79 vesico-vaginal fistulas. If these two figures are combined, a crude prevalence rate for catastrophic obstructed labor can be estimated at 1,238 cases per 100,000 births, with an obstetric fistula rate of 350 fistulas per 100,000 deliveries. These figures are astonishingly high, but they reflect the dismal reproductive circumstances for Hausa women. The outpatient gynecology clinic at Ahmadu Bello University saw more than 300 new obstetric fistulas during the period in which Harrison's study was conducted, in addition to the 79 patients who developed fistulas after delivering in that institution. In Sokoto in northwestern Nigeria, uterine rupture during labor occurs as often as 1 in 74 deliveries, a statistic that has been confirmed in two separate studies.

The prevalence of obstetric fistulas in northern Nigeria is striking and has been repeatedly confirmed by many different studies. These studies find the overwhelming cause of vesico-vaginal fistula to be untreated, prolonged obstructed labor (particularly in first-time mothers) that has lasted at least two days (sometimes more), with extremely high rates of fetal death.

Obstructed Labor and Obstructed Care

At least 75 percent of all maternal deaths are due to direct obstetric causes such as hemorrhage, infection, hypertensive disorders of pregnancy (preeclampsia/eclampsia), complications of unsafe abortion, and obstructed labor. The occurrence of such complications cannot always be prevented, but each one of these complications can be treated effectively, particularly if treatment begins promptly after their onset. The dramatic declines in maternal mortality and morbidity that took place across the industrialized world in the twentieth century are testimony to that fact. It was access to lifesaving technologies when they were most needed that transformed maternal mortality. Maternal mortality and childbirth injury have fallen promptly and dramatically wherever and whenever this has been done, yet even today thousands of women in northern Nigeria labor for days without relief and either die or suffer devastating injuries while giving birth. The delivery of effective medical care is obstructed at many different levels.

Delay means disaster, but both temporal and spatial constraints must be overcome to avert a poor obstetric outcome. Although this sounds simple, most commonly it is not. Conceptual, educational, economic, political, physical, and social barriers exist at every decision point along the way.

The first major obstacle in Hausaland is conceptual and social. It arises from the limited self-agency and restricted decision-making capacities under which Hausa women must live, and this, in turn, is further compounded by the burden of *kunya*, or shame. Particularly for adolescents, *kunya* presents a barrier even to the acknowledgement of the pregnant state, much less calling attention to the development of complications of this embarrassing condition.

Professor Kelsey Harrison's research group was shocked to discover in their series that all of the pregnant women from Zaria who died without proper prenatal care (and 82 percent of the unbooked pregnant women from outside Zaria who died) had ready access to transportation and lived within two kilometers of an all-season road. Because the movements of Hausa women are closely controlled by men, the determination that a woman has a serious medical problem requiring care at a hospital is a male responsibility, but Hausa men are woefully ignorant of women's reproductive affairs. With their low position in the social hierarchy, pregnant Hausa women must have male permission to seek medical care, and usually this means that they must be accompanied on their journey by their husband or other male relative. In first pregnancies (where obstetric fistulas most commonly occur) the situation is made worse by the Hausa tradition in which the young pregnant bride is expected to deliver her first child at her parents' home, even though the husband maintains "total control of his wife's spatial mobility."

The decision to seek care is also influenced by the family's distance from the healthcare facilities, their perception of the costs involved, their previous experience with the healthcare system, the belief that a problem does, in fact, exist, and the perceived quality of the care available to them should they seek it. Because of the overwhelming emphasis placed on *kunya*, or "modesty," for Hausa women, women in difficult labor may be too frightened, too ignorant, or too fearful of being seen as "immodest" to seek help. The prevalent traditional view that a woman should "go it alone" during labor whenever possible may preclude assessment of the situation by a skilled observer who can tell that a serious problem is developing. Ekwempu and colleagues found that the imposition of fees for healthcare services necessitated by reduced government funding for healthcare in Zaria was correlated with a 56 percent increase in maternal mortality between 1983 and 1988, largely because pregnant women could not afford to go to the hospital when emergencies arose except as a last resort. They also found a steady decrease in the percentage of obstetric admissions coming from farther away over this same period: in 1983, 52 percent of cases admitted to Ahmadu Bello University Teaching Hospital came from more than 30 kilometers away, whereas the percentage had dropped to only 18 percent in 1988, a fact attributed to the combination of the rising price of transportation coupled with increases in healthcare costs. Over this same period the case mix of patients with complicated obstetric problems rose steadily. Only the most severely ill patients were going to the hospital, but by then it was often too late.

Factors influencing the decision to seek care were explored in detail at the local community level by Kisekka and colleagues in a study of the determinants of maternal mortality in Giwa District, Zaria. The authors carried out a household survey of 400 compounds and held 12 focus group discussions in five villages in Giwa District, a rural area approximately 60 kilometers from Zaria. Interviews were carried out with 878 women aged 10–44 years of age, 86 percent of whom were illiterate. The area was served by 10 dispensaries, two maternity centers, and one comprehensive health center, staffed by a total of 27 trained health workers. The maternal mortality ratio in the area was estimated by these investigators to be high, at 940 per 100,000 live births. In spite of the presence of local health facilities and a tertiary care teaching hospital 60 kilometers away (Ahmadu Bello University Teaching Hospital in Zaria), 41 percent of these women said they never attended prenatal clinics, and the vast majority (608 out of 878) delivered their last child at home. In descending order of importance, the factors hindering prenatal clinic attendance were disapproval by one's mother or mother-in-law, cultural barriers (*kunya*), excessive cost, husband's disapproval, transportation problems, and long lines or maltreatment by clinic staff. Similar findings among patients who developed obstetric fistulas from prolonged obstructed labor have been reported from Jos by Wall and coworkers.

In addition to these reasons for nonattendance, Kisekka and coworkers also found a tendency to attend for prenatal care only when problems (such as bleeding) arose but to discontinue attendance once such problems disappeared. There was also a strong belief that pregnancy and childbirth are "natural" and that clinical supervision was therefore unnecessary. This, coupled with the equally strong belief that what happens in pregnancy must be accepted because it is the will of God, strongly discouraged both clinic attendance and seeking medical care during labor.

Delay in reaching a healthcare facility is influenced by the cost and time of travel, the distribution of hospitals and dispensaries, the condition of roads, and the reliability of the transporting vehicles—all of which are extremely bad in northern Nigeria. Delay increases morbidity, which produces bad outcomes, which reinforces negative views of hospital care, which in turn increases the reluctance of patients to seek it. If a patient is in labor for three or four days but finally goes to a hospital, where she has a Cesarean delivery of a dead baby and then develops a fistula, the hospital is likely to be blamed for both the fetal death and for the bladder injury. Never mind that it was three days of obstructed labor that killed the child and destroyed the base of her bladder: for the patient, perception is reality in such cases.

An analogous situation can be found in other areas of Hausa healthcare-seeking behavior. Hausa villagers are very reluctant to seek orthopedic care for fractures from hospitals in northern Nigeria, generally preferring to use traditional bonesetters. Not only are bonesetters familiar and sympathetic figures, but they use familiar ingredients when they set bones and they tend to keep limbs immobilized for less time than do orthopedic surgeons. Since the fractures that are seen in hospitals tend to be complex fractures that have failed traditional treatment, they generally have high rates of infection and gangrene. The prognosis for recovery in such cases is relatively poor when compared to uncomplicated fractures. This results in high rates of limb amputation. It is not difficult to see how the view takes hold that if you go to the hospital with a broken limb, they will simply cut it off. This reinforces the preference to use traditional practices that have contributed to a high rate of gangrene in the first place, and so the cycle continues.

For similar reasons, delay in seeking obstetric care is common. In Rahan and Sani's study of Hausa obstetrics in Katsina, 13 percent of deliveries occurred en route to the hospital. Among women who arrived at the hospital undelivered, 31 percent were in the second stage of labor with the cervix fully dilated and the baby in descent through the vagina. In Harrison's study of deliveries in Zaria, there were an average of 18 deliveries per day, but there were only 33 beds available for all pregnant and puerperal patients, and the daily bed-occupancy rate was 120 percent. Patients were almost stacked on top of one another. To make matters even worse, the entire 250-bed hospital had only one operating theater with two operating tables, and all emergency obstetric cases had to compete with other emergencies for surgical time, a problem that is nearly intractable in West African obstetric units. Seventy percent of women who delivered in a hospital went home within 24 hours, and 38 percent were discharged within 12 hours. Among singleton births that took place in the hospital, the operative delivery rate was 10 percent among women receiving prenatal care, but 31 percent among unbooked women, including a Cesarean delivery rate of 18.2 percent in the latter group, due mainly to patients arriving with complications of obstructed labor.

Throughout Hausaland the birthrate is high (contraceptive prevalence is extremely low), the maternal healthcare infrastructure is inadequate to meet the needs placed upon it, there is a profound shortage of skilled birth attendants, and the hospital systems are dysfunctional. These facts reflect society's views of the value of women. When a patient with an obstetric emergency finally reaches a health center or hospital, she must often contend with shortages of supplies and equipment, lack of trained (and often lack of caring) personnel, and the interminable internal delays that plague a system that doesn't work very well even at its best. The maternal healthcare systems throughout Hausaland—on both sides of the Niger-Nigerian border—still suffer from the legacy of misplaced political priorities (going as far back as colonial rule), disorganization, chronic underfunding, thoroughgoing mismanagement, an inability to manage logistics and supplies, rampant corruption, and a view that women are just not very important. To worsen matters further, the structural readjustment programs imposed on Africa by the world financial community in the 1980s have had a devastating impact on economic growth, which in turn has affected the ability of these countries to devote adequate resources to maternal healthcare.

You have obstructed labor? Good luck with that. "Allah maganin kome," as the proverb says: "God is the remedy for everything."

Learning to Value Women's Lives

At the end of his exhaustive, paradigm-shifting analysis of obstetrics in northern Nigeria—the study that launched the Safe Motherhood movement in the 1980s— Professor Kelsey Harrison summarized the situation of the female patients he had spent years caring for in the northern part of his country: "Large numbers of women are born into a cycle of deprivation where they will remain uneducated; where their religion and culture encourage child marriage so that they may begin childbearing while still children themselves; and where they are systematically neglected both physically and emotionally. Moreover, they may be denied access to effective medical care when they need it, and the consequent damage by neglect is compounded by inappropriate and exceedingly harmful traditional medicine."

While it is true that much of the maternal morbidity and mortality is due to the inadequate healthcare facilities in northern Nigeria and an unreliable system of transportation, the situation is made vastly worse by the position of women in Hausa society. Cut off from formal education, undervalued in the eyes of the law, exhorted to assume a subordinate and servile position in life by their religion, regarded primarily as vehicles for the production of children rather than as individuals to be loved and cherished in their own right, often married without choice at a remarkably early age and forced to begin childbearing before they are physically mature enough to do so easily, restricted in their movements by the practice of wife seclusion, devoid of personal autonomy and tightly controlled by a social structure that requires the permission of a male authority figure before action can be taken even in life-threatening circumstances, Hausa women are trapped behind social barriers that prevent easy access to lifesaving medical care when they are pregnant or when they develop a catastrophic complication in childbirth. Furthermore, Hausa traditional culture also supports practices that are objectively harmful to maternal and newborn health: *gishiri* cutting in cases of difficult labor and the belief that newly delivered women should be loaded with salt, kept warm, and subjected to frequent hot baths. These are formidable obstacles to overcome. Together they produce a clear pathway that leads to obstetric fistula (figure 5.3).

The solution to these problems will come only through fundamental social change. Such change requires elevating the status of women and improving their education while simultaneously empowering them to take control of their own reproductive lives. Such changes will face bitter opposition from many quarters. Providing universal access to trained delivery attendants and prompt referral of childbirth complications to functioning emergency obstetric centers must become a top government healthcare priority in both Nigeria and Niger. Improved economic circumstances will help alleviate some of the misery, but the most important development will be improving the status of women. This will require courageous political change in the face of dogmatic opposition, which will arise particularly from the most conservative corners of the Muslim community.

Recent trends suggest that opposition to such needed changes is becoming more ferocious and entrenched. Hausaland has a long history of Islamic fundamentalist revivalism, going back to Shehu 'Dan Fodio at the beginning of the nineteenth century. The utter corruption of the Nigerian government, its failure to provide functioning public services for its people, its rampant cronyism, and the failure of the economy to provide jobs and a decent standard of living for the population have led many northern Nigerians to take refuge in a truculent and often violent Salafist Islamic fundamentalism. One of the strongest memories I have of my return to northern Nigeria in the summer of 2001 was the presence of veiled women (some in total body burqas) on the streets of Kano—a new phenomenon—and the striking presence of posters and bumper stickers glorifying Osama Bin Laden on the ubiquitous white vans that serve as cheap public transportation. What this really signified became apparently only on September 11 of that year.

The terrorist group Boko Haram is deeply entrenched in northern Nigeria, particularly in the impoverished northeastern region of the country. This group, which has pledged its allegiance to the terrorist Islamic State organization in the Middle East, seeks the overthrow of the corrupt Nigerian government and its replacement with a new Islamic caliphate. Among its strongest operational values is a contempt for women,

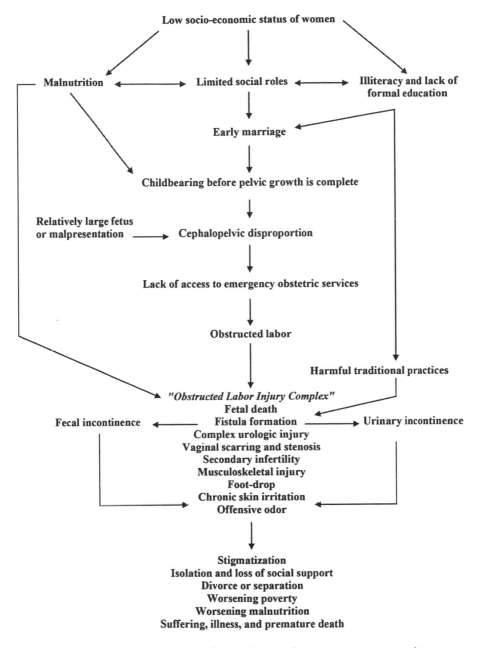

FIGURE 5.3. The pathway to obstetric fistula, showing how circumstances combine to create a fistula and the consequences that result from this injury. © *Worldwide Fistula Fund, used by permission.*

manifested in the kidnapping and enslavement of the Chibok schoolgirls and a subsequent policy of using young adolescent and preadolescent girls as involuntary suicide bombers. One can hardly expect immediate improvements in maternal health services in such an environment.

Still, there is little question but that the most important tool for raising the status of women in this part of the world will be the education of girls and young women. Harrison's own data from Zaria (now confirmed by other studies) showed a direct link between the level of maternal education and steadily decreasing maternal mortality. While the overall maternal mortality ratio was 1,050 maternal deaths per 100,000 births in the Zaria study, it was 1,154 deaths per 100,000 births for illiterate women, 400 deaths per 100,000 births for women who had some primary education, and none at all for women with postprimary education. The question remains open as to whether northern Nigeria will embrace this obvious pathway to social development.

Nigerian obstetrician-gynecologist Nimi Briggs, who worked with Harrison on the Zaria study, has eloquently stated this link in his paper "Illiteracy and Maternal Health: Educate or Die": "To reduce deaths and improve maternal health, the sub-Saharan woman must be helped to enhance her own self-esteem and the worth she places on her life. At the same time we need to create an enabling environment where access to functional and basic but professional medical care is readily available. There is now overwhelming evidence that, in the long term, no approach will be as successful as universal formal education."

A country cannot flourish if it wastes one-half of its available brainpower, as the Hausa are now doing. Perhaps the single most important aspect of improving maternal health in Hausaland will be to educate men in the important stake that they themselves have in women's reproductive health, for only when Hausa men appreciate this will the status of their wives, their mothers, their sisters, and their daughters start to improve. As the proverb says, "Duniya mace da ciki ce" (The world is a pregnant woman), and when obstetrics goes well, there is nothing better, but when obstetrics goes bad, nothing is worse.

CHAPTER 6

Deadly Delays in Deciding to Seek Care

An obstetric fistula results from a crush injury to the soft tissues of a woman's pelvis during obstructed labor. The threshold at which tissue death and fistula formation occurs is unpredictable and varies from woman to woman, from case to case, and from labor to labor because it is influenced by the interplay of multiple factors (see figure 2.10). For this reason, there is no minimum time after which an obstetric fistula will be produced. Relatively short labors may result in a fistula if the conditions for "a perfect storm" are present, whereas other prolonged labors end without producing a fistula. In practical terms this means that *all* cases of obstructed labor must be regarded as emergencies. As Thomas Addis Emmet recognized nearly 150 years ago, "The amount of injury is by no means in proportion to the length of labor. Therefore, the only safety consists in as speedy a delivery as the circumstances of the case will admit." It is delay in receiving proper treatment after labor becomes obstructed that causes obstetric fistulas; tens of thousands of fistulas occur every year in the world's poorest countries because women do not get the treatment they need in a competent and timely fashion.

Reduction in the total worldwide number of obstetric fistulas can only occur through three mechanisms. These mechanisms are also the only ways by which childbirth-related deaths and other severe maternal morbidities can be avoided.

First, the risk of getting an obstetric fistula can be reduced if a woman's risk of becoming pregnant is reduced. This means that family planning programs, which reduce the number of pregnancies occurring in a particular population, can reduce fistulas by reducing the number of "at-risk" (i.e., pregnant) women. Unfortunately, once a woman becomes pregnant, family planning does nothing to reduce her risk of a fistula in the current pregnancy: that ship has already sailed.

Second, the risk of a woman developing an obstetric fistula might be reduced if the risk of her developing obstructed labor could be reduced. This can partially be achieved by promoting good nutrition during girlhood and postponing marriage until late adolescence when pelvic growth has been completed. In addition, it requires a sensitive and specific screening test that could be applied to women early in their pregnancies to assess their risk of developing obstructed labor. Unfortunately, there is no accurate, practical, reliable test that does this.

Small women and short women appear to be at higher risk of obstructed labor, but, since small women and short women may also have smaller babies, they may escape the perils of cephalo-pelvic disproportion and fistula formation. The best predictor of subsequent pregnancy outcome turns out to be prior obstetric performance, and this is absolutely useless as a guide to the risks a woman faces in her first pregnancy, which is when most fistulas occur. And, even if a woman has delivered successfully before—even many times before—she is still at risk for developing obstructed labor in a subsequent pregnancy if the shape of her pelvis has been altered by disease or environmental circumstances, if the baby is especially large or has some developmental abnormality, or if the fetus presents abnormally. (There are well-documented cases of women in Africa developing a fistula during their fourteenth deliveries.) In spite of decades of effort applying both high- and low-technology approaches to this screening problem, there are still no screening tools suitable for routine clinical use that have adequate sensitivity and specificity in predicting which women will develop obstructed labor. Obstructed labor remains a clinical diagnosis that is made during labor.

The third and final way in which the risks of developing an obstetric fistula might be reduced is by improving the outcome of labor after it has become obstructed. It has been said in politics that "eternal vigilance is the price of liberty." In an obstetric context, eternal vigilance *is* the price of obstetric fistula prevention. Because there is no good way of accurately screening for obstructed labor in advance of labor itself, the only way to prevent obstetric fistulas is to detect obstructed labor early in its course and to intervene to improve obstetric outcomes and to prevent maternal injuries. The cornerstone of current attempts to reduce maternal mortality focuses largely on improving the outcomes for women who develop pregnancy complications such as hemorrhage, sepsis, hypertensive crises in pregnancy, and other problems. Prompt, effective treatment of complications when they arise is the main way to avoid death or serious morbidity; this is the rationale for enhancing rapid access to emergency obstetric services in developing nations. In cases of relatively obstructed labor, assisted vaginal delivery with forceps or a vacuum extractor will relieve the obstruction and terminate a prolonged labor, but when cephalo-pelvic disproportion is absolute, the treatment most likely to improve both maternal and fetal outcomes is Cesarean section, which bypasses the obstruction in the birth canal that is impeding delivery and creates an abdominal alternative to vaginal delivery. It was the development of safe, effective Cesarean section toward the end of the nineteenth century that allowed the Western world to conquer the problem of obstructed labor. Therefore, the key to obstetric fistula prevention is prompt diagnosis and competent treatment of obstructed labor.

The Three Phases of Delay in Obstetric Emergencies

In their groundbreaking article "Too Far to Walk: Maternal Mortality in Context," Sereen Thaddeus and Deborah Maine proposed a three-part framework for evaluating delays in accessing emergency obstetric care. This framework is based on the understanding that most life-threatening emergencies cannot be predicted and that, once a complication arises, a bad outcome can be avoided only by the prompt provision of effective treatment. In any emergency scenario, a similar series of steps occurs: development of a complication, recognition that a complication has arisen, a decision to seek treatment for the complication, movement to a center where emergency obstetric services are provided, and delivery of care that resolves the complication. Not all cases of maternal death or serious maternal injury can be prevented, but if the time between the onset of the complication and the delivery of appropriate treatment is minimized, overall outcomes will be dramatically better. This is particularly true in cases of obstructed labor, where it generally takes several hours of maternal tissue compression by the fetal head before the injury threshold is crossed. Of all of the major complications that a woman could develop during labor, the formation of an obstetric fistula should be among the most preventable.

Thaddeus and Maine articulated three principal "phases of delay" impacting the successful resolution of life-threatening obstetric emergencies: (1) delay in deciding to seek care, (2) delay in arriving at a suitable obstetric care facility, and (3) delay in receiving appropriate care at that facility. The three phases of delay are each influenced by different factors, and the solutions to these impediments can be provided by different actors during each phase. In this scheme, phase 2 and phase 3 delays appear to be the most amenable to solution.

There is abundant evidence that maternal death and serious birth injury rise with increasing distance from medical facilities. Most travel delays (phase 2 delays) can be overcome by a combination of community mobilization and the establishment of emergency obstetric transportation networks (ambulances, etc.) linked by an effective communications system that ties the various components of the healthcare system together. This is the kind of project that people can reasonably demand from their governments and healthcare systems as an essential public service. Sustained efforts to develop infrastructure in this way have played a major role in improving maternal health in countries such as Honduras, Sri Lanka, and Malaysia.

The problem of phase 3 delays (delays in the delivery of competent emergency care) properly falls within the purview of public health officials, hospital administrators, physicians, midwives, and their professional organizations. Deaths and injuries that occur after a woman has arrived at a hospital are often due to incompetence, neglect of patients, shortages of supplies and personnel, or other logistical factors. Instituting tight administration, vigilant oversight, protocols for the treatment of common problems such as obstructed labor, and ongoing professional development and self-criticism will go a long way toward resolving phase 3 delays. People should rightly demand timely delivery of competent medical care and accountability from the hospitals and health centers that serve them.

Overcoming Phase 1 Delays: The Critical Component of Obstetric Fistula Prevention

In both phase 2 and phase 3, it is at least theoretically possible to allocate responsibility for poor system performance and to demand accountability for the high rates of maternal death and disability that result. Improved performance can be leveraged for the public good. This is primarily a political problem but one that can be overcome even in low-resource countries. The more complicated problem appears to be changing the causes of phase 1 delays, because these depend largely upon individual behavior. For this reason phase 1 delays can be seen as the critical component in obstetric fistula prevention.

If the process of accessing emergency care outlined by Thaddeus and Maine is to function effectively in the first phase, several things must happen in rapid sequence: a problem must arise, it must be recognized as requiring action, the action needed to solve the problem must be identified and agreed upon (usually invoking some conception of cause and effect or at least identifying the "repository of knowledge" where the solution to the problem can be found), and a decision to act must be made that moves the process into the second and third phases of care-seeking. The factors that impact attitudes and decisions in this critical first phase are far more diffuse, intangible, and difficult to control than those impacting delays in the second and third phases because these factors operate at the level of individual and family dynamics. As Edward de Bono has written, "Most of the mistakes in thinking are inadequacies of perception rather than mistakes in logic." In the first phase of delay, perception is everything. Understanding that a problem is present, understanding what the problem is, and understanding how the problem may be solved are absolutely critical for the successful resolution of obstetric emergencies.

Obstetric fistula has been eliminated as a public health problem in wealthy countries where educational standards are good and prompt access to emergency obstetric care is the cultural norm. In contrast, there are millions of unrepaired obstetric fistulas in sub-Saharan Africa and South Asia. The epidemiology of obstetric fistula clearly indicates that women who develop this condition come predominantly from poor communities, usually located in the rural areas of resource-poor nations, where women have limited access to formal education, marry early (often while still children themselves), have high rates of fertility, and usually lack employment opportunities that would generate a significant cash income and lead to greater personal autonomy. For example, among 899 women who developed an obstetric fistula and presented for care at Evangel Hospital in Jos, Nigeria, studied by Wall and colleagues, the mean age at marriage was 15.5 years, most were illiterate, 78 percent had no formal education, only 4.5 percent had ever used contraception, and only 10 women had any kind of regular paid or salaried employment. The rest were all housewives, agricultural workers, menial laborers, or earned what little income they could through petty trading.

Because fistula patients tend to be poor, uneducated, and immersed in rural African or Asian culture, there are deep social components to the obstetric fistula problem that have not yet been adequately explored by researchers. Although all three phases of delay are influenced by cultural factors, these influences appear to be most pronounced in the first phase of delay during which the problem is perceived, the possible solutions are debated, and a decision is made to seek a solution to the problem as understood.

The most fundamental point to be made is that the decision to seek therapy is not simply a decision either "to do nothing" or "to go to a hospital." Women with pregnancy complications in rural African and Asian communities can utilize many competing therapeutic options, albeit of greatly differing therapeutic efficacy, especially when it comes to obstructed labor. Therapeutic pluralism is the norm in these communities, and the quest for therapy often involves the concurrent use of multiple healing pathways, depending on how the presenting problem is understood and how the efficacy of competing therapies is evaluated. From the standpoint of bioscientific obstetrics, obstructed labor is a problem of faulty obstetrical mechanics—the fetus will not fit through the birth canal—but those most intimately affected by a case of obstructed labor may be more worried about social factors than about simple mechanics. Their concerns may lie more with metaphysics than with physics proper. They may be more interested in placating the supernatural forces they fear may be responsible for the delay in delivery than with understanding and rectifying the faulty obstetrical mechanics involved. Such motivations have significant implications for what happens next.

How Long Should a Normal Labor Last?

The critical problem in the first phase of delay is recognizing that labor is prolonged. By WHO standards, labor is prolonged if it lasts more than 24 hours. There is an old adage in tropical obstetrics that "the sun should not rise twice on a laboring woman." If a woman is laboring under the supervision of a skilled birth attendant, the diagnosis of prolonged/obstructed labor should not be difficult to make, but in parts of the world where fistulas are common most women deliver by themselves, in the company of family members, or using other forms of traditional birth assistance. Under these circumstances, what is regarded as the "normal" length of labor may be quite different from accepted obstetrical norms. For example, the Prevention of Maternal Mortality Network in West Africa found that in Bo, Sierra Leone, and in the Nigerian cities of Sokoto and Zaria, prolonged labor was not considered a problem of sufficient importance to seek medical care until two to five days had elapsed. As Douglas and Wildavsky have pointed out, "risk" is constructed differently in every culture, based on local perceptions and values, and "substantial disagreement remains over what is risky, how risky it is, and what to do about it." The concepts of risk and blame are deeply anchored in local cultural constructs and underlying assumptions about the nature of the world. Determining when labor is actually prolonged depends very much upon local notions of what the "normal" length of labor might be. Anthropologists are only just beginning to investigate cross-cultural notions of time in relation to pregnancy, labor and delivery—concepts that are critical to obstetric fistula prevention. Added to the problem of determining the "normal" length of labor is the difficulty of distinguishing "false" labor (irregular uterine contractions that may mimic labor but that do not produce cervical change) from "true" labor (uterine contractions of sufficient force, duration, and frequency to produce effacement and dilatation of the cervix)—a diagnosis that is difficult to make without performing serial cervical examinations. Distinguishing labor that is prolonged by ineffective uterine contractions from labor that is truly obstructed also takes obstetrical experience. Tracking the progress of labor with a partograph (a simple graphic depiction of the progress of labor) is extremely effective in determining when labor is prolonged. Intensive and ongoing community education programs that emphasize the importance of seeking skilled care if labor lasts more than 24 hours are likely to be fundamental in altering traditional attitudes about the "normal" length of labor.

What Is to Be Done?

Once it has been determined that labor is prolonged, a solution to this problem must be proposed. For effective fistula prevention, the laboring woman should be transported rapidly to an emergency obstetric care facility where proper treatment can be provided. At this point, however, there are many divergent therapeutic pathways that can be chosen by the actors involved. Some of these pathways—perhaps many—will lead to adverse outcomes including death or severe morbidity when labor is obstructed.

One decision is simply to do nothing. In clinical medicine this is referred to as "watchful waiting," and while avoiding *unnecessary* intervention is often a virtue in obstetric practice, this approach can be disastrous if it allows labor to drag on for several days. In some cases the decision to do nothing is based on religious fatalism—if God so wills, the problem will resolve itself. In other cases the parties involved simply have no idea of what to do or where to turn, and so do nothing. In the study of 899 fistula cases from Jos, Nigeria, by Wall and colleagues, 6.5 percent of patients reported that they were unaware of the availability of hospital obstetric care, and nearly 27 percent could not give any reason as to why they delayed seeking help.

In some cases an intervention *other* than transporting the patient to an obstetric emergency care facility will be chosen. One common therapeutic option is to seek help from a local authority on problems associated with childbirth. Such individuals function as repositories of "authoritative knowledge" with respect to childbearing difficulties, "the source" in which solutions can be found within the local cosmology. These authorities may be midwives or shamans or religious figures (pastors, priests, imams, etc.) who are thought to possess special skills or information that may be of therapeutic utility in difficult cases of labor. In Christian Africa, churches are often the first place of refuge in cases of dystocia. Therapy typically consists of prayer and religious rituals that do not effectively address the problem of mechanical obstruction. Muslims often resort to versions of Islamic folk medicine, attempting to harness the power they believe resides in the Koran. In northern Nigeria, for example, a common treatment for many ills is writing out on a wooden slate a verse from the Koran that is thought to be "therapeutically potent," washing off the ink that has been used to write (and therefore embody the power of) God's words, thereafter drinking the inky water as a medicine. In other parts of Africa, traditional lineage priests or clan elders may be convened to discuss the case, particularly if there is suspicion that the pregnant woman has committed adultery or other sins that are blocking her delivery. The Prevention of Maternal Mortality Network found:

> In all of the areas studied, certain behavior (including infidelity and disregarding the authority of one's husband or elders) is believed to lead to obstructed labor and hemorrhage. Women in Accra, Benin, Bo, Calabar, and Freetown reported that when complications arise, the oracles are consulted, and if, for example, the oracle says the complication is due to the woman's insubordination to her husband or elders, she has to apologize and perform cleansing rites before she is taken for treatment. Similarly, in Bo, a woman suffering from a complication thought to be due to infidelity is forced to confess her sins, and her husband must spit water on her abdomen to appease the gods; only then is she taken for further help, if the complication is thought serious enough to warrant hospital treatment. In most of the communities studied, people believe that the will of God, heredity, and evil spirits can cause obstetric complications. In such situations, the care of traditional healers and diviners is sought, and the modern health-care system is used only as a last resort.

Beliefs that problems in labor arise from disturbances in the social environment rather than as simple problems of obstetrical mechanics are common in many cultures, and women are often blamed for these, and other, health misfortunes. Among the Esan people of Edo State, Nigeria, "It was observed from discussions with both men and women that illnesses in adult women are mostly caused by offenses against tradition or custom. In contrast, the illnesses of adult males and children are seldom self-inflicted but are often caused by the misdeeds of women. In essence, a woman is blamed for disasters to her child, her co-wives' children, and her husband; but she alone must bear the responsibility for her own state of health." Obstructed labor—recognized as a condition potentially fatal to both mother and child—is thought to be caused by factors such as "having sex in the afternoon or in the fields, incest, adultery, practicing witchcraft and taking a husband's property (such as money) without his knowledge or permission. Most of these supernatural factors can be brought promptly under control when the woman confesses her offence, which is necessary before ritual can be successful; otherwise, no cure can be provided and death becomes inevitable."

According to Monica Wilson, the Nyakyusa of East Africa believe that "a delayed delivery is commonly attributed to the woman's adultery, and she is pressed by the midwife to confess the name of her lover or lovers, but it is also believed that it may be due to *imindu*, that is the shades [ancestral spirits]. The husband consults a diviner who indicates whether the *imindu* is on his side or that of the woman's father and the one who is thus indicated should pray. 'Sometimes the woman herself tells of a quarrel which would lead to *imindu* and then her husband or father goes to pray.'"

Denise Allen described a belief called *usangalija* among the Sukuma of west-central Tanzania. *Usangalija* is the Sukuma term for prolonged or stalled labor. It refers to the phenomenon of "mixing," when a woman allows "foreign" sperm to enter her while pregnant with a baby fathered by a different man. This "mixing of men" is potentially fatal for both the mother and child. It is said to produce a sort of revulsion on the part of the fetus, who "instead of moving down the birth canal, . . . moves up in uterus instead." Allen recounted several stories of women who were accused of adultery after they experienced difficulties during childbirth. The proposed local treatments of *usangalija* included such therapies as taking a pinch of sand from the exact spot where a dog—a notoriously promiscuous animal species—had previously given birth, mixing it with water and giving it to the laboring woman to drink, or taking a root found growing in the middle of the road—a place through which much traffic has passed—grinding it, mixing it with water, and giving to the woman to drink.

In other cultures sexual misbehavior on the part of the husband is also thought to affect a pregnancy. According to Rachel Chapman, among the Shona of Mozambique, "adultery on the part of the husband can also kill his pregnant wife: if the woman with whom he has had the affair comes near the wife while she is in labor, the wife will begin to sweat and then die." More commonly, however, the problem is attributed to infidelity on the part of the pregnant woman. This has profound implications for family dynamics. As Chapman writes:

> In a patrilocal marriage, where a wife moves to live with her husband and his patrikin, a mother-in-law [*sogra*] can also exercise considerable influence over her son's wife if she experiences trouble with childbirth. Infidelity on the part of the pregnant woman is

widely believed to cause problems during childbirth, especially prolonged or blocked labor, and it is the right and duty of a mother-in-law to extract this information from her daughter-in-law. Armed with such a confession, the *sogra* can inform her son, often initiating a break in relations between the young couple or even catalyzing divorce proceedings, thus fortifying her own position of influence with her son. Senior women's power in this setting is linked to their ritual control over certain diagnoses in pregnancy and birthing that carry social meaning.

It is critical to understand that, for women in many cultures, obstetric problems such as prolonged labor are not viewed as random physiological events but rather are tied directly to their unique individual relationships with their family and community. Anthropologist Nicole Berry recounted the following explanation from one of her Mayan informants in rural Guatemala:

> Sandra told me that one of her births had taken more than five days. Why did it take so long, I asked? Probably, she said, because she had been fighting a lot with her sisters-in-law during the pregnancy. As the birth is a family event, if things are not going well within the family, they might not go well within the birth. A bad relationship between a husband and wife, the central actors in the birth narrative, can be the root of even worse problems. Husbands who don't take care of their wives and fight a lot with their wives while they are pregnant were also blamed for causing birthing problems.

When traditional midwives are consulted for obstetrical problems, they follow their own culturally derived diagnostic and treatment logic, which is usually quite different from that advocated by biomedical obstetrics. This may lead to therapeutic decisions that seem logical within the local context but that are ineffective or even directly harmful to the laboring woman. For example, it may be decided that the uterus is not contracting strongly enough. To combat this, an oxytocic drug may be administered, either in the form of a traditional recipe using locally obtained bioactive materials or in the form of a standard pharmaceutical preparation obtained on the black market or elsewhere. In obstructed labor this will usually increase the force applied to the impacted fetal part, thereby increasing the likelihood of uterine rupture or fistula formation. In some cases violent external force—such as pushing or sitting on the pregnant woman's abdomen—may be applied to try to force the baby out, with disastrous consequences. In other cases crude attempts may be made to release "the obstruction" by cutting inside the vagina, such as the practice of cutting for *gishiri* among the Hausa. This practice itself frequently creates a fistula through direct urethral or bladder injury.

Who Decides What . . . and Why?

Because traditional ethnomedical therapies have little efficacy in relieving obstructed labor, the most critical decision in the prevention of obstetric fistulas is the decision to seek help from a biomedical facility that provides competent emergency obstetrical services, including Cesarean delivery. It is the decision to seek help in such a venue that starts the laboring woman down the therapeutic pathway that may save her life as well as prevent the development of a fistula. Who decides this? In many cases the woman herself may have little or no say in this critical decision.

In many societies where obstetric fistulas are common, women have scant independent agency. They may have little choice as to when they have sexual relations and whether to use contraception when they do. Contraceptive agency is affected strongly by male attitudes but also by social factors unknown in the West such as the presence of cowives in polygynous households. When women in fistula-prevalent areas become pregnant, they may have little say as to whether or not they get antenatal care—and where and under what circumstances they deliver their children. In many societies "proper" social relationships require that female reproductive capacity is always under clearly delineated male control, usually by the girl's father before marriage and by her husband after marriage. Money and material goods ("bridewealth," in anthropological parlance) are transferred by the husband and his family to the girl's family as part of the marriage contract in exchange for the use of her reproductive capacity and the assumption of other obligations on their part. The rights and obligations entailed by such practices vary enormously from society to society, but male belief in ownership of a woman's reproductive capacity may significantly impact decision making during obstetrical emergencies. Analogies of children being the "harvest" obtained by a man as the result of "tilling" his wife's "field" are explicit agricultural analogies in many countries. The control of such a valuable resource is not easily relinquished, and if wife-seclusion (purdah) is the prevailing cultural practice (as it is among the Hausa), a woman may not be allowed to leave her family compound without explicit permission from a controlling male authority. The consequences can be devastating. There is a famous anecdote concerning a woman from northern Nigeria who lived a 10-minute walk from the hospital, but, because her husband was away on business and could not give her permission to travel, she labored at home for several days only to deliver a dead child and develop a fistula. Lack of formal education further increases this sense of helplessness in the face of obstetrical complications. Fistula patients almost invariably have low educational attainments, as noted previously.

Weeks and colleagues interviewed 30 Ugandan women who had near-miss obstetrical experiences at Mulago Hospital that might have proved fatal if circumstances had been different. In analyzing the recurrent themes in their interviews, they noted, "The most striking feature is the women's descriptions of their powerlessness, which was seen in all aspects of their lives." The authors explained, "Traditionally in Ugandan culture, the roles of men and women are strictly defined with men being breadwinners and the women homemakers. Their background of poverty and limited education restricts their ability to control their own lives. For many families, this places women in a subservient role within relationships, relying heavily on their male partner for financial support and decision-making, and being sexually compliant and looking after the home and family in return. A dysfunctional form of this arrangement was seen in many interviews, with women left hungry, ignorant, or even raped."

The Power of Fear in Promoting Delay

Fear of the biomedical healthcare system is also a potent factor that delays the decision to seek help when labor is obstructed. There are many different facets to this fear: fear of the unknown, fear of ridicule and abuse by the hospital staff, fear of economic exploitation, fear of receiving poor-quality care, and fear of being forced to undergo an unwanted—and perhaps unnecessary—surgical operation, all fears that may be justifiable, depending on the locale and the context. For women (and their families) who live in rural areas with little formal education and limited interaction with more cosmopolitan communities, the prospect of going to a biomedical health facility may be daunting.

In many cultures where a woman's status is determined primarily by her reproductive capacity, the ability to deliver a baby "on her own" is important in validating her status as a fully adult woman. Failure to deliver vaginally may be stigmatized as a form of reproductive failure. The fact that Cesarean delivery may be lifesaving is not always widely understood. In a study of the use of maternity services in Uganda, Grace Kyomuhendo reported that Ugandan women regarded pregnancy and childbirth as a journey "on a thorn-strewn path," the successful traversal of which entitles a woman to be praised as *garukayo* (dare to go back). She writes:

> The traditional praise *garukayo* far supercedes mere praise of the new mother, but is also meant to remind her that the hardships experienced notwithstanding, she has no option but to prepare to get pregnant again. . . . The way a woman endures pregnancy and birth therefore has implications for her position in her household and community. One who experiences no problems and needs no assistance is held in much esteem, having walked bravely and emerged unscathed. One who experiences a difficult pregnancy, perhaps requiring hospitalization, an episiotomy or caesarean section, is not respected and is referred to as *omugara* (lazy), though the circumstances are beyond her control. To seek external help is to stumble and such women even after delivery do not deserve a genuine *garukayo*.

Attitudes of this kind are very common in parts of the world where obstetric fistulas are prevalent.

Aside from the belief that Cesarean delivery is somehow "unnatural" and therefore represents a failure of womanhood at the most elemental level, a Cesarean section is also a major abdominal operation. It inevitably causes pain and may be accompanied by complications, particularly when the surgery is performed for difficult cases of obstructed labor in low-resource settings by surgeons who may not have top-notch obstetrical skills. The likelihood of recurrent dystocia and the risk that the uterine scar may rupture during labor means that many women have already been told that if they have the operation they will need a repeat Cesarean later. The combination of unfavorable attitudes toward Cesarean section and dissatisfaction with earlier experiences may contribute to delay until catastrophe strikes in subsequent pregnancies.

Fear may be compounded by linguistic confusion. As Nicole Berry points out in her study of maternal health in Guatemala, "Operations have no parallels in 'traditional' medicine that Kaqchikel villagers used, and on an intuitive level it is not difficult to understand why they are so unpopular. Cutting a body open seems inherently invasive and dangerous, and it is difficult to imagine that anyone weak, sick, or compromised could have the strength to survive such an ordeal." Blood is often needed and frequently is not available. Constant requests to donate blood for operations make villagers leery of being exploited by having a valuable resource extracted from their bodies by powerful government officials and the word *operacion* was frequently used to refer both to Cesarean delivery as well as to tubal ligation, which would end a woman's chances of having further children. The result of this situation was that "women and their families feared that if they went to the public hospital for a c-section, they might come out unable to have more babies."

The conditions under which care is provided and the attitudes of hospital staff toward patients may create a situation in which going to the hospital or health center is seen as a decision of "last resort." Many healthcare facilities in low-resource countries are understaffed, poorly supplied, and overwhelmed with patients, thereby producing highly stressful conditions in which, even with the best of intentions, adequate care cannot be provided. Abuse and neglect of patients by underskilled and overworked doctors and nurses is commonplace in such circumstances. One study in Gabon documented a much higher case fatality rate among women seeking care for abortion complications compared to other obstetric emergencies, a fact that was linked to a delay between diagnosis and treatment that was 20 times longer for abortion complications than for postpartum hemorrhage or eclampsia. This was attributed by the authors to cultural stigmatization of patients by healthcare personnel. In these cases, disdain for patients turned out to be fatal. In China, where the government has adopted a rigorous policy of limiting family size, women who become pregnant "outside permitted limits" (perhaps in quest of a son) often avoid institutional maternity care so that they will not be abused, harassed, stigmatized, or punished for their pregnancies, sometimes with fatal results.

Economic Constraints on the Decision to Seek Care

Even when the problem is clear, when the location at which help may be obtained has been identified, and when the fears surrounding possible treatments (such as Cesarean section) have been overcome, there may still be substantial economic barriers that delay or prevent access to necessary care. The economic costs of obtaining medical care at a hospital or clinic derive from many sources, and the sum of these costs may be beyond the budget of all but the most affluent families. Particularly in remote areas, the costs of transportation required to reach a hospital may be substantial, sometimes more than the cost of care itself. There are costs not only for the patient herself but also for accompanying family members. There are food costs for the patient and her family members both while traveling and during the period of hospitalization. There are opportunity costs that result from going to the hospital rather than selling goods in the market, working in the fields, or engaging in other forms of economic activity. In Tanzania, Kowalewski has reported that women over age 35 and women with more than four children actively avoid hospital delivery because they need to provide farm labor and childcare, and nobody else is free to provide these necessary services. For people in subsistence or marginal economic circumstances, such opportunity costs may be an insurmountable barrier.

Emergency obstetric care often involves both "formal" charges from the healthcare system, as well as "unofficial" (but still very real) costs incurred for necessary goods and services. In many cases healthcare institutions have instituted user fees to help recoup the costs of providing services, but such fees disproportionately affect women, children, and the poor, with adverse health consequences. Such charges also diminish the utilization of services, adversely affecting the most vulnerable population groups. But even if care is ostensibly free, the patient and her family may still incur substantial informal charges—costs of supplies and medications as well as bribes and gratuities for access and services—that may dwarf other expenditures. As Afsana wrote of her research on obstetric costs in Bangladesh, "When emergency surgical procedures such as caesarean sections were required, the urgency put poor villagers under tremendous stress to secure the money. Families would arrive at the hospital with some cash, but the amount of money required was beyond their imagination." Furthermore, "Collecting the required money was difficult for poor villagers, who usually had no assets or savings. No one wanted to loan them money either. Some families borrowed money from moneylenders at very high interest rates, which tripled within six months. Some raised money by selling domestic birds, cattle or land or even a tin shed roof."

These combined costs—opportunity costs, formal charges, and informal payments— often reach catastrophic levels that may consume over half of a family's annual income. Nahar and Costello found that more than 20 percent of families were spending between 51 percent and 100 percent of their monthly income to pay for a "free" delivery in Bangladesh and that 27 percent of families were forced to spend between two to eight times their monthly income to cover the costs of complicated maternity care. A Pakistani study by Khan and Zaman on obstetric costs found that both vaginal delivery and Cesarean section were beyond the limits of what three-quarters of households could afford. Similar results have been found in Ghana and Benin, leading Josephine Borghi and coworkers to conclude that, "for those women who require hospital delivery, accessing sufficient cash to cover the bill can cause significant delays in receiving treatment." Among the poorest of the poor, the need to finance expenditures of such magnitude may result in permanent financial struggles and submersion in a cycle of debt and impoverishment from which they cannot escape. After investigating the costs of emergency obstetric care in Burkina Faso, Storeng and colleagues wrote, "A pervasive theme in in-depth interviews was anxiety about the costs of care. . . . A caesarean section, which in Burkina Faso is performed almost exclusively as a life-saving intervention, was widely held to presage unaffordable costs, potentially accompanied by social calamity if it meant that a woman was divorced or abandoned on account of being 'too expensive.'" The result of these economic factors is that large segments of the population in the world's poorest countries have almost no access to Cesarean section, and it is among these women that the obstetric fistula problem is most pressing. While many women are *willing* to pay to receive lifesaving care, even under the best of circumstances they may simply not be *able* to pay. The consequences of this economic situation are tragic. The terse observation made by Storeng and coworkers from Burkina Faso that "inequities in maternal mortality are largely shaped by social, economic and political vulnerabilities that disproportionately affect the world's poor" is quite accurate.

If all of these obstacles can be overcome, if the determination has been made that something is wrong and that help is needed, the next challenge is to identify the location at which help can be obtained and to get the laboring woman there in a timely fashion. This, too, is difficult for women living in the bottom billion.

CHAPTER 7

Deadly Delays in Getting to a Place of Care

When labor is prolonged or when a complication occurs, how does a laboring woman get to a place where effective help can be provided? Where should she go? How will she get there? How will she pay for the cost of transportation? Who should go with her? The answers to all of these questions depend on the social, economic, and geographic context in which her labor is taking place. Phase 2 delays describe the barriers that must be overcome in getting to a healthcare facility once the decision to go has been made.

In the best of situations, the pregnant woman is registered in a prenatal clinic, is seen regularly (at least four times) during her pregnancy, plans to deliver in a community health center under the care of a trained midwife, and has formulated an emergency plan of what to do should an emergency arise. The emergency plan should include a specified location at which she can receive emergency care as well as a transportation plan to get there. Under ideal circumstances, the pregnant woman is cared for by a skilled birth attendant from the moment she goes into labor. A skilled birth attendant can assess her progress and deliver her safely if labor is normal but also can determine when labor is not normal and recognize any danger signs that might indicate a looming catastrophe. Such a person should be so placed as to intervene directly or to refer her to a higher level of care if needed. Sadly, most women in poor countries do not deliver their babies under these circumstances. What to do when things go awry?

Delay in arriving at a suitable healthcare facility when labor is prolonged or an obstetric emergency arises is partly an infrastructure problem. The family must identify a "target" healthcare facility and transport the laboring woman to it. How does laboring "Patient A" get to "Facility B," and will Facility B actually be a place where the care she needs can be delivered?

To deal effectively with cases of obstructed labor, Facility B must be able to provide Cesarean delivery. It is true that some cases prolonged labor will be due to uterine inertia—uterine contractions inadequate to move the fetus through an otherwise adequate birth canal. In other cases the fetus may be extracted vaginally (sometimes alive, but often dead and macerated) using instruments, but cases of obstructed labor generally require surgical delivery by Cesarean section. If Facility B cannot provide the necessary services, the patient must be transferred to Facility C. Many times it will turn out that Facility C cannot provide the care that is needed either and will refer the poor woman to Facility D. Sometimes this process is repeated many times, and the suffering patient bounces from place to place while valuable time is lost. Sometimes there is no alternative.

In a landmark 1987 paper, A. M. Greenwood and colleagues described the clinical situation around the town of Farafenni in the tiny West African country of the Gambia. They looked at 41 villages between 12 and 35 kilometers from Farafenni. There were no paved roads. Occasional taxis traveled on dirt roads between the larger villages and Farafenni town, but in the more isolated villages the only way to reach Farafenni was on foot, by bicycle, or by horse or donkey cart. When a patient with a medical problem reached Farafenni, the only healthcare facilities there consisted of a small government dispensary staffed by a health auxiliary and a midwife, one doctor in private practice, and several small, poorly equipped pharmacies. The only prenatal clinics in the area were held every other week and required pregnant women to make a 20-kilometer journey. If complications arose, patients were referred from the Farafenni dispensary to the government hospital in the capital city of Banjul, the only place with emergency obstetric services and the capacity to transfuse blood. This involved a 200-kilometer journey that took hours to complete and required a ferry crossing of the Gambia River. Any Farafenni woman with an obstetric complication was in serious trouble.

This situation is not unusual for poor women in poor countries. A recent study from Tanzania by Claudia Hanson and colleagues found that maternal deaths from direct obstetric causes were strongly related to distance from hospital, with a maternal mortality ratio of 111 per 100,000 live births among women living 5 kilometers or less from a hospital, but rising to 422 deaths per 100,000 live births if women lived more than 35 kilometers away. The same story repeats itself over and over, around the world.

In an article with the ominous title of "Where Giving Birth Is a Forecast of Death," Linda Bartlett and the Afghan Maternal Mortality Team described the obstetric situation in Rāgh, Badakshan Province, Afghanistan. Badakshan is located in the Hindu Kush mountains in the far northeast of the country. It is a remote rural area, largely buried in snow for six months of the year. The people live by subsistence farming, and healthcare services are almost nonexistent. It can take up to 10 days by walking or riding to reach the hospital in Faīzābād, which is the only location that provides comprehensive emergency obstetric care. In Rāgh 65 percent of deaths among women of reproductive age were from obstetric causes. The maternal mortality ratio in Rāgh was 6,507 deaths per 100,000 live births, meaning that over 6 percent of all pregnant women could be expected to die from a complication during a single pregnancy or delivery. In this part of the world, a woman's lifetime risk of maternal death is 1 in 3, and the most common cause of maternal death is obstructed labor, accounting for 30 percent of maternal mortality. Among the women who died, none was accompanied by a midwife or physician. Skilled attendance at birth simply does not exist for these women.

In Zambia, there are supposedly 1,131 health facilities at which deliveries take place, but only 135 (12 percent) provide any form of emergency obstetric care. In rural areas in Zambia, less than a quarter of the population lives within 15 kilometers of an emergency obstetric care facility. It is no surprise that only a third of births in rural Zambia take place in a healthcare facility. As the distance to the closest health facility doubles, the likelihood of delivery taking place there decreases by 29 percent. Lack of geographic access to skilled care is one of the major reasons why the majority of births in rural Zambia continue to take place at home.

The first problem in overcoming phase 2 delays, then, is the way healthcare facilities are distributed, the capabilities that those facilities have, and how effective is the communication between facilities, particularly when dealing with complications. In other words, can Facility B communicate with Facility C when Patient A arrives with a complication beyond its clinical capabilities?

The Distribution of Emergency Obstetric Care Facilities

Emergency obstetric services are generally divided into two categories, called "basic emergency obstetric services" and "comprehensive emergency obstetric services." The difference between the two levels of care is the ability to transfuse blood and to perform Cesarean sections (which also implies the ability to administer anesthesia). The World Health Organization recommends that there should be a minimum of four centers providing basic emergency obstetric services and one center providing comprehensive emergency obstetric services for every 500,000 people around the world. The geographic location and accessibility of such services is critical to their being utilized. In most developing countries (such as the Gambia, for example) comprehensive emergency services are clustered in urban areas—sometimes only in the capital city—and this produces marked discrepancies in the availability of care between rural and urban areas. This also tends to skew maternal mortality and morbidity statistics, with rural areas faring much worse. In obstetric emergencies, the time-to-access is critical in preventing maternal death or serious maternal injury such as a fistula. This is seen most clearly in the case of obstetric hemorrhage, where a delay in treatment of only a few hours may be fatal. In obstructed labor, the great risk is uterine rupture, which is often fatal without immediate surgical intervention. With women in obstructed labor whose uterus does not rupture, the consequence may well be an obstetric fistula. As noted, there is no magical window of time within which obstructed labor is safe.

In the early 1990s, Deborah Maine carried out an exercise to evaluate the costs of preventing maternal deaths. Her model used a hypothetical rural population of 1 million people producing 46,000 births per year with a postulated maternal mortality ratio of 800 maternal deaths per 100,000 live births. After analyzing various scenarios, Maine found that the most cost-effective strategy for preventing maternal deaths (measured in terms of cost per maternal death averted) in this hypothetical population was a system of 5 health centers (providing basic emergency obstetric care) linked by a transportation system to five small rural hospitals that provided comprehensive emergency obstetric care. The next-most cost-effective scenario was a system of 10 health centers with basic emergency obstetric services linked with transportation to one large urban hospital that provided comprehensive obstetric care.

Mahmud Khan and colleagues carried out an innovative study to assess the need for comprehensive emergency obstetric care in Bangladesh. They used a model that attempted to minimize the social costs associated with delivering emergency obstetric care. In their model social costs were calculated based on two components: the cost of providing emergency obstetric care at a comprehensive obstetric care facility and the costs incurred by households accessing these facilities (including the costs faced by households associated with the nonavailability of services in the area). Social costs vary with the radius of the catchment area served. In general, the costs of providing care per pregnant woman served decrease as the radius increases (due to increasing catchment population and the consequent decreasing need to construct and operate more facilities); but the costs per household increase with increasing radius to a facility as the travel time and travel costs (including opportunity costs) increase with distance. Using this model it should be possible to find a point at which cost intersects most favorably with the radius of the catchment area of each emergency obstetric facility. Based on their analysis, the authors estimated that minimizing the social costs associated with pregnancy and pregnancy-related deaths in Bangladesh would require 450 emergency obstetric care facilities. Unfortunately, at the time of their writing there were only 90 such facilities in the country, 20 percent of what was required.

Transportation, Communication, and Planning

Assuming the obstetrical need is present, that a decision has been made to seek help, and that a target health facility has been identified, the question becomes: How do we get there? The "we" is important, since it is both unlikely and unwise for a woman in obstructed labor to attempt to travel to a hospital by herself, particularly if she is a poor woman in a poor country. Companion or family transport increases the complexity and the cost of transportation; and because most obstetric emergencies in resource-poor countries begin at home, the first transportation barrier is getting from home to a health facility, rather than transfer from a health post to a more advanced center that offers basic or comprehensive emergency obstetric services.

The first consideration is overcoming geographical challenges. In the Gambian example given earlier, getting to the hospital involves both road transport and a river crossing. What are the weather conditions? Many parts of Africa are totally inaccessible during heavy rains (and often at night, due to safety concerns). For example, in the village of Danja in southern Niger, the designated hospital for obstetric emergencies in is Madarumfa, only a few miles away; but in the rainy season a trip from Danja to Madarumfa becomes a 65-mile journey because seasonal flooding blocks the direct roads, requiring alternate routes of travel.

Improvements in basic transportation infrastructure could alleviate many of these problems, and such improvements are the kind of projects that citizens should reasonably demand from their governments and healthcare systems. For example, in the 1990s the government of Honduras discovered that maternal mortality was a far bigger problem in the country than it had realized and implemented policies that dramatically reduced the rates of maternal death. At that time maternal mortality was highest in the department of Intibucá, an inaccessible mountainous region in the west of the country along the border with El Salvador. To meet the healthcare challenges in Intibucá, the Honduran government constructed additional hospitals and health centers there, linked them together with an ambulance service, and created a radio network to improve communication. In the case of San Francisco de Opalaca (which had the highest maternal mortality in the country and was accessible only on foot), the government built a new road to reach the town and open the community to outside access. Sustained efforts to develop transportation and other critical infrastructure in this way have also played a major role in improving maternal health in countries such as Sri Lanka and Malaysia.

What transportation resources are available? Is a vehicle of any kind available? In Zambia, for example, it is estimated that only 1 percent of households own any form of motorized transportation. In Ethiopia women are often carried on stretchers by a party of friends and relatives, sometimes for days, before they can reach a hospital (or, in some cases, before they can even reach a road). Bicycles may be the only form of transportation available in some places, and few of those will be equipped with a mobile stretcher attached to its rear wheel. Imagine the panic, difficulty, and distress involved in a husband trying to take his pregnant wife in obstructed labor to a hospital 20 miles away while balancing her on the handlebars of his bicycle—yet such attempts to get help are not uncommon. Donkeys, horses, and motorcycles may all be used, if available.

Reliable availability and reasonable cost of transportation are key factors in getting women the care they need during obstetric emergencies. Individuals or families may struggle to come up with viable solutions to this kind of sudden, unexpected problem within a rapidly closing time frame. Numerous anecdotes report women with dire obstetric emergencies being refused help for fear that the owner or driver of a vehicle will be blamed if something disastrous occurs while en route to the hospital. Worse still are those unscrupulous individuals who, having access to a means of transportation, exploit the emergency at hand by demanding exorbitant payment.

Systematic solutions to these problems must begin at the community level. The first step is to heighten a community's understanding and awareness of the nature of obstetric emergencies such as prolonged labor. The importance of registering women within the health system for antenatal care must be emphasized, so that a clear plan for what to do in an emergency is already in place. The development of individual birth plans should be encouraged. What will be needed for a normal delivery? Where is the birth planned to take place, at home or in a health facility? Who will attend the birth? Do those involved understand the signs and symptoms that suggest that an emergency is developing and immediate medical attention is needed? Are supplies for a clean delivery and the routine needs of newly delivered mothers and their babies at hand?

What will happen if an emergency arises? Who can accompany the pregnant woman and help make decisions for her if she is unable to do so? Where will emergency funds come from? How will emergency transportation be arranged and paid for? What are the communication plans—how will the request for assistance be made? If blood donors are needed, who will respond? Where should they go if and when an emergency arises? Because the time-to-action interval is often very short in obstetric emergencies, not having an advance plan in place can lead to fatal delays. Not many pregnant women in the Third World have carefully developed plans of this kind, and a fatalistic worldview often becomes a self-fulfilling prophecy, with deadly results.

Because these risks are potentially faced by all pregnant women, and because it is difficult to predict in advance who will develop a complication of labor and delivery, communities should be encouraged to develop their own agreed-upon protocols for how to provide transportation in obstetric emergencies. Local solutions should be encouraged. These may involve schemes such as setting up a system of motorcycles to summon an ambulance from a district hospital or constructing specialized motorcycle ambulances for patient transport using a sidecar. (Motorcycle ambulances have the advantage of being less likely to be diverted to other, nonemergency, social purposes than are regular motorcycles). In Sierra Leone, an all-wheel drive vehicle was posted to Bo Government Hospital, and a network of motorbikes was set up involving eight local primary health centers to be used to summon the vehicle. In northern Nigeria, a community loan program limited to obstetric emergencies was established with compulsory contributions and community oversight and administration, which charged no interest with a 6-month grace period and a 24-month repayment plan. This was instituted in conjunction with a community-based emergency transport plan that used private vehicle owners who agreed to charge only a previously set, agreed-upon fee.

In Sokoto in northwestern Nigeria, one group helped organize local transportation workers to create a revolving emergency fuel fund to support the transportation of obstetric emergencies. Many possible solutions exist to overcoming transportation delays, but they require community engagement and leadership.

It is almost impossible to underestimate the communication difficulties that confront poor women living in the rural areas of resource-poor countries who develop obstructed labor or some other obstetric emergency. Farafenni in the Gambia serves as one example, but there are many others. A recent paper on Malawi by Jan Hofman and colleagues provides several striking examples of the obstacles confronted by three rural health centers in Makanjira, Mase, and Phirilongwe served by a car ambulance at the Mangochi District Hospital. The car ambulance took three hours to reach Makanjira (four hours in the rainy season, when the road was passable), about 20 minutes to Mase, and an hour to Phirilongwe one way (both of which were often inaccessible by road during the rainy season), plus any additional time picking up an emergency patient at the health center. However, much of the time there were unbelievable communication delays in summoning the car ambulance. In Makanjira, for example, someone from the health center would have to go to the post office to phone the district hospital to request the ambulance, a 15-minute trip. At night, the post office was closed, so contact would have to made through a radio link to the Mangochi police station, which was asked to relay the request to the district hospital. Usually messages were not received for one or two days after they were sent, making the system almost worthless. The Mase Health Center had no means of transportation to or communication with Mangochi, and there was no public transportation. In fact, there was very little motor traffic on the road to Masse at all, so if an ambulance was needed, someone would be sent by bicycle from Masse to Mangochi (a three-hour trip) to request that the ambulance be sent. If the attempt was made to transport the patient by bicycle, it would take six hours. Phirilongwe was in a similar situation: there was no public transportation, motor vehicle traffic was sporadic and sparse, and if the ambulance was to be summoned, someone would have ride 20 kilometers by bicycle to the Chiliipa Health Center to make radio contact with Mangochi, a two-hour trip. The acquisition of motorcycle ambulances at each health center significantly reduced referral time. On average, it took an hour and a half to transport a patient by motorcycle ambulance from Mase Health Center, two hours from Phirilongwe, and five hours from Makanjira. Use of the motorcycle ambulances reduced referral time by as much as 35–76 percent, depending on the site.

It is clear that an efficient referral system is a mission-critical part of an effective system of emergency obstetric care. The system cannot work without effective communication between its component parts, particularly when it comes to getting lifesaving emergency interventions for critically ill patients. This communication must be of two kinds: communication at the level of policy formation and process management and ongoing communication with respect to individual patient emergencies.

Maternity care referral systems in any country need referral centers that are adequately staffed, equipped, and supplied; active collaboration between and among centers with good documentation and record keeping; formalized arrangements for communication, transportation, referral, and acceptance of patients; supervision and accountability as well as systems to monitor performance; affordable costs; and political and policy support. In Guinea, for example, improvements in referral management led to a dramatic decrease in the number of uterine rupture cases that were referred to the teaching hospitals in the capital city of Conakry.

Uterine rupture is one of the deadliest consequences of prolonged obstructed labor; therefore, decreasing these cases is a good marker for improvements in the management of obstructed labor. To tackle the problem of maternal mortality generally, and the problem of uterine rupture specifically, the two teaching hospitals in Conakry began a collaborative program with seven peripheral health units. The protocol involved making systemic changes to improve organization and communication. They instituted a common prenatal record so that information flow was enhanced among the centers. Likewise, a common transfer record was created so that important patient information was accurately transmitted from the referring clinic to the receiving hospital. Care for known high-risk pregnancies was centralized for efficiency, and experienced pediatricians were assigned to the peripheral units to improve newborn care. Monthly meetings were established with representatives of all nine institutions involved to determine policies and procedures for transfer, delivery methods, use of medication, and other clinical issues. These changes were combined with twice-monthly training sessions to improve emergency medical skills among the staff. The outcome of the program was a decline of nearly 50 percent in the number of uterine rupture cases, combined with earlier transfer of high-risk pregnancies to the referral centers and an increasing number of high-risk deliveries taking place in the teaching institutions. The number of Cesarean sections increased, as would be expected, and maternal mortality improved.

By definition, resource-poor countries lack infrastructure development. One of the common manifestations of this in the past was extremely poor telecommunications infrastructure, such as that already noted in Malawi. Landline telecommunication requires an extensive infrastructure, which takes a long time to develop. There are a few ways to overcome this lack of infrastructure. In remote areas of Niger (the world's poorest country) where infrastructure development is unlikely to occur rapidly, the deployment of solar-powered shortwave radio units linked to a rudimentary ambulance system and hospital upgrades has dramatically improved communications within the healthcare system. As Bossyns and colleagues noted, "Before the introduction of the radio-ambulance system, the only way for a woman with obstructed labour to get to the hospital was to walk 75 kilometers or go by camel." The critical factor in the success of this program, however, was upgrading hospital facilities so that the care provided was seen as being credible. Fewer patients died. Communication between health centers and the district hospital improved and became more frequent, occurring many times each day. Staff morale also improved, as they no longer felt as isolated at the periphery as they had been. One staff member exclaimed to the researchers, "We now all live together in one big building, each one with our own office!" The local people also applauded the improvements.

Solar-powered radios, however, have been dwarfed by the explosive growth of mobile phones in Africa. It is estimated that there are now more than 600 million mobile phone users in Africa. The presence of inexpensive, widely available mobile telecommunications has the potential to revolutionize communication in maternal healthcare. Not only is the increasing availability of mobile phones likely to improve communication between referring and receiving healthcare facilities, thereby helping to triage patients and improve care by long-distance "mentoring" of less experience health workers in real time, but it also improves the ability of pregnant women to contact midwives and health centers. One recent study from Zanzibar evaluated a program called "Wired Mothers," in which automated health education and appointment reminders were sent to enrolled pregnant women throughout pregnancy, along with a modest phone voucher to enable recipients to contact their local primary healthcare provider in case of questions. Compared to a control group, those among the "Wired Mothers" were more than twice as likely to receive four or more prenatal visits. Furthermore, 60 percent of women in the "Wired Mothers" group had skilled attendants at birth, compared with only 47 percent of the control group. Another study in Tanzania explored the use of mobile phone banking technology to wire funds to patients to enable them to get transportation for healthcare. The prospects for mobile phone technology to further improve maternal healthcare in resource-poor countries are exciting.

Maternity Waiting Homes

The major risk factor for an obstetric fistula is prolonged obstructed labor. Because obstructed labor cannot be managed effectively by untrained birth attendants, the most effective way to prevent a fistula is through early monitoring and continuous evaluation of the progress of labor by a skilled birth attendant who has access to emergency obstetric services. Because skilled birth attendants are often in short supply and are distributed unevenly throughout the population, one potential remedy for this problem is to concentrate women who are at risk for obstructed labor in maternity waiting homes close to hospital facilities toward the end of their pregnancies, to assure that they will have immediate access to skilled care. This is particularly important for women who have had a Cesarean section because of obstructed labor and for women who have had a previous fistula. Both of these groups are at risk for recurrent obstructed labor in subsequent pregnancies, and women who have had a prior Cesarean delivery are much more likely to develop a uterine rupture if labor becomes obstructed.

The success of the maternity waiting home approach depends upon two factors: (1) accurate assessment during pregnancy of the risk of obstruction when labor begins and (2) convenient, welcoming, affordable places for such women to stay while awaiting delivery. In theory, this paradigm seems like it could prevent many obstetric fistulas and other complications. For this strategy to work, however, several preconditions must be met. These are not so simple. There must be a good, relatively inexpensive screening test for the likelihood of developing obstructed labor. Ideally, this test should have high sensitivity and high specificity, meaning that it accurately detects women at high risk for obstructed labor while at the same time eliminating "false positives," that is, women who do not develop obstruction during labor. The test should have a "high positive predictive value"; in other words, a positive test should carry with it a high likelihood of labor being obstructed. For the prenatal risk assessment and referral strategy to work, the total population of pregnant women must be screened accurately and referred promptly to the maternity waiting home before labor begins. And, of course, the maternity waiting home must be supervised so that women actually get to the hospital when they go into labor. Unfortunately, there are serious problems with the maternity waiting home strategy at all levels of operation.

The "risk approach" to reducing maternal mortality was strongly pushed by the World Health Organization in the 1970s and 1980s, but, unfortunately, it did not work. Allan Rosenfield and colleagues later described this approach as a "strategic misstep," one of many that were made early on in the international attempts to reduce maternal death and disability. The basic problem is that "the majority of obstetrical complications occur in women categorized as having low risk"; that is, they are unexpected, unpredictable complications. The screening methodologies so far have not worked. As Yuster summarized the problem of antenatal risk assessment, "The risk approach identifies a large number of women who do not go on to develop complications, and at the same time, misses or bypasses an equal or greater number who do." One study from Zimbabwe that used a "risk approach" for screening found that nearly three-quarters of all pregnant women were "high risk" using their guidelines. This is not particularly helpful, since it is not feasible to send three-quarters of all pregnant women to stay in a maternity waiting home. The logistics, as well as the social displacement and family disruptions such a policy would cause, would be unmanageable.

The fundamental problem with antenatal risk screening for obstructed labor is that most of the risk factors that are commonly utilized to make the assessment (such as age, number of previous deliveries, height, and so on) are not the direct causes of poor outcomes themselves; rather, they are only indirectly linked to such problems. Obstructed labor is influenced by many different cofactors that vary simultaneously: the size of the mother, the shape of her pelvis, the size of the fetus, the presentation of the fetus, the strength of uterine contractions, the point at which obstruction occurs, the resilience of maternal tissues, and the duration of labor. Only some of these factors are detectable before labor begins, and this greatly compromises the ability to predict which women are at high risk of obstructed labor.

More than 20 years ago Judith Fortney looked at the predictability of obstructed labor by analyzing data collected by the Kasongo Project Team in central Africa. She examined the predictability of feto-pelvic disproportion / obstructed labor using the commonly collected obstetric risk factors and found the sensitivity and specificity of these factors were uniformly poor. For example, first pregnancies predicted only 27 percent of feto-pelvic dystocia in this dataset, and fewer than 1 percent of these women developed obstructed labor. Measurement of height (which has a relation to pelvic size) was no better at predicting obstructed labor, but did predict the absence of this complication with good reliability. Among the cases of obstructed labor that did develop in Kasongo, 73 percent were recognized in advance of labor by screening (good sensitivity) but only 1 percent of the screened women identified as being "at risk" for obstruction actually developed the condition (poor specificity). A height measurement of 155 centimeters or less had a specificity of 86 percent in detecting obstructed labor, but a sensitivity of only 46 percent. "But," as Fortney commented, "notice that only 15% of women are shorter than 155 cm, and that most of the [Cesarean] sections for CPD [cephalo-pelvic disproportion] occur in women 155 cm or taller, simply because 85% of women are 155 cm or taller." These screening criteria would not only be inaccurate; they would overwhelm maternity waiting homes with women who would probably deliver just fine.

A large collaborative study conducted by the World Health Organization on the relationship between maternal anthropometry and birth outcomes (using nonspontaneous deliveries as the outcome measure for obstructed labor) analyzed 16 different anthropometric variables and found that only maternal height showed a small but significant increase in the relative risk for instrumentally assisted vaginal delivery or Cesarean section, but this did not meet criteria for use as a screening test. Numerous other studies have found a similar relationship between short maternal height and cephalo-pelvic disproportion, but none have good sensitivity and specificity, even when combined with high-technology imaging studies such as CT scanning or magnetic resonance imaging. At present there are no accurate ways to predict obstructed labor with any reliability in advance of the event itself. There are no accurate screening tools suitable for general use in obstetric practice in those parts of the world where fistulas are prevalent.

This means it is difficult to make recommendations as to who should be sent to a maternity waiting home because of risk of developing obstructed labor. Because skilled birth attendance and institutional delivery of complicated cases are so important in reducing maternal death and severe obstetric morbidity, some observers still see maternity waiting home as a key pathway to achieving these goals. One enthusiastic advocate of maternity waiting homes, J. K. Knowles, of Ekwendeni Hospital in Malawi, went so far as to write, "Clearly, it is important to persuade all pregnant women, including those who are well but possibly at risk"—a category that would include all pregnant women everywhere—"that they should use the antenatal shelter, rather than concentrate exclusively on those who are unwell." Although the intentions are good, implementing such a program would be impossible, even if it worked. The only clear candidates for utilizing a maternity waiting home because of a fear about obstructed labor are women who have had a previous Cesarean delivery (because of the risk of possible rupture of the uterine scar), women who have had a vesico-vaginal fistula from obstructed labor, and perhaps a few women with obvious pelvic pathology, such as some of the historical cases described in chapter 3. But there are still other problems with which to contend.

As with other healthcare institutions, the utilization of a maternity waiting home will depend on a pregnant woman's personal cost-benefit analysis. For women with a prior Cesarean section, a previous obstetric fistula, or a pregnancy occurring after a uterine rupture, the benefits of staying at a maternity waiting home (if carefully explained) will certainly outweigh the potential costs of going into labor in a village remote from good obstetric care. But waiting homes must be seen as welcoming places that offer high-quality care in pleasant surroundings if patients are to leave home and family (and possibly numerous small children) to stay there for weeks before their labor begins. The opportunity costs can be substantial, and not all maternity homes work out.

In the late 1980s when the maternity waiting home concept was becoming popular, a team from Korle Bu Teaching Hospital in Accra, Ghana, conducted research in the community of Nsawam, about 37 kilometers outside of Accra. After discussions with the local community about the health problems that pregnant women were encountering (such as poor local roads that were impassable in bad weather, lack of accessible transportation except on market days, surly drivers who charged exorbitant fees to transport women with pregnancy complications to hospital, etc.), they decided to develop a maternity waiting home. Financial resources were limited, but the team located a ward in the old hospital that was not being used and decided it was suitable for renovation. Cracks in the walls were repaired, old wiring was replaced, new ceiling fans and lights were installed, new water and sewer pipes were laid, beds were refurbished and given new mattresses, doors and windows were repaired, and a new cooking area was renovated and roofed to keep out the rain. At the end, they had an eight-bed maternity waiting home that was opened amid much fanfare, attended by high-level government officials, staff from the Ghana Ministry of Health, community leaders, and traditional chiefly dignitaries. The use of the home was to be free of charge.

Perhaps the most remarkable thing about the Nsawam maternity waiting home was that after it opened, it was unused. In the first year, 25 women were referred to the home, but only one woman used it, and she stayed only one night. When the team investigated what was going on, they found that educational outreach programs in the community had generated considerable awareness about the maternity waiting home, but few women were enthusiastic about using it. Most women wanted to deliver at home because it was cheaper and they thought they could not afford the costs of an institutional delivery. The costs of cooking for themselves away from home, the costs of being away from their families, and the costs of having to forego working in their fields and gardens were just too burdensome.

The biggest problem, however, appeared to be the social isolation of the maternity waiting home, which was admittedly a nice facility. The surrounding buildings were mainly offices, which were unoccupied at night. The waiting home was too far from the maternity unit in the new hospital for easy access, and there was no easy way of getting taxi transportation, especially at night, if labor started. Furthermore, the maternity waiting home was not staffed by doctors or nurses on site, so the women would be largely left by themselves. This caused some women to remark that if they had to stay by themselves anyway, they would rather be at home. Combined with these factors, it turned out the maternity waiting home had been built near an old mortuary—hardly an auspicious location. What pregnant woman would want to stay by herself in unfriendly surroundings on the outskirts of the hospital, alone and unattended except, perhaps, by unfriendly ghosts?

Phase 2 delays are the result of lack of convenient access to obstetric care, coupled with poor communication and unreliable transportation. People will make the effort to get to hospitals when they realize there is a serious clinical problem if they have confidence that they will be treated fairly, respectfully, and competently when they finally arrive. Unfortunately, that is not always the case.

CHAPTER 8

Deadly Delays in Receiving Care

In 2002, Dr. Sarah Kilpatrick and colleagues published an illuminating comparison of maternal deaths in Zambia and the United States. They compared maternal mortality at a referral hospital in Zambia (Kabwe General Hospital) with maternal mortality occurring within the University of Illinois at Chicago's perinatal network. The differences in maternal deaths were staggering: 108 maternal deaths within a population of 7,014 births in Zambia but only 33 pregnancy-related deaths among 161,814 live births in Chicago. The maternal mortality ratio in Zambia was 1,540 maternal deaths per 100,000 live births, compared to 20.4 maternal deaths per 100,000 live births in Chicago, a seventy-five-fold difference. What accounted for these huge discrepancies?

One factor was that African patients were sicker on arrival: nearly 40 percent of the maternal deaths at Kabwe General Hospital occurred within 24 hours of arrival, showing how critically ill these patients were by the time they arrived at the hospital. This represents the cumulative effect of the first two delays. Although hemorrhage was a major contributor to death in both countries, in Zambia most of the hemorrhagic deaths were due to uterine rupture from prolonged obstructed labor—something that did not occur at all in Chicago. The major difference was the high level of serious infection in Zambia, whereas infection was the least common cause of direct maternal death in Chicago. In Chicago, 48 percent of direct maternal deaths were regarded as being preventable, but in Zambia this number was 98 percent. Having arrived at a referral hospital, these Zambian women should have lived, but instead they died. Why?

In Chicago, with its low number of maternal deaths, the most common factor linked to a fatal outcome of an otherwise preventable death (86 percent) was an error made by physicians, nurses, or other caretakers. In Zambia more than 70 percent of the preventable deaths were caused by systems failures rather than clinical mistakes: chronic shortages of critical supplies and drugs (antibiotics, blood, surgical sutures, intra-venous fluids, etc.), failures of the referral system, lack of emergency transportation (broken ambulances), poor communication (no telephone or radio service in critical circumstances), lack of staff (including anesthesiologists for emergency surgery), nonfunctioning equipment in the operating room, and so on. The major problem was bad management and poor institutional governance. The working environment was terrible; good clinical practice could not flourish.

Surveying the Battlefield of Emergency Obstetric Care

The obstetric carnage that characterizes so much of women's reproductive lives in poor nations is, in T. K. Sundari's words, "the untold story" of the toll taken by dys-functional healthcare systems. What is it like to try to work in this kind of setting? One of West Africa's most distinguished obstetricians, the Nigerian Dr. Kelsey Harri-son, provided a piercing view of systematic hospital dysfunction in his autobiography, *An Arduous Climb*. He described the clinical conditions that existed at Emuoha Hospi-tal when he arrived at the University of Port Harcourt in Nigeria in October 1981 to become the senior lecturer in the Department of Obstetrics and Gynaecology. Emuoha Hospital was run by the university and was used as its teaching hospital while a per-manent clinical facility was being constructed. Emuoha was a fairly typical African hospital, located in a rural village about 7 kilometers from the main university cam-pus. It was accessible only by dirt roads. In the rainy season, the roads were virtually impassable—not the ideal location for an emergency health facility. Harrison de-scribed what he found:

Its inadequacies were frightful. There was an absence of basic needs that would make the hospital qualify to function as a teaching hospital. For example, the bed complement of 76 fell far short of the 300 required and there was absence of a functioning 24-hour casualty department. The professional administrative and technical staff needed had not been assembled, except for one administrative officer and a principal accountant. . . . My clinical duties brought me face to face with the full horrors of the place. The problems resulted from poor accessibility, grossly inadequate infrastructure and utilities, inefficient security, and acute shortages in personnel with generally low morale. . . . Electric power supply was not from the national grid (NEPA), rather it was from one stand-by generator, an arrangement that meant that the whole hospital functioned on intermit-tent rather than continuous power supply. Interruptions lasting for longer than 24 hours were common events. On one occasion there was no power or running water for two days. . . . Laundry of hospital linen was by hand washing. The wet linen was left to dry outside either on washing lines or the hospital's grass lawns. The hospital had a plumber but no tools for him to work with. Medical records were poorly kept, haphazardly stored, and difficult to retrieve. Frequently used drugs were often out of stock in the hospital's pharmacy. There were periods when the hospital was without sterile wound dressings, because power and piped water were interrupted so that the hospital's autoclaves would not work. . . . [T]he restriction on water and electric power and in autoclave function resulted in most surgical wounds becoming infected. . . . [T]here was no telephone in the hospital. . . . The cancellation of planned operations due to power failure was commonplace. For me there was another source of irritation. It was domestic animals—sheep, goats and chickens—left free to wander in the hospital's corridors and wards, increasing the risk of spread of tetanus and other infections.

Things were even worse at night, when staff left the hospital and often could not be called back in. Harrison describes a case of labor involving the wife of a high government official who arrived halfway through the first stage of labor with ruptured membranes, the baby in a breech presentation, and a prolapsed umbilical cord. An immediate Cesarean section was indicated, but the operating room was locked and nobody knew where the key was kept. The nurse in charge lived in Port Harcourt and could not be contacted because there was no phone service. An attempt to break in to the operating theater was contemplated, but since nobody knew where any of the emergency supplies were kept, the attempt was abandoned. The woman was forced to labor for hours in a knee-chest position with an attendant's hand inside her vagina pushing the fetal head up off of the umbilical cord so the baby would not die from asphyxiation. When she was finally fully dilated, Harrison managed to perform an assisted vaginal breech delivery under exhausting conditions and was lucky to deliver a living child. Other cases did not end happily. One obstetrician was forced to carry out an emergency Cesarean section for prolonged obstructed labor in the middle of the night using only a two-cell battery flashlight because of the lack of electrical power. Both the mother and baby died from complications that were the direct result of the appalling circumstances in which they had received care.

In a famously disheartening letter to his colleagues Sereen Thaddeus and Deborah Maine, Farhang Tazhib of the University of Sokoto in northwestern Nigeria, once wrote:

Today, Mary, the lady who helps us in the house, came late to work. I told her off for being late and asked why. She said that one of her townswomen . . . had died in the hospital while giving birth to a baby. This was her fifth delivery. She was not from a far off village but from Sokoto City itself. She had not gone too late to hospital but rather [had] gone on time. . . . By the time they found a vehicle to go to hospital, by the time they struggled to get her an admission card, by the time she was admitted, by the time her file was made up, by the time the midwife was called, by the time the midwife finished eating, by the time the midwife came, by the time the midwife examined the woman, by the time the bleeding started, . . . by the time the doctor was called, by the time the doctor could be found, by the time the ambulance went to find the doctor, by the time the doctor came, by the time the husband went round to look for blood bags all round town, by the time the husband found one and by the time the husband begged the pharmacist to reduce the prices since he had already spent all his money on the swabs, dressings, drugs and fluids, by the time the haematologist was called, by the time the haematologist came and took blood from the poor tired husband, . . . by the time the day and night nurses changed duty, by the time the midwife came again, by the time the doctor was called, by the time the doctor could be found, by the time the doctor came, by the time the t's had been properly crossed and all the i's dotted and the husband signed the consent form, the woman died. Today the husband wanted to sell the drugs and other things they never used to be able to carry the body of his wife back to their village, but he could never trace [the body] again in the hospital.

Why are so many hospital systems in poor countries dysfunctional? How can this be changed?

The Requirements for Responsive Emergency Obstetric Care Systems

The "third delay" refers to the interval between when a patient arrives at a health facility and when she receives effective treatment. The first two delays may mean a patient arrives at a hospital after days in labor and with the damage already done, but even in poor countries a Cesarean delivery for obstructed labor should be done within two hours of hospital admission. Sooner is better, but as Tahzib's anecdote describes, there are often interminable delays because the system of care itself is broken. The Hausa proverb says "Hakuri maganin duniya" (Patience is the world's medicine)—unless, of course, the delay ends up killing you.

Hospitals are complex social organizations. Nine essential components for a smoothly functioning emergency obstetrical unit are listed in table 8.1. The ability to provide prompt emergency care is influenced by each one of these factors, and each factor is intimately intertwined with the others.

Table 8.1. *Components of effectively functioning emergency obstetrical services*

- Absence of economic barriers to emergency obstetrical care
- Effective referral systems: communication and transportation
- Adequate facilities and infrastructure
- Adequate access to supplies, drugs, and equipment
- Adequate numbers of competent, motivated staff
- Adequate clinical and administrative management, guidelines, and policies
- Adequate institutional finances
- Adequate political and governmental support
- An institutional ethic that promotes a flourishing work environment

Economic Barriers to Care

A crucial driver of healthcare utilization is cost. There are many economic barriers to care, and these are well known to women and their families in poor countries. I touched on these barriers in chapter 6. A fundamental principle of effective (and equitable) obstetric services is that there should be no obstacle to lifesaving emergency care anywhere in the health system. Although many government healthcare programs have abolished user fees and made maternity care free (in theory), in practice there are substantial economic barriers to emergency services. These may be as small as the cost of a hospital registration card (a nominal expense, unless you live among the bottom billion), but there may also be substantial expenses for surgical supplies, drugs, blood, intravenous fluids, needles, and such (which may not even be available in the hospital because of inefficient or corrupt logistical practices). Desperate poor families lose precious time trying to raise money and purchase such items in the market. The worst abuses come from corrupt healthcare workers who demand bribes to perform necessary or even lifesaving procedures. In Zaire (now the Democratic Republic of the Congo) many years ago, I was told numerous stories of midwives who refused to repair lacerations occurring at delivery unless they were paid in advance. Behavior of this kind is beneath contempt, but the prevalence of such practices hinders many women from delivering in institutions or seeking help there when complications arise.

Adequate Facilities and Infrastructure

Comprehensive emergency obstetric care (table 8.2) requires a hospital. The word "hospital" itself conveys a special meaning. The *Oxford English Dictionary* says that the English word "hospital" is derived from the medieval Latin word *hospitale*, "a place for the reception of guests," which is also the root of the English word "hospitality"— "the reception and entertainment of guests, visitors or strangers, with liberality and goodwill." Hospitals should be welcoming places, havens from illness and distress. In poor countries, hospitals are usually not very welcoming.

The physical environment of a medical institution has a direct impact on the quality of clinical care that can be provided there. Here is Kelsey Harrison's graphic description of obstetric care at Ahmadu Bello University Teaching Hospital in Zaria, northern Nigeria, in the late 1970s, when he carried out his epochal survey of 22,774 consecutive deliveries:

> In the labour ward, as elsewhere in the hospital, there were acute shortages of space, materials and personnel. . . . During the first half of the period of this survey, there were only nine beds in the actual delivery suite, two in the second-stage room. . . . [W]orking conditions were very austere and all equipment was of the most basic kind. . . . With an average of 18 deliveries daily and with 10 percent of the pregnant women arriving in the

Table 8.2. Components of emergency obstetric care (signal functions for essential obstetric services)

Basic emergency obstetric services	Comprehensive emergency obstetric services
• Ability to administer antibiotics by intramuscular or intravenous injection • Ability to administer drugs by intramuscular or intravenous injection to make the uterus contract (oxytocic drugs) • Ability to administer drugs by intramuscular or intravenous injection to control blood pressure and to prevent or control seizures • Ability to extract a retained placenta by hand after delivery • Surgical ability to remove retained products of conception by curettage or aspiration with a suction device • Ability to perform an assisted vaginal delivery, with a vacuum extractor or forceps	• All basic emergency obstetric services, plus: • Ability to administer anesthesia and perform Cesarean delivery • Ability to provide blood transfusions

Source: From Deborah Maine, Tessa M. Wardlaw, Victoria M. Ward, James McCarthy, Amanda Birnbaum, Murazt Z. Akalin, and Jennifer E. Brown, *Guidelines for Monitoring the Availability and Use of Obstetric Services*, 2nd ed. (New York: UNICEF, 1997).

second stage of labour and 4 percent in the third stage, there was much overcrowding. Rarely was the daily bed-occupancy rate under 120 percent. The entire hospital of 250 beds was served by one operating theatre with two operating tables. All operations whether surgical, obstetric, or gynaecological including operative deliveries took place in it. This arrangement led to further congestion, confusion, and overcrowding. The resulting delay in carrying out emergency surgery increased maternal and fetal risks. . . . There was only one all-purpose maternity ward of 33 beds for all pregnant and puerperal patients, no matter how septic they were or how great their need for intensive care. . . . The maternity ward was always grossly overcrowded and attempts at decongestion failed. Restriction on the number of visitors to the ward was impossible to enforce for cultural reasons. Many defects in the construction of the ward itself could not be rectified, and in their presence, keeping the ward clean and tidy was a major task. Ceiling fans provided the only additional ventilation. In these circumstances, strict barrier nursing was impracticable.

A hospital is a specific physical space configured for the provision of healthcare services. Effective emergency care for women in obstructed labor requires functional buildings in which to carry out the necessary activities. Laboring women need shelter from the external environment. There must be adequate electric power, clean water, sinks, toilets, showers, and places to wash both people and clothes. There must be adequate space for the preparation and distribution of food. There must be places to accommodate the family members who accompany patients. There must be storage for clinical supplies and space in which to perform administrative and logistical functions.

The physical plant must be laid out so that critical clinical activities are performed smoothly and efficiently. There must be at least one functioning surgical theater. There must be labor and delivery rooms, a blood bank, outpatient clinics, and inpatient beds so that women in labor or recovering from surgery have a comfortable place to rest and sleep. The bottom billion often have no such places to go when labor becomes obstructed.

Adequate Drugs, Supplies, and Equipment

Effective obstetrical care requires supplies and equipment. Effective treatments for the major causes of maternal mortality—hemorrhage, infection, complications of high blood pressure, and obstructed labor—have been widely available for more than 75 years. The costs of these treatments are modest, but each treatment requires bedside intervention with some kind of technology. Hemorrhage requires blood transfusions and drugs (such as ergometrine, oxytocin, or prostaglandin preparations), which in turn require sterile tubing and intravenous fluids, blood bags, needles, and syringes. The treatment of puerperal infection requires antibiotics and the surgical capacity to remove infected tissue from the uterus. Hypertensive obstetrical crises require the administration of drugs to lower blood pressure and to prevent or treat eclamptic seizures (such as magnesium sulfate). Performing a Cesarean section for obstructed labor requires sterile drapes, injectable anesthetic agents, sterile surgical instruments, sutures, catheters, dressings, and more. Operations must be carried out through a sterile field, on a functioning operating table, with the patient properly positioned under good lighting, with blood pressure and oxygenation monitors. Even in relatively unsophisticated general hospitals at the district level, there is a list of "mission-critical" supplies without which the lifesaving functions of the institution are impaired or curtailed completely.

In many countries, having an uninterrupted stock of vital supplies (such as drugs, laboratory testing reagents, intravenous tubing, needles, and surgical sutures) requires careful long-term planning. These items must often be ordered in quantities that will last for an entire year, and the order must be placed up to a year in advance. Purchasing bureaucracies are often inefficient and corrupt. Many necessary items are not made in-country and may not be available for purchase in local markets even in emergency situations. When found locally, such items are often of poor quality or even completely fake. There is a growing problem of counterfeit pharmaceutical products in the world's poorest countries, which results in precious funds being spent on bogus drugs, with deadly consequences for patients. In many hospitals, equipment is poorly maintained. When it breaks or is damaged, repairs may not be possible for months, if at all. Preventive maintenance is generally neglected, and best of luck to you in finding a biomedical engineer to repair broken sophisticated medical equipment even in a capital city in sub-Saharan Africa. The ability to provide effective care is often thwarted by poor inventory control, bad maintenance practices, ineffective budgeting, theft of supplies, corruption, and indifference.

Adequate Numbers of Competent, Motivated, Caring Staff

Every practicing clinician knows that it is not the building but the quality of the staff that defines a hospital. Fabulous things can be done by competent, motivated people even in less-than-ideal physical surroundings; however, the staffing challenges faced by healthcare institutions in poor countries are daunting at all levels. In an ideal setting, hospitals providing comprehensive emergency obstetric care would be staffed by well-trained doctors, nurses, and midwives who have adequate equipment and supplies; work in safe, comfortable physical surroundings within a fair and efficient management structure; receive good pay and benefits; have a clearly defined pathway for professional growth and development; participate in ongoing educational and training programs; carry out their duties with a strong commitment to professional behavior and high ethical standards; treat patients fairly and compassionately; and carry a workload that is challenging but reasonable. Most healthcare institutions providing obstetric services to the bottom billion of the world's women meet few, if any, of these criteria for success.

The first problem is a shortage of personnel: there are simply not enough trained doctors, nurses, and midwives to provide healthcare in these countries. According to the World Health Organization's *World Health Statistics 2015*, low-income countries face appalling deficits in the number of healthcare workers they have to meet the needs of their populations. For example, in sub-Saharan Africa there are 2.7 physicians and 12.4 nurses and midwives per 10,000 population, compared to 28.7 physicians and 88.2 nurses and midwives for the same number of people in affluent countries. The maternal mortality ratio (maternal deaths per 100,000 live births) is 450 in low income countries globally (500 in sub-Saharan Africa) compared to 17 deaths per 100,000 live births in high income countries. In poor countries, only 51 percent of births are attended by skilled personnel, compared to 99 percent of births in rich nations. The Cesarean section rate is 6 percent in poor countries (only 4.1 percent in sub-Saharan Africa as a whole and even lower in many places) compared to 28 percent in the affluent world. These are huge discrepancies.

The shortage of trained healthcare workers results from two factors: inadequate educational and training infrastructure in poor countries coupled with the "brain drain" of skilled personnel who leave to seek better professional lives for themselves elsewhere. In many countries there are few (if any) opportunities for specialist training after basic medical education. That means doctors must go elsewhere. If they go to a neighboring (poor) country, the education they receive may well be substandard. If they go to an affluent country, they are unlikely to return after completing their residency program.

Ghana can be used as an example of this problem, but also as a potential solution. As late as the 1980s there were no specialty programs in Ghana for medical graduates who wanted to train as obstetrician-gynecologists. Those who wished to pursue such a career usually went to Britain or the United States for specialty training—and then stayed in those countries. Between 1960 and 1980, only 3 of the 30 specialists who trained abroad returned to Ghana. However, in the late 1980s, a unique residency training program was established as a collaborative effort by the American College of Obstetricians and Gynecologists and the Royal College of Obstetricians and Gynaecologists in Britain, funded by a generous grant from the Carnegie Corporation of New York. The project was spearheaded by the late Dr. Tom Elkins. The curriculum was five years long and was developed specifically with the needs of Ghana in mind. Among its unique characteristics was a fourth year that included three months of training in hospital management, a three-month observership at a specialist unit in Britain or the United States, and six months of mandatory clinical practice in a rural district hospital in Ghana. Almost every graduate of this program has remained in Ghana to practice obstetrics and gynecology, and many have now become academic and professional leaders in Ghanaian and West African medicine. Perinatal outcomes have improved for the babies delivered and maternal mortality has decreased steadily as these practitioners have taken on clinical responsibilities. The number of obstetrician-gynecologists in Ghana is still smaller than it should be for the needs of the country and the program has not been replicated elsewhere to the extent that it should have been, but it demonstrates the feasibility of creating ingenious local solutions to the problems of medical education in resource-poor countries.

There continues to be a shortage of adequately trained staff in most African hospitals. Lack of clinical personnel combined with low levels of technical competence leads to high rates of bad outcomes. Bad outcomes combined with heavy workloads (including around-the-clock emergency call for obstetrics), lack of supplies and equipment, and poor pay contribute to poor morale. The indifference that develops accelerates the downward spiral of clinical care. Add bad management, lack of opportunities for continuing education, the temptations of private practice, and it is easy to see how the system can break down completely. Worse still, these factors may also lead to mistreatment, abuse, neglect, or exploitation of patients by hospital staff. The poorest of the poor will not be a high priority in a system like this.

Labor is difficult. It is also involuntary. Often it is unpredictable, and frequently it deviates from expected routines. Labor is also painful. For many women—particularly those who are frightened, alone, and unsupported—labor may be overwhelming. Untreated obstructed labor is exhausting, and, by definition, it cannot run normally and smoothly because of the obstruction. After two days or more, the laboring woman will be weak and exhausted, dehydrated, possibly infected, definitely in pain, disoriented, and probably not cooperative. By almost any criterion, she is likely to be a "difficult patient" because of her clinical condition and her personal circumstances, all the more

Table 8.3. *Typology of the mistreatment of women during childbirth*

Third-order themes	Second-order themes	First-order themes
Physical abuse	Use of force Physical restraint	Women beaten, slapped, kicked, or pinched during delivery Women physically restrained to the bed or gagged during delivery
Sexual abuse	Sexual abuse	Sexual abuse or rape
Verbal abuse	Harsh language Threats and blaming	Harsh or rude language Judgmental or accusatory comments Threats of withholding treatment or poor outcomes Blaming for poor outcomes
Stigma and discrimination	Discrimination based on sociodemographic characteristics Discrimination based on medical conditions	Discrimination based on ethnicity/race/religion Discrimination based on age Discrimination based on socioeconomic status Discrimination based on HIV status
Failure to meet professional standards of care	Lack of informed consent and confidentiality Physical examinations and procedures Neglect and abandonment	Lack of informed consent process Breaches of confidentiality Painful vaginal exams Refusal to provide pain relief Performance of surgical procedures without consent Neglect, abandonment, or long delays Skilled attendant absent at time of delivery
Poor rapport between women and providers	Ineffective communication Lack of supportive care Loss of autonomy	Poor communication Dismissal of women's concerns Language and interpretation issues Poor staff attitudes Lack of supportive care from health workers Denial or lack of birth companions Women treated as passive participants during childbirth Denial of food, fluids, or mobility Lack of respect for women's preferred birth positions Denial of safe traditional practices Objectification of women Detainment in facilities
Health systems conditions and constraints	Lack of resources Lack of policies Facility culture	Physical condition of facilities Staffing constraints Staffing shortages Supply constraints Lack of privacy Lack of redress Bribery and extortion Unclear fee structures Unreasonable requests of women by health workers

Source: From M. A. Bohren et al., "The Mistreatment of Women during Childbirth in Health Facilities Globally: A Mixed-Methods Systematic Review," *PLoS Medicine* 12, no. 6 (2015): e1001847, doi:10.1371/journal.pmed.100187.

if she is a frightened, first-time mother. If you add poorly trained nurses and doctors to this mix, who are underpaid and overworked, who feel socially superior to their patients, and who are forced to carry out their clinical duties in unpleasant surroundings with unclear administrative guidance and little accountability, it should be no surprise that many obstetrical patients are neglected or mistreated (table 8.3).

The prevalence of patient abuse and neglect varies considerably from country to country, but the accumulated evidence suggests that these are common experiences for birthing women among the bottom billion of the world's population. In one study from Enugu State University Teaching Hospital Parklane in Nigeria, 98 percent of 446 women interviewed after delivery reported at least one form of abusive or disrespectful care during their last delivery. In a study from the Morogoro Region of Tanzania, McMahon and colleagues found that "all respondent groups regardless of gender, distance to facility, or district reported negative experiences . . . of abuse or disrespectful care." Moyer and colleagues quoted one Ghanaian woman from the Kassena-Nankana District of northern Ghana as having said, with regard to the difference between home birth and hospital delivery, "In the house the old women will pamper you, but in the hospital they will be shouting on you, treating you as if you are not a human being." In Addis Ababa, Asefa and Bekele found that 79 percent of respondents experienced at least one form of abuse or disrespect during childbirth. Interestingly, however, only 16 percent of women reported feeling abused or disrespected, which the Ethiopian authors interpreted as reflecting a cultural expectation by women to be treated indifferently (or worse) by the healthcare system. This must change.

Management, Guidelines, and Policies

Providing competent clinical care in a timely fashion requires organization and good management. Providing high-quality care requires adequate numbers of competent staff, who work in a safe, efficient, and adequately equipped environment, and are motivated to provide emergency obstetric services in a timely, effective, and respectful manner to all pregnant women on the basis of their medical needs.

These goals can only be achieved when each member of the obstetrical team understands his or her role and carries it out promptly and reliably. Each person must understand what to do, how to do it, and be motivated to do it whenever the need arises. This requires training, preparation, performance monitoring, outcomes analysis—and perhaps most importantly, good clinical communication. Written clinical protocols that are emphasized, reviewed, monitored, and enforced are critical to achieving these goals, particularly in environments in which staff is in short supply and educational levels are lower than ideal. Two clinical examples demonstrate the importance of effective management: the partograph for diagnosing abnormal labor and a specific clinical protocol for the management of obstructed labor when it has been diagnosed.

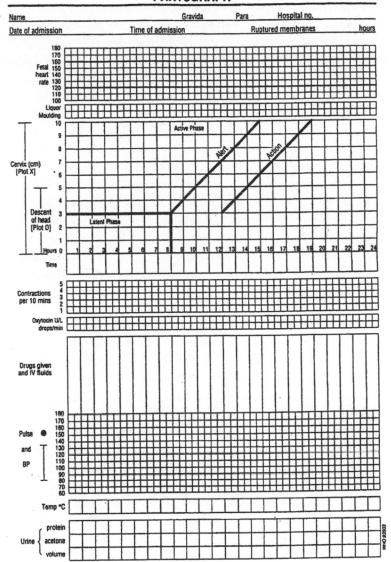

FIGURE 8.1. The partograph, a standardized method for tracking the course of labor to determine if it is normal or abnormal. Obstructed labors, if plotted correctly, will rapidly cross both the alert line and the action line. If used properly, the partograph will detect obstructed labor early and will insure that patients are referred to a higher level of obstetric care in a timely fashion. *From the World Health Organization, Maternal Health and Safe Motherhood Programme; Preventing Prolonged Labour: A Practical Guide. The Partograph, Part II: User's Manual. Geneva: WHO, 1994.*

The first step in preventing a fistula is the detection of obstructed labor. This requires the evaluation of abnormal labor and the determination that labor is abnormal due to obstruction, rather than from weak, irregular, or inadequate contractions. If labor does not progress normally in the presence of strong uterine contractions, it is obstructed. The evaluation of abnormal labor is facilitated by a simple technique in which the progress of labor is charted on a graph. This graphic representation of the course of labor is called a "partograph" or a "partogram"—from "parturition," the act of bringing forth young (figure 8.1).

The partograph is based on a simple principle: normal labor proceeds in a straightforward fashion that can be measured and plotted. Abnormal labor falls outside the expected parameters and requires further investigation to determine why it is not progressing normally. Abnormal labor usually occurs either because the contractions are too weak, too ineffective, or too inefficient for labor to proceed, or, because even though the contractions are strong, forceful, and regular, an obstruction (feto-pelvic disproportion) is present. Cases of the former kind usually require the use of uterine-stimulating drugs; obstructed labor requires intervention using forceps or a vacuum extractor, or Cesarean delivery, depending on the level and nature of the obstruction. A partograph is simply a tool to help determine when labor is abnormal and what the abnormality is.

Labor occurs when uterine contractions of sufficient frequency, duration, and intensity propel the fetus from the uterus through the cervix and vagina into the outside world. The first stage of labor begins when uterine contractions of sufficient magnitude begin to cause cervical change (dilation and effacement—or "thinning"— of the cervix to open it for delivery). This continues until the cervix is completely opened and thinned out (10 cm) to allow the fetus to pass into the vagina. In women who have had a baby previously, the fetus usually starts to descend through the birth canal during the first stage of labor; in women having their first baby, descent may not start until the cervix is fully opened. In normal labor once the active phase is reached (at 3 cm dilation according to the WHO partogram), the cervix should continue to open at a rate of at least 1 centimeter per hour, so full dilation should occur within seven hours. This can be recorded on a partograph, plotting effacement and dilatation with respect to descent of the fetal head against time. Normal labors thus plotted should always be to the left of the "alert line" drawn on the graph. If a labor plot crosses the alert line, immediate assessment must be made, and if a labor further falls off the normal labor curve and crosses the "action line," action must be taken. The concept is simple and powerful.

The World Health Organization carried out a multicenter clinical trial of the partograph in Southeast Asia in 1990–1991, tracking the labors of 35,484 women. The partograph was used in conjunction with an agreed-upon protocol for the management of labor, and the results were impressive. The protocol cut the number of prolonged labor cases in half (from 6.4 percent to 3.4 percent of labors), reduced the proportion of labors requiring the use of uterine-stimulating drugs from 20.7 percent to 9.1 percent, and reduced the number of emergency Cesarean deliveries from 9.9 percent to 8.3 percent. There was also a dramatic reduction in stillbirths from 0.5 percent to 0.3 percent. Among pregnancies with only one fetus and no complications, the Cesarean section rate fell from 6.2 percent to 4.5 percent.

Some of these outcomes seem counterintuitive, but the reasons for the results are straightforward. Proper and consistent use of the partograph not only identifies abnormal labors in which intervention is needed, but it also identifies normal labors that can be left to run their natural course. Using the partograph and a labor management protocol, unnecessary interventions are avoided and necessary interventions are directed more precisely. The partograph system properly used also makes nursing and midwifery staff pay regular attention to their patients and to the progress of their labors.

Constant monitoring of patients and prompt intervention during emergencies is a fundamental principle of good obstetric care, but in many hospitals in poor countries, women may be left alone and neglected in labor. In an article reviewing rupture of the pregnant uterus at Kenyatta National Hospital in Kenya, for example, V. M. Lema and colleagues sadly noted that 59 percent of the uterine ruptures occurred because of inadequate monitoring of women who were in labor in the hospital; some of them died. In another article by Umeora and colleagues that described uterine rupture at a hospital in southeastern Nigeria, more than half of the patients with this life-threatening condition waited at least 14 hours before undergoing surgery, and a quarter of them died. Better emergency preparedness and a standard emergency protocol for obstructed labor could prevent such catastrophes.

When obstructed labor is diagnosed (particularly in neglected cases that arrive by referral from outlying areas), the likelihood of a good outcome is greatly enhanced by the use of a standard emergency protocol that is implemented promptly and efficiently (table 8.4). All patients should be thoroughly evaluated as soon as they arrive at the hospital. If labor is obstructed, the goal should be to deliver the fetus immediately, and certainly within two hours, since the total duration of obstruction will often not be known and every wasted minute increases the likelihood of a bad outcome. A line for intravenous fluids and medications should be placed and rehydration should be started. Many women in obstructed labor—particular from remote rural areas in tropical countries—will have been in the first or second stage of labor for several days, and they are often severely dehydrated (fluid deficits are large as 3 liters are not uncommon). Many of these patients will be infected and bleeding; some will be profoundly anemic. Restoration of circulating fluid volume is a key component in the resuscitation of patients in obstructed labor, as in other obstetric emergencies. Hemoglobin levels should be assessed, and blood should be typed and cross-matched. Many patients will require transfusion, especially if an emergency Cesarean section is performed. A clinical flowchart should be created at the bedside to record vital signs and to track the patient's condition. Her pulse, blood pressure, temperature, and urine

Table 8.4.   Management of obstructed labor

- Placement of an intravenous line and immediate hydration of the patient upon her arrival
- Blood typing and cross-matching for possible transfusion
- Catheter placement to drain the urinary bladder
- Administration of broad-spectrum antibiotics
- Delivery of the fetus within two hours, usually by Cesarean section; immediate surgical operation to explore the abdomen if uterine rupture is suspected
- Establishment of clinical flowchart for observing vital signs (temperature, pulse, blood pressure, urine output)
- Prompt and appropriate interventions thereafter in accord with changing clinical circumstances

---

Source: Based on Eugene J. Kongnyuy, Grace Mlava, and Nynke van den Broeck, "A Criterion Based Audit of the Management of Obstructed Labour in Malawi," *Archives of Gynecology and Obstetrics* 279 (2009): 649–654.

output should be measured at frequent intervals and recorded. Broad-spectrum antibiotics should be administered as soon as possible since prolonged obstructed labor involves prolonged rupture of the membranes with greatly increased risk of intrauterine infection. Many of these women will have undergone multiple vaginal manipulations (often with the insertion of herbal remedies by local healers), which further increases the risk of ascending infection into the pelvis and abdomen. In some circumstances even worse treatments may have been tried, such as the brutal *gishiri* cuts in the vagina sometimes given to laboring women in northern Nigeria (see chapter 5).

One of the most important procedures in obstructed labor is prompt drainage of the bladder to minimize further damage and to avert the formation of an obstetric fistula. When the fetal head is wedged deep in the pelvis against the maternal pelvic bones, the soft tissues of the urethra and bladder neck are often compressed so tightly that voluntary urination is impossible (see figure 2.8). Bladder outlet obstruction prevents urination, but not urine production. The constant production of urine by the kidneys leads to a continuous flow of urine into a grossly overdistended bladder that may already contain several liters of urine, depending on how long labor has been obstructed. Not only is this excruciatingly painful for the woman in labor, but the increasing distension also stretches the bladder wall, making it progressively thinner and ever more vulnerable to ischemic injury, increasing the chances of a fistula. The urethra may be compressed so tightly that passage of an ordinary catheter is impossible. If this happens the bladder must be decompressed from above by aspirating urine with a needle and syringe or even by placing a suprapubic catheter into the bladder through the belly wall. Prompt decompression of the bladder during labor, after delivery, and for a week after obstructed labor in the postpartum period may facilitate bladder healing and even stave off the formation of a fistula.

Following delivery, each patient will require an individualized plan of care, based on her own clinical circumstances and mode of delivery. Treatment of urinary, uterine, or surgical-site infections may require prolonged antibiotics. Transfusions may also be needed, along with treatment of accompanying medical comorbidities. In most cases prolonged catheter drainage will be required to allow the bladder to recover from the trauma sustained during labor and delivery. In some cases in which a fistula develops, prolonged catheterization may allow the fistula to heal spontaneously. Women who develop a fistula in spite of all attempted interventions will need evaluation for surgical correction of their injuries by a skilled fistula surgeon.

A Responsive Institutional Ethic of Care

The quality of care provided by a hospital is the operational expression of its underlying value structure. It is the ultimate expression of an institution's organizational culture. How hospitals function in real time is the only meaningful expression of what the institution stands for. As Campbell and colleagues have written in the Lancet, "Making strategic choices requires decision-makers to be explicit about the values attached to alternative outcomes, since such values affect the target group and the packages of appropriate interventions." A commitment to values of operational efficiency, clinical competence, and respect for patients will show up in how well a hospital runs, the clinical outcomes that result, and in how the institution is viewed by the local community. As Peter Singer has argued at some length, "ethics" is nothing more than an answer to the question "How ought we to live?" and clinical ethics is the answer to the question, "How are patients to be treated?" Do they receive timely and appropriate care when they arrive in labor? How can that be assured?

The third delay is substandard obstetric care, which is a reflection of the organizational culture of the institution. Improving substandard care requires analysis of everything that contributes to delays in providing proper care. The establishment of a system to analyze these problems requires the embrace of an institutionalized ethic of introspection, self-criticism, and a willingness to change. This is not easy, particularly in highly dysfunctional settings, but it is possible. The model for creating a culture of critical obstetric introspection has developed from the analysis of maternal deaths.

A clinical audit is an audit of clinical practice. Just as an audit of a hospital's books by a certified public accountant is a systematic evaluation of its finances, a clinical audit is a systematic evaluation of an institution's experience with a clinical problem, such as maternal mortality. A maternal death audit involves a careful examination of all maternal deaths occurring at a hospital over a specified period to ask, what was done well, what was not done well, and where can care be improved in the future? There is a long history of maternal mortality reviews in obstetrics, and they have been instrumental in reducing childbirth-related deaths.

The same approach could be used for conditions other than maternal death. In Europe, the United States, and other resource-rich countries, maternal mortality ratios have now reached such low levels that clinical audits are starting to look not at maternal deaths (which are rare) but rather at what are called either obstetric near-miss events, or the more cumbersome "severe acute maternal morbidities." These are cases in which a woman develops a potentially fatal complication (such as uterine rupture, obstetric fistula, or even for all cases in which a diagnosis of obstructed labor was made) but survives. Detailed evaluation of such cases allows doctors, nurses, midwives, and administrators to take a close look at how clinical processes have functioned in specific cases and to improve what is done in the future. As Kongnyuy and van den Broek noted, "The success of audit largely depends on the motivation of the healthcare providers themselves. If they are able to evaluate the care they are giving, and willing and able to give praise where this is due, as well as make amendments where needed, then this should lead to improved motivation, ownership and sense of responsibility for delivering good quality care."

In practice, things are never this simple. Especially when staff shortages are common, critical supplies are missing, facilities are run down and inadequately maintained, training is substandard, pay is low, professionalism is poor, and motivation is lacking, clinical audits can turn into vehicles for the attribution of blame, public shaming, denial of responsibility, and acrimony. To avoid harmful behavior like this, strenuous attempts must be made to ensure confidentiality and to focus on the process of improving care, rather than ascertaining fault for clinical omissions or mistakes. The difficulty of questioning clinical practice through the audit process was described in detail for the maternity unit of a hospital in Ouagadougou, Burkina Faso, West Africa, by Richard and colleagues. Introduction of an ongoing audit process readily identified problems with staff negligence, poor maintenance or lack of equipment, lack of emergency medical supplies, lack of or disregard for clinical protocols, organizational difficulties with transmission of information, and communication problems both within clinical teams and between clinical staff and patients and their families. But failure to maintain adequate confidentiality and anonymity, staff fears of being blamed for poor outcomes, difficulty in undertaking self-criticism (which was seen as an admission of inadequacy, rather than an opportunity for improvement), and an unsupportive environment that often lacked adequate levels of human and material resources, made it difficult to create systematic improvements in care.

The Importance of Champions

Leadership in improving poor obstetric services lies with the midwives and obstetricians who set, maintain, uphold, and elevate the standards of maternity care. These individuals must be the champions for change in fixing the dysfunctional health systems serving the women of the bottom billion. Because a multitude of factors influence poor performance by health workers in impoverished settings—from low pay to overwork to lack of supplies to poor organization—change must improve the entire context in which obstetric care is delivered.

The ancient Roman philosopher Lucius Annaeus Seneca famously wrote, "The larger part of goodness is the will to become good" (Epistle 34). The creation of an environment in which high-quality obstetric care flourishes depends on the motivation of those involved in providing care; in other words, it depends on their will to become good. Interventions that improve motivation—such as better pay, more respect, better working conditions, opportunities to improve one's knowledge and skills, and increased job satisfaction—are key determinants in improving care for women with obstructed labor and other pregnancy complications. Instituting meaningful change invariably requires supervision based on a thoughtful plan; most importantly, constructive change requires the presence of a champion.

In 1987, a young and recently trained obstetrician named Godfrey Mbaruku was posted to the regional hospital in Kigoma, on the shore of Lake Tanganyika in western Tanzania, a country well known for its large number of fistula cases. What he found in his new hospital was disheartening. The scenario he faced was similar to that described by Dr. Kelsey Harrison for the hospitals at Emuoha and Zaria in Nigeria. The maternal mortality ratio was extraordinarily high: nearly 1 percent of pregnant women were dying (933 maternal deaths per 100,000 live births). Staff morale was terrible. There were extreme shortages of personnel and supplies. Equipment did not work. Case records and statistics were both deplorable and deplorably kept. Uterine rupture from prolonged obstructed labor was the most common cause of maternal death. It was enough to make most people throw up their hands in despair. But Godfrey Mbaruku was a tenacious and committed doctor. He wanted to understand why the situation was so bad and what could be done to fix it.

He undertook a systematic review of the maternal deaths during the three years prior to his arrival in Kigoma (1984–1986). He found many overlooked cases that had not previously been recorded; the hospital's statistics were even worse than people had thought. The high rates of maternal death were reflective of very poorly functioning obstetric services.

Having ascertained the scope of the problem, Mbaruku set about determining what the contributing factors were. He looked at equipment, personnel, patient attitudes, and departmental operations. He found huge problems with equipment on the maternity wards and in the operating room. There were major shortages of basic equipment. Much of the newer equipment was nonfunctional. There were acute and chronic shortages of water due to the absence of a reserve tank. He also began confidential assessments of staff attitudes, which were terrible. He noted "a deplorable indifference" among the staff and listened to frequently voiced frustrations over living conditions, inefficient hospital bureaucracy, and interpersonal squabbles. Patients were dissatisfied with the quality of care they received, the frequent absences of staff, the unavailability of essential care after regular hours, and lack of transportation to bring on-call personnel to the hospital when needed. The administration of mission-critical departments in the hospital was also poor. The pharmacy frequently lacked intravenous fluids, antibiotics, anesthetic agents, and other essential drugs, in part because these items had to be obtained from a central warehouse in the capital city, 400 miles away. Resupply was difficult, and transportation was often sporadic and unreliable. The blood bank had a chronic shortage of blood, which contributed to catastrophic outcomes during acute emergencies. The operating theater had shortages of equipment and supplies and no trained anesthetist. Lack of lifesaving skills was often a critical problem in patient care.

At this point Mbaruku set up a prospective study to see whether obstetric care could be improved and maternal mortality reduced. He developed a 22-item list of specific interventions to correct the problems he had uncovered, and he then set about putting his solutions into practice. His effort was comprehensive—and heroic.

First, he clarified and reorganized the professional responsibilities of the staff. This required overturning many traditional roles in the hospital hierarchy and the delegation of much responsibility downward to nurses and midwives. He arranged regular monthly staff meetings to review the events of the previous month and to discuss problems and their management. An attempt was made to reach consensus whenever possible.

At the same time, he began a push to use local resources rather than relying on support from the capital city. Staff members were encouraged to come up with their own solutions to local problems. Many of these were ingenious. He created and nurtured a repair and maintenance system using local carpenters and mechanics. By doing this, he was able to return much damaged and unused equipment (including sphygmomanometers, sterilizers, and suction machines) to service at surprisingly low cost. He created preventive maintenance schedules for equipment and on-the-job training that emphasized the importance of adhering to the manufacturers' instructions in the proper use of equipment. He found an old reservoir tank that was rehabilitated to provide a reserve water supply for the maternity ward.

Continuing education programs were established for all personnel involved in obstetric care to improve the management of specific medical conditions, particularly those contributing to maternal deaths (such as hemorrhage, infection, hypertension, and obstructed labor). Drills on the application of lifesaving skills were implemented; training was particularly targeted to lower-level auxiliary staff (who were often the first to see critically ill patients upon admission to the maternity unit). Follow-up sessions were introduced to let staff know about patient outcomes and to stress the importance of early diagnosis and intervention. The importance of sterile technique, disinfection and sterilization of equipment, prompt administration of broad-spectrum antibiotics before surgery, and the management of anemia were emphasized. Sanctions were imposed on staff who failed to meet expectations and to cooperate with the new regime, and new procedures for dealing with patient complaints were instituted.

Shortages of supplies were addressed. Priority lists of essential drugs were drawn up. A small backup store of critical emergency supplies was created in the maternity ward. A small unit was established to produce sterile intravenous fluids on site, and the blood bank was reorganized. A public relations campaign was instituted to recruit blood donors, and the relatives of women receiving blood were encouraged to replenish the units that had been transfused in the blood bank. A microbiologist was hired to create a facility for bacterial culture and antibiotic sensitivity testing. The operating theater was repaired and refurbished using local funds.

Perhaps most importantly, housing was obtained for all essential staff members within the hospital compound, so that the prompt attendance of midwives, nurses, and doctors who were on call could be assured.

As a result of these changes, the annual number of hospital births increased steadily after 1987, rising from 3,000 per year to nearly 4,300 per year. Not only did the absolute number of maternal deaths decline substantially, but the maternal mortality ratio also dropped from an average of 849 per 100,000 live births in the period 1984–1986 to an average of 275 per 100,000 for the period 1987–1991. Although this is still roughly 10 times the maternal mortality found in resource-rich countries, the change was dramatic.

Staff attitudes improved substantially, while patient complaints fell. The community recognized Kigoma Regional Hospital as a safe place to give birth, and the number of deliveries increased by more than 40 percent. As Mbaruku wrote, "Our limited experience revealed that many of the factors contributing to maternal death were staff-related. Prior to the intervention most of the staff were convinced that the maternal deaths were due to circumstances beyond their control, such as delayed arrivals for medical care, cultural factors such as use of local drugs, lack of drugs and equipment, and a non-helpful administrative system. All these reasons tended to justify passivity, especially when coupled with very low remunerations. The staff tended to forget their potential capacity to solve visible problems. Few or no attempts were made to look for appropriate solutions to obvious problems"—until a champion arrived on the scene.

Generating Political Will

In a provocative editorial in the British medical journal *BMJ*, obstetrician-gynecologist Tarek Meguid bluntly declared that "lack of political will is a clinical issue." "A clear link exists between the practice of medicine and politics," he wrote. "The task in front of every clinician is to advocate for change where such change is needed to prevent ill health and disease. Disease and ill health do not start or stop at the clinic." The high levels of maternal death, obstetric fistula, and other forms of severe maternal morbidity in poor countries are reflections of the values that dominate healthcare systems. Clinicians—like Godfrey Mbaruku or Catherine Hamlin (whom we shall meet a bit later)—understand this and respond to the challenges. Putting the best interests of patients ahead of all other considerations and advocating relentlessly on their behalf is the ethical soul of medicine. Clinicians—be they doctors, nurses, midwives, or others—have a moral obligation to generate the political will to change the nature and quality of the healthcare that is being provided to the bottom billion of the world's population. As Meguid wrote, "Women and girls and their babies have a human right to life and health, and this right must be protected. Those who protect these rights must have the power to live up to that responsibility." Such power can only be achieved by generating the political will to tackle obstetric health problems such as obstructed labor and the other causes of maternal death and disability. The structures that produce these outcomes can be changed, but doing so requires political will. How can the necessary political will be generated?

Political scientist Jeremy Shiffman has spent a large portion of his career studying the political environments in poor countries that make their governments responsive to maternal health needs like obstetric fistula. He argued that for a problem to be addressed, it must emerge as a priority on the nation's policy agenda. It is only when leaders believe an issue is worthy of sustained attention that they will mobilize the resources to deal with it. Shiffman's research has identified three major factors that get issues like maternal mortality and severe childbirth injuries onto national policy agendas: transnational policy influences, the national political environment, and effective domestic advocacy.

Transnational influences are the norms promoted by international health advocates and policy makers who agree (for example), that obstetric fistula and maternal death are unacceptable outcomes of childbirth that must be reduced to the lowest possible level. These norms emerge through consensus-building processes carried out internationally by obstetrician-gynecologists, public health workers, aid agencies, and researchers. Formal position statements are frequently produced as concrete articulations of such consensus, such as the UN Millennium Development Goals (one of which was the reduction of maternal mortality by 75 percent by the year 2015). In the best cases such policy positions are accompanied by external financial resources provided by the World Bank, individual nations, aid agencies, private donors, and other charities. In this way financial and technical resources become available to change the clinical realities on the ground in line with these articulated goals. Advocacy for patients is one of the most important ethical responsibilities of the healthcare professions. The existence of an internationally recognized, explicitly articulated ethical obligation to advocate for the best interests of childbearing women can (and should) be a powerful unifying force in such policy debates.

The political environment in any nation is a crucial factor in developing effective policy agendas. The late Speaker of the US House of Representatives, Tip O'Neill, is famous for saying, "All politics is local." This means that the local political stage is crucial in determining which causes rise to the top of the policy agenda. There are always competing problems that can divert attention from obstetric fistula or maternal health. Therefore, effective, persistent advocacy by domestic groups for maternal health issues like obstetric fistula is a key factor in how the policy agenda gets set.

Successful advocacy requires unity among groups promoting a cause. It requires effective use of evidence to support the advocacy position; the organization of forums to promote the cause; and advocacy of clear, convincing, practical policies to solve the problem. Most importantly, it requires the emergence of effective champions to lead the cause. These champions must be people who hold moral authority because of their commitment to the eradication of obstetric fistula, the reduction of maternal birth injuries, and lowering the rates of death in childbirth.

Successful champions are effective political entrepreneurs who are knowledgeable, credible, persistent, and effective coalition builders. They can articulate their ultimate vision: a world without obstetric fistula in which all women deliver safely, are respected as human beings, and have access to the reproductive healthcare that they need. They marshal resources effectively while avoiding political pitfalls. They are able speakers and can lead their followers effectively. Such champions must also be opportunistic, in the sense of being able to seize the moment when a "focusing event" occurs that highlights their concerns.

The natural place to start building political will for such changes is within the medical community. Obstetricians, midwives, and nurses are natural allies in solving the problems of phase 3 delays. These groups have the technical understanding of the clinical problems involved and a moral commitment to provide sound care for women with obstetric problems. Shiffman correctly notes that the problem is not lack of knowledge. Straightforward, effective treatments for all the major causes of maternal death and disability have been known for 75 years. The problem is ineffective management at the institutional level, and champions like Godfrey Mbaruku demonstrate how this can be changed.

In his book *The Honor Code: How Moral Revolutions Happen*, the Ghanaian philosopher Kwame Anthony Appiah discusses the role of honor as a motivating force for moral change. Honor is a broad concept but one that is probably understood intuitively by almost everyone around the world as it involves universal attitudes of respect, esteem, or even reverence, for those individuals reflecting a society's finest values. Members of the medical profession are generally held in high regard. They are given esteem based on their professional achievements and the positions of care and responsibility that they hold. They also tend to have a strong sense of personal and professional honor.

Appiah argues that honor is not just about being esteemed; rather, it is in large part about the *worthiness* of being held in esteem, about being *justifiably* esteemed. His book examines several historical examples of how moral revolutions to overturn awful human practices (such as dueling, the foot binding of Chinese women, and human slavery) were spurred by concepts of honor and the call to justice that it provoked. Can a medical profession that tolerates the abuse and disrespect of laboring women be worthy of esteem? Can a medical profession that tolerates organizational cultures in healthcare institutions that allow the persistence of the third delay be worthy of esteem? Are such low standards of performance worthy of honor and respect? Appiah writes, "One day, people will find themselves thinking not just that an old practice was wrong and a new one right but that there was something shameful in the old ways. In the course of the transition, many will change what they do because they are shamed out of an old way of doing things."

National associations of obstetrician-gynecologists, nurses, and midwives can (and should) be motivated by their sense of personal and professional honor to campaign for improved systems of maternity care. The third delay is incompatible with such honor. Because of the honor to which these professionals are entitled, they can be highly effective advocates for improved obstetric outcomes. They should forcefully seek to capture the attention of the government ministers and prominent politicians responsible for overseeing health-related matters. In the countries in which maternal death and disabilities like obstetric fistula are common, most of these individuals are male, so one potentially effective route to moving these problems up the political agenda is to gain the ears of these men's wives and mothers. An advocacy toehold within the domestic sphere of such officials, from which they cannot easily escape and which relentlessly appeals to their sense of honor, could be quite effective. Exposure to shame in a society bound by codes of honor can be powerful. (I have often wondered what leverage might be exerted by a group of unrepaired fistula victims taking over a health minister's office and staging a "wet-in" to protest the lack of attention given to their condition.)

Healthcare professionals should demand the resources they need to do their jobs properly. The people of their communities should back them up. The people of these countries—even the poorest countries—should demand that government-run institutions function effectively. They should demand decent infrastructure for roads and transportation. They should demand clean, efficient, effective healthcare facilities. They should demand competent and respectful treatment within those institutions. They should demand the removal of economic barriers to essential obstetric care. And they should demand an end to the corruption and abuse that permeates their healthcare systems. This is their fundamental human right. The most important factor in creating systems that meet the healthcare needs of pregnant women in the bottom billion is the development of systematic accountability for healthcare services among doctors, nurses, midwives, administrators, politicians, and the communities they are meant to serve.

The Importance of Trust

There is abundant evidence that women with obstetrical problems such as obstructed labor will use healthcare facilities when they and their families value the services provided by these institutions more than they value the competing choices offered in a pluralistic medical system. Kruk and colleagues, working with Godfrey Mbaruku in Tanzania, found that women were more likely to have a facility-based delivery if they had a high opinion of the skill level of doctors and nurses who worked there compared to that of local traditional birth attendants. For obstetric services to be valued in obstructed labor, the community must understand that obstructed labor is only a physical impasse resulting from abnormal obstetrical mechanics that can be corrected by appropriate interventions such as instrumental vaginal delivery and Cesarean section. The community must also understand the potentially devastating consequences of not intervening quickly when labor is obstructed. The care that patients receive must be perceived to be both effective and of high quality. Care must be socially as well as physically accessible, and it must be regarded as affordable within the local socioeconomic context. However, care does not necessarily need to be free. As Kruk and colleagues noted in a study of maternity services in rural Tanzania, "The fact that at least some women in this population were willing to pay more than twice as much to deliver in mission facilities rather than government facilities underlines the importance of quality of care to women in rural areas." Indeed, bypassing local facilities is common and is closely associated with perceptions of quality and a sense of trust in the distant but more highly valued institutions. Another study from Tanzania by McMahon and colleagues found that the most common response to disrespectful, abusive, and low-quality care by pregnant women and their families was simply to stay home and avoid institutional delivery altogether—a strategy that could prove fatal.

None of these conclusions is particularly striking by itself. What is striking are the ways in which all three phases of delay are linked. Delays in obtaining effective emergency care depend largely upon the feasibility of getting to an appropriate facility in a timely fashion (phase 2 delay), but the decision to set out on such a journey in the first place is tied directly to the perceived quality of the care and its expected cost (phase 1 delays). Effective and satisfying treatment of obstructed labor (or any other obstetric complication) depends on health facilities being properly staffed, properly equipped, and willing to treat patients in a compassionate and respectful manner (phase 3 delays). Each type of delay is related to the others in complex, but perfectly understandable, feedback loops. At the most fundamental level all effective healthcare systems are driven by trust, which must be earned.

Phase 1 delays occur when the decision to seek effective institutional care is postponed. There is abundant evidence that emergency obstetric care is sought more quickly and is rendered more effectively to women who are registered in an antenatal care system. Prenatal care plays a crucial role in obstetric fistula prevention, not because those women who will develop obstructed labor can be predicted accurately in advance but because women who are already booked in the system are more likely to get emergency care promptly than are unregistered women. Kelsey Harrison's magisterial study of nearly 23,000 hospital births in Zaria, northern Nigeria, demonstrated the dramatic effects of antenatal care and formal education in improving maternal and child health in resource-poor settings. Among illiterate, unbooked women (33 percent of his study population), the maternal mortality ratio was a stunning 2,900 maternal deaths per 100,000 deliveries with a perinatal mortality of 26 percent. Among educated women registered for antenatal care (10 percent of the study population), the maternal mortality ratio was more than 10 times lower (250 deaths per 100,000 deliveries) with a similar reduction in perinatal mortality (only 3 percent). Multiple studies of uterine rupture from prolonged obstructed labor show similar outcomes: delay and disaster are far more common among unbooked pregnancies than they are among women who are registered for and who attend antenatal clinics. Taken together, the data indicate that competent obstetrical care that is delivered respectfully, promptly, and at affordable cost is the key to obstetric fistula prevention, but such care will not be effective unless it is utilized by the women who need it.

Overcoming the cultural barriers to the utilization of care requires a multifaceted approach. Intensive community education about obstructed labor combined with an efficient, welcoming system of prenatal care and competent, accessible emergency obstetric services is fundamental to reducing the burden of obstetric fistulas. Particularly in the rural communities where fistulas are prevalent, it is critical that men understand the vital stake that they themselves have in the health of their mothers, wives, sisters, and daughters. Men can play an extremely important role in making the system of maternity care function effectively. Thoughtfully structured programs that increase the availability of skilled midwifery care at the local level can be particularly effective in raising awareness of these issues, especially if such programs are combined with a vigorous, ongoing social marketing and community education campaign. Even in circumstances in which skilled midwives cannot be placed in local communities due to logistical barriers, lack of financial resources, or shortages of trained personnel, it may still be possible to reduce the consequences of obstructed labor by training, supporting, and utilizing local childbirth monitors who can at least ensure that the sun does not rise twice on a laboring woman without her being sent for competent evaluation and treatment.

CHAPTER 9

Compassion, Respect, and Justice

The previous several chapters have discussed the three delays that lead to severe child-birth injuries such as vesico-vaginal fistula and even to maternal death. The first delay—delay in deciding to seek care—is largely a problem of individual and family decision making. The second delay—delay in arriving at an appropriate healthcare facility—is mainly a problem of inadequate infrastructure for transportation and com-munication (even within the healthcare system). The third delay—delay in receiving needed interventions after a woman in obstructed labor reaches a hospital that provides emergency obstetric services—is the problem of substandard obstetric care. Patients with obstetric emergencies who arrive at a hospital should receive prompt, competent, effective emergency treatment. The delivery of substandard obstetric care results from infrastructural deficits and the way those deficits are handled within the organizational culture of the hospital. In psychologist Edgar Schein's influential model, organizational culture is composed of the external artifacts of the organization (physical structure, visual and verbal behavior, etc.), its expressed values (which may not correlate very well with its actual behavior), and the organization's deep-level, un-questioned assumptions about the world and the "unspoken rules" of behavior that result. It is how these deep-level values are expressed in organizational behavior that really drive the way the system operates. Actions speak louder than words.

Hospitals and the healthcare systems of which they are a part are forms of orga-nizational culture. They are institutionalized reflections of the values that govern partic-ular human societies. Healthcare systems are structures that result from the choices made by the governing elites in charge of them. These choices reflect both professed values as well as the deep-level, hidden assumptions that lie behind them. Professed val-ues are commonly articulated in formal statements of an organization's mission, vision, and values, but the deep-level, hidden assumptions—the real operational values of the institution—are more influential but are usually harder to uncover, as they usually are not expressly articulated. Many hospitals (including many in which I have worked) see their mission statements as little more than marketing tools for public consumption, not governing philosophies that are actualized and taken seriously. The real values governing any healthcare system are shown by how patients are treated and by the actual clinical outcomes that result from the care provided, from tertiary-care referral hospitals down to rural health posts in remote villages. This is the fundamental point behind the concept of structural violence discussed in chapter 5.

Substandard obstetric care—the phase 3 delay—is a direct result of the values that govern actual clinical behavior within an institution. Meaningful change occurs when the operative assumptions underlying the process of caregiving change. Actions speak louder than words. This is hugely important for the women of the bottom billion because the values that drive behavior in healthcare institutions have an immediate impact on the delivery of acute clinical care and the outcomes that result (the phase 3 delay).

This chapter explores the values that ought to guide the provision of medical care for patients who arrive at hospitals in obstructed labor as well as for patients who develop an obstetric fistula and subsequently seek to have their injuries repaired. This chapter—which emphasizes the importance of compassion, respect, and justice—is a natural bridge between chapter 8 (which described the problem of poorly functioning obstetric services in low-resource countries) and chapter 10 (which describes the development of the Addis Ababa Fistula Hospital). Just as Dr. Godfrey Mbaruku was able to transform Kigoma Regional Hospital in Tanzania into an effective obstetrical referral center, so too Drs. Reginald and Catherine Hamlin created a model institution to care for women with obstetric fistulas. Champions like these are driven by compassion, respect, and justice.

These values are important because they have a direct impact on the clinical experience of patients. The most important lesson of chapter 8 is that patients want to be treated empathetically, with compassion, to be treated with dignity, and to be treated fairly and competently. The women who are the innocent victims of obstructed labor are poor and are now overwhelmingly from non-Western cultures, but anyone in their position would want to be treated in this way. Those institutions that treat women with compassion, respect, and justice are valued, respected, and utilized—and they are also more effective.

In this chapter I will explore the issues surrounding these values in more detail because the obstetric fistula problem is, in the final analysis, a human rights issue. The treatment (or neglect) of obstructed labor and the availability of surgical repair for obstetric fistulas are direct reflections of the way women are valued and how they are treated in the societies where fistulas are common. To make these issues more concrete, I will frame much of the discussion that follows around a hypothetical patient from northern Nigeria whom I will call Safiya, a common Hausa woman's name. The closest equivalent English name for Safiya is Dawn, an appealing name that reflects a new beginning, hope, expectation, and promise. Social scientists talk about the "modal personality" within a particular culture as a collection of traits that, taken together, represent a typical personality found among persons residing in that society. Safiya represents a modal fistula sufferer. In constructing her case I have pulled typical findings from numerous series of fistula cases to produce a compelling narrative, while at the same time acknowledging that fistula patients come from all walks of life, with many different personal and familial experiences. Safiya is a heuristic device to help us think through some of the practical and ethical questions surrounding obstructed labor and the treatment of women with obstetric fistulas.

Safiya's Story

Safiya is the firstborn child of Binta, her mother, and Muhammadu, her father. She was born in northwestern Nigeria in a rural village about 50 miles from Sokoto, the ancient capital of the Fulani caliphate of Usman 'Dan Fodio. Her father is a peasant farmer. The family is poor, barely scraping by financially. The land is poor, rainfall is marginal and often unpredictable, and life is hard. Safiya had her first menstrual period at the age of 15. Unfortunately, just as Safiya was becoming a woman herself, her mother died during the delivery of her seventh child. She had never used any form of contraception and she had never received any prenatal care during her last pregnancy. She bled to death from a postpartum hemorrhage the day after delivering a son. Lacking a mother's care, the child died three weeks later.

Safiya was a slim, attractive, and well-behaved girl. She was noted for her *kunya*, her female modesty. She had never been to school but had received several months of Koranic education from one of the village religious teachers. With his wife's death and five other children to support, it was therefore with some relief that Muhammadu agreed to give Safiya in marriage to Alhaji Arziki, a (relatively) prosperous farmer and trader from a village several miles away. Alhaji Arziki was in late middle age and already had one wife. Her name was Mairamu (Miriam), a word that rather ominously also means "little scorpion" in Hausa. Mairamu was older and "battle-hardened," with five children of her own. Alhaji Arziki had prospered and now felt affluent enough to demonstrate his increasingly prominent position in the village community by taking another wife. Safiya, his bride, became the newest member of his household—and Mairamu resented her presence.

Mairamu was not an evil woman, but she felt threatened by Safiya. Mairamu had proven her loyalty to her husband and her worth as a woman by producing five children of her own, which she had raised by herself uncomplainingly under less than ideal circumstances. Now, when she had become firmly installed as the *uwargida*, the "mother of the house," this new girl was entering the picture. It was unsettling. In Hausa a co-wife is called *kishiya*, "the jealous one." There is even a common appellation in Hausa applied to cowives: *kishiya mai ban haushi*, which may be loosely translated as "cowife, here comes trouble."

Alhaji Arziki tried to treat both wives fairly. He slept with them in regular rotation as he was obligated to do by Islamic tradition, but Mairamu noted both his pride in and his extra attentiveness to his new bride, and she bristled. *Bora* and *mowa* are two Hausa words of great importance in the domestic affairs of polygynous households. A *bora* is a disliked wife; a *mowa* is a favored one. As the new bride, Safiya, was a *mowa*, and Mairamu had become a *bora*. This was a recipe for strife, and it was not long in coming. Safiya's cowife Mairamu was about to live up to her name as the "little scorpion."

It only took a few months after her marriage for Safiya to become pregnant. This was a source of pride and pleasure for Alhaji Arziki but one of irritation to Mairamu. Safiya had some idea of what to expect, as she had been present for many of her mother's pregnancies, but, of course, she had never been pregnant herself. She did not register for prenatal care; nobody could really see the point in it, since everything belonged in God's hands anyway. In any case, the nearest health center was more than 20 miles away. It was poorly equipped and was staffed by an indifferent health auxiliary worker who was not particularly well liked by the community.

Safiya went into labor early one morning when Alhaji Arziki was away on business in city of Gusau. She was too embarrassed to tell Mairamu about her pains. Mairamu had been increasingly unfriendly toward Safiya as her pregnancy advanced. Traditionally, many young Hausa girls return to the home of their mother to deliver their first child, but as her father was a widower who lived a long distance away, the plan had always been for Safiya to stay in her husband's compound, assisted by her cowife and a traditional midwife named Bokiyar Gari, if any help was needed. Mairamu had grudgingly acquiesced in this.

First labors take longer to complete than do subsequent ones; unfortunately, Safiya's labor was not only long, it was also obstructed. The first several hours were only moderately uncomfortable, but the pains gradually grew worse. Safiya drank some water and ate some porridge, but she wasn't very hungry. She stayed in her room. By nightfall her pains were regular and hard. Occasionally she cried out, on the verge of losing her modesty. Mairamu sat with her, dutifully as was expected of her but somewhat resentfully. She worried about how a new child would impact her own children's share of the family resources. Safiya was unable to sleep. Her pains grew progressively more intense.

The next day was worse. Safiya felt tremendous pressure. She pushed as hard as she could, trying to force the baby out, but nothing happened. The pains were becoming unbearable. She tried to urinate, but couldn't pass anything. Mairamu fetched the *ungozoma*, the traditional midwife, Bokiyar Gari, who sat with Safiya as well. The baby's head was wedged tightly into the pelvis and had taken on an odd cone-shape, but it was still lodged in the midvagina. When the midwife looked at Safiya's genitals, she couldn't see anything yet. The baby was not yet ready to be born. So they waited.

Bokiyar Gari gave Safiya a concoction to drink made from a collection of roots, leaves, and herbs that had been steeped in salty water over the cooking fire. It was vile. It made Safiya vomit. Normally the rise in abdominal pressure produced by vomiting would have helped force the baby farther down through the pelvis, but in this case there was no progress. The pain was unbearable. Safiya badly needed to urinate, but not a drop would come out.

The midwife left the compound and went across the village to the local mosque. The imam who led the Friday noontime prayers listened to her story. He took out a wooden slate and wrote some Arabic on it in ink. These were powerful verses from the Koran, well known to help women in difficult labor. He washed the ink off the slate into a bowl and gave it to the midwife. She returned to the compound, where she washed Safiya's abdomen with the blue-black water. Then she forced Safiya to drink the rest of it, but all she did was vomit again. She was delirious with pain. Still no progress. The hours passed.

Alhaji Arziki returned from Gusau at noon the following day. On arriving in the village, he had been excited to hear that Safiya was in labor, but when he reached his compound, he was disappointed to find that he did not have a new son to greet him after two and a half days of labor. What was wrong with her? Mairamu never had labors that took this long. He thought Safiya must be guilty of some wrongdoing, but it was in God's hands. "Ha'kuri maganin duniya" (Patience is the world's medicine). You just never knew with women. He would wait and see what happened.

By the afternoon Safiya was very ill. Even Alhaji Arziki could see this. There was a dark, foul-smelling discharge from her vagina. Maybe they should take her somewhere? Alhaji Arziki was the wealthiest man in the village. He owned a Honda 250 motorcycle. That would have to do. So they put Safiya on the motorcycle behind her husband. His eleven-year-old son climbed on precariously behind Safiya to help hold her on the seat and the unwieldy family trio set off down the dirt road out of the village to seek medical care.

Since nobody liked the health worker at the nearest clinic, they decided to go straight to the district hospital, which was more than 40 miles away. It took them nearly five hours to get there because of the condition of the roads, which were uneven, unpaved, and full of potholes. Safiya fell off the motorcycle twice, spilling the party onto the side of the road. Once she burned her leg rather badly on the overheated exhaust pipe. It was after dark when they finally arrived.

They carried Safiya into the hospital, bumping her buttocks on the steps as they did so, and laid her on the floor. It took some time before they could find a nurse. Eventually, they found an unoccupied bed in the corner of the female ward and put her into it. There was a dirty mattress and no sheets. It would have to do. Nobody examined her. She spent the night unattended and in pain.

Late the following morning a midwife came and examined her. Nobody had bothered to call her during the night. The midwife was irritated by this—and many other things. She was not paid much, and most women preferred to deliver in their villages by themselves, rather than come to the hospital. The villagers did not give her the respect she deserved, and when they finally did come in, it was always because of some problem that probably could have been avoided. They were all so stupid.

The baby's head was now visible. It was also soft. This was not a good sign. "Push, you stupid girl!" the midwife said crossly. "Have this baby!"

Safiya pushed, weakly. Her strength was gone.

"Push you stupid girl! Have this baby! Are you a child or a woman?" the midwife shouted.

Safiya just lay there, exhausted.

The midwife slapped her in the face. "Push!" she yelled. "Push, you stupid girl! Don't you know how to have a baby? You are a stupid 'bush-girl'! Push! Push! A real woman knows how to have a baby! Are you stupid?"

The midwife called for a helper, whom she sent to the head of the bed. "OK. We will help you 'express' this baby," she said. To herself she muttered, "Whether you like it or not." With the next contraction both the midwife and her assistant pushed down on the top of Safiya's uterus as hard as they could, hoping to force the baby through the pelvis. Safiya screamed in agony. "Be quiet!" the midwife shouted. "Have this baby!"

They kept this up for nearly an hour, but there was still no progress. At least Safiya's uterus had not ruptured, a common complication of this popular but extremely risky obstetrical technique. The midwife left, angry and annoyed. "This is too much work," she muttered to herself as she walked away. "Stupid 'bush-girl.'"

Eventually the midwife returned carrying an instrument, a *venteuse*, or vacuum extractor. Roughly, she inserted her hand into Safiya's vagina and placed the soft plastic cup of the *venteuse* against the now-macerated fetal head. She pumped the handle on the extractor several times to create the vacuum that would secure it against the back of the baby's skull. Once it was firmly attached, the midwife glared at Safiya and said, "Now PUSH!" She pulled as hard as she could, yelling at Safiya all the while. With a deep sucking sound and a gush of blood, the head of the now-dead fetus slid through the vagina. The baby had been dead for two days and had started to decompose. The head was mushy and the parietal bones easily slid over one another with the vacuum extractor attached. The midwife released the vacuum, disengaged the *venteuse*, and pulled the head downward, bringing out the one shoulder; then she pulled upward, guiding the other shoulder over the perineum. The rest of the body followed easily. She wrapped the limp, lifeless, and decaying corpse (it had, in fact, been a boy) in a towel, cut the umbilical cord, and placed the small enshrouded body on a table. A few minutes later, the placenta delivered spontaneously. Safiya started to bleed, but the midwife massaged her uterus firmly (and oh so painfully) for several minutes, and the bleeding subsided.

Exhausted, Safiya fell asleep.

The next morning the urine started to come away. Safiya now had a fistula.

Compassion

Compassion is the genuine wish to relieve the suffering of others. Compassion is an outgrowth of empathy, the ability to understand and sympathize with the circumstances in which others find themselves. Empathy exists within each one of us. It is not a "gift" or a "talent" distributed randomly and inexplicably to some but not to others; rather, it is an integral part of our biological heritage as a social species. We have empathy because it is a prerequisite for social cooperation. Without empathy, we could not understand others, interpret their feelings, or anticipate appropriate actions in response to their circumstances. Empathy is the foundation upon which both morality and common social endeavors rest.

This was well understood by Adam Smith and David Hume, the great Edinburgh moral philosophers of the eighteenth century. In his book *The Theory of Moral Sentiments*, Adam Smith described the importance of sympathy (or "fellow feeling") in human affairs. Sympathy (what we call empathy today) is produced, according to Smith, "by changing places in fancy with the sufferer, that we come either to conceive or be affected by what he feels." "Whatever is the passion which arises from any object in the person principally concerned," Smith wrote, "an analogous emotion springs up, at the thought of his situation, in the breast of every attentive spectator." This capacity for fellow feeling, Smith declared, was innate in every human being. "The greatest ruffian, the most hardened violator of the laws, is not altogether without it," he wrote.

Smith's close friend and colleague David Hume (the greatest of British moral philosophers) shared these sentiments, declaring that the "tender sympathies" aroused by this mental process formed the soil from which all morality ultimately springs: "No qualities are more entitled to the general good will and approbation of mankind, than beneficence and humanity, friendship and gratitude, natural affection and public spirit, or whatever proceeds from a tender sympathy with others, and a generous concern for our kind and species."

These authors both understood that through fellow feeling, or empathy, an understanding of the situation of others arises (based on analogy with our own similar experiences). The emotional resonance that results generates concern to alleviate the suffering of others. Smith expressed it eloquently and succinctly: "By the imagination we place ourselves in his situation, we conceive ourselves enduring all the same torments, we enter as it were into his body, and become in some measure the same person with him, and thence form some idea of his sensations, and even feel something which, though weaker in degree, is not altogether unlike them."

The origins of this empathetic fellow feeling go back deep into evolutionary time. Empathy probably originated in tandem with related mammalian behaviors concerning maternal care. By producing relatively small numbers of live-born offspring who developed through internal gestation (rather than hatching from eggs) and who required nourishment through breast milk, mammals generally (and primates particularly) had to invest considerable time and energy in the care and rearing of their offspring. Compared to the thousand-fold spawn of fish, for example, each mammalian child was a precious commodity who needed care and nourishment since a far greater share of the well-being and ultimate survival of the group depended upon each individual. As primatologist and philosopher Frans de Waal has written, "Whether a mouse or an elephant, a mother needs to be exquisitely in tune with the indications of hunger, danger, or discomfort in her young. Sensitivity to emotional signals confers a clear adaptive value." And Adam Smith was even more eloquent in his description of this phenomenon: "What are the pangs of a mother, when she hears the moanings of her infant that during the agony of disease cannot express what it feels? In her idea of what it suffers, she joins, to its real helplessness, her own consciousness of its disorder; and out of all these, forms, for her own sorrow, the most complete image of misery and distress."

As social animals, humans must communicate with one another to coordinate group activities. Empathy is a fundamental precondition for such communication, and this, in turn, produces important secondary effects, like helping members of our group who are in need, just as we would like (and need) help if we were in similar circumstances. Empathy generates compassion, which in turn produces altruistic behavior, which improves group cohesion and survival.

De Waal argues that "empathy automatically produces a stake in another's welfare." Not only does the group as a whole benefit from this mutual caring, but we ourselves as individuals also get an internal reward—a "warm glow"—from such behaviors. The mechanisms that produce this effect were "hardwired" into our nervous systems eons ago. We are only just beginning to understand the complex neurological mechanisms that lie behind these phenomena. So-called mirror neurons may be fundamental to the generation of such feelings because these neural structures allow us to "match" the states, emotions, and behaviors of those around us. This generates sympathetic concern, allows us to take or see the perspective of our fellows, and generates altruistic behaviors that help those we perceive to be in need. Mirror neurons are likely the mechanism that allows us "to change places in fancy with the sufferer," as Adam Smith conceived it more than two hundred years ago.

Morality probably had its origins in such neurophysiological processes. These same mechanisms were likely also at work in the origin and development of the world's great religions. These neural mechanisms of sympathy, empathy, fellow feeling, and concern for "the other" can be seen as a kind of "divine spark" glowing deep in the evolutionary past, fanned into flames in the teachings of the great religious visionaries of the past. Variants of the Golden Rule—"Do unto others as you would have them do unto you"—hold a prominent place in all of the universalizing world religions. Sympathy generates compassion, and compassion mandates altruistic helping behaviors. It is no wonder that if you drill down into the core sentiments of the great world religions, you find compassion as the foundation upon which to construct a good and meaningful life.

Compassion also lies at the root of medical practice. Above all, medicine is a "helping profession" built around other-oriented behaviors. In one of the most famous medical essays of the twentieth century, Harvard professor Dr. Francis W. Peabody wrote, "One of the essential qualities of the clinician is interest in humanity, for the secret of the care of the patient is in caring for the patient." For the care of the patient to be most effective, it must be founded upon compassion.

This should be intuitively obvious, but often it is not. Medicine and surgery had relatively few effective treatments to offer patients prior to the end of the nineteenth century. Most drugs were ineffective (if they were not actively harmful). Antibiotics did not exist; patients survived infectious diseases largely through luck and their own hardiness. Blood could not be transfused safely and reliably. Surgery was largely experimental, and operations had high case fatality rates, especially in complicated procedures. Anesthesiology was still in its infancy, and critical care medicine and intensive care units did not exist. But, in spite of these limitations, physicians could still do a great deal for patients if they were compassionate. Indeed, prior to the twentieth century, compassion was probably the single most effective therapy that physicians had at their disposal—and this was true for the healing traditions in all of the world's cultures. The same neurophysiological processes involved in the generation of empathy and compassion are also linked to the therapeutic benefits that result from receiving compassion.

This can be demonstrated through what is known as the "placebo effect." In popular perception a placebo is nothing more than a "sugar pill" given to an unsuspecting patient in lieu of an actually effective treatment, but in reality, a placebo is much, much more. The word *placebo* is Latin for "I will please," and placebos have been shown to have remarkably powerful therapeutic effects. For example, in therapeutic drug trials in which some patients are given active drugs and others are given pharmacologically inactive placebos, *both* groups may show substantial improvement. Grant Thompson has defined the placebo effect as "a beneficial effect on a patient's symptoms or pathological abnormality that is not accounted for by the properties of the treatment itself, nor by the natural history of the symptom or disease."

The explanation for this positive therapeutic effect that seemingly comes out of the blue lies in the complex neurophysiology of our perception of well-being and our response to caring. As social animals we are deeply interconnected. Our feelings of health and happiness, distress and sorrow, pain and suffering, pleasure and well-being are tied together in complex ways. Our responses to clinical situations of pain and suffering are deeply affected by anxiety, our interpretation of the meaning of a particular event, the expectations we have concerning the event, conditioned responses, specific clinical circumstances, and, perhaps most importantly, by our culture and its symbolism, which creates the framework in which our clinical experience is interpreted and understood.

To give a dramatic example, consider a case of snakebite. There are some 3,000 species of snakes in the world, but only about 15 percent are considered dangerous to humans; yet most people regard all snakes as dangerous, if not lethal. When bitten, the immediate reaction of a snakebite victim is terror. The extreme fear produced at the perceived prospect of a rapid and potentially horrible death itself produces violent physiological reactions. A major task for clinicians treating snakebite victims is trying to sort out the "autonomic" reactions produced by fear from the systemic effects of the venom. Terror-related symptoms are almost universal, but only about a quarter of bites from venomous snakes actually involve envenomation; the rest are "dry bites" from snakes that have lashed out in fear themselves as they try to escape from what they also regard as a life-threatening situation.

The first task in dealing with a victim of snakebite is reassurance (along with trying to determine the species involved and stabilizing the patient's vital signs). The symptoms of terror—clammy skin, rapid shallow breathing, a weak pulse, fear—resolve dramatically after a placebo injection. Here the presence of a reassuring, compassionate, culturally sanctioned therapeutic activist and healer—the doctor—is the treatment. The effects on the patient are dramatic and immediately beneficial.

Since each of us has been ill at some point in our lives (even if we have never been bitten by a snake), we know these facts intuitively, even if we can't articulate them fully. As Tenzin Gyatso (the fourteenth Dalai Lama) has written:

> If one is sick and being treated in hospital by a doctor who evinces a warm human feeling, one feels at ease, and the doctor's desire to give the best possible care is itself curative, irrespective of the degree of his or her technical skill. On the other hand, if one's doctor lacks human feeling and displays an unfriendly expression, impatience, or casual disregard, one will feel anxious, even if the person is the most highly qualified doctor and the disease has been correctly diagnosed and the right medication prescribed. Inevitably, the patient's feelings make a difference to the quality and completeness of the recovery.

These same influences can also work negatively through a reverse phenomenon called the "nocebo effect." *Nocebo* is Latin for "I will harm," and it refers to the activation of these same powerful neurophysiological responses when they act in a deleterious way. Nearly 75 years ago, in a classic anthropological paper with the provocative title "Voodoo Death," physiologist Walter B. Canon explored the question of "whether an ominous and persistent fear can end the life of a man." "Fear," he wrote, "as is well known, is one of the most deeply rooted and dominant of the emotions. Often, only with difficulty can it be eradicated. Associated with it are profound physiological disturbances, widespread throughout the organism." These disturbances could, he postulated, if prolonged and unchecked, lead to death, and he described the mechanisms by which this could occur.

What do placebos and nocebos, empathy and compassion, have to do with obstructed labor, vesico-vaginal fistulas, and healthcare systems? They influence our perceptions of and attitudes toward laboring women. Imagine what Safiya's experience would have been like had she been treated with compassion and concern instead of indifference from the start of her labor. Safiya suffered from both obstructed labor and obstructed care.

Consider this rather puzzling fact: alone among normal physiological processes, the muscular contractions of the uterus during labor are *painful*. In the scheme of biology, this is unusual: muscular contractions are not normally painful. The body has three types of muscle: the striated muscle in the arms, legs, torso, and so on; the specialized pumping muscle of the heart (cardiac muscle); and the smooth muscle of internal organs like the bladder, gut, and uterus. In every instance, the normal physiological functions of these muscles occur painlessly. If pain occurs in our calves, in our chest, or in our bladder, we know intuitively that something is wrong. Why is the uterus different? The normal physiological function of the uterine smooth muscle is to contract during labor to expel the fetus—and this is painful. Is there an adaptive benefit to labor pain?

I believe that labor pain does have an adaptive evolutionary benefit. Human labor is long and difficult compared to birth in other species. The tight fit of the fetal head through the maternal pelvis predisposes human females to arduous deliveries and obstructed labor. Few creatures are as vulnerable as a woman in the second stage of labor, her cervix fully dilated and all of her efforts concentrated on pushing the fetus through the birth canal. At that moment, a woman's capacity to do anything other than labor is greatly reduced, irrespective of whatever external circumstances might arise.

One of the most important functions of pain is to serve as a signaling device. Pain tells the body that all is not well. In social species such as humans, pain generates external signals that allow other members of the species to know that one of their fellows is distressed. These distress signals summon help and support from others. Because each of us has experienced pain, we recognize its manifestations in others through Smith's process of fellow feeling. This is a perfect evolutionary example of empathy generating compassion that results in altruistic action: providing aid to a distressed woman in childbirth.

This probably explains why human childbirth is generally a social event rather than a solitary process. The parturient woman is surrounded by others (usually, but not always, other females) who gather and sympathize, support and care for her during labor and delivery (and frequently afterward as well). Human societies have always recognized that birth is stressful, often dangerous, and sometimes fatal for the mother and child. It is therefore not surprising that women in travail commonly receive significant support from other women (who are more keenly attuned to the fellow feeling that arises from labor than are men, especially in patriarchal societies). While little could be done for obstructed labor throughout most of human history except to watch, wait, and sympathize, social support by female peers brought the internal coping mechanisms surrounding the placebo phenomenon into play during labor, with distinctly beneficial results for the birthing woman. There is ample evidence from modern obstetrics and midwifery that the presence of a supportive companion (commonly referred to as a doula) is profoundly beneficial for the woman in labor. Such a presence adds much to what advanced obstetrical technology can achieve, and such a presence actually lessens the need for intervention compared to women who labor without this support.

In the late 1920s Finnish anthropologist Hilma Granqvist carried out ethnographic studies of Arab villages in Palestine, in which she documented and described childbirth customs. Her narrations portray small villages that were deeply involved in the communal support of women during birth. Men left the house in which a woman was laboring while her relatives and neighbors gathered around her. There was a constant stream of village women coming to greet and support her. The attention of the entire village was focused on the woman in labor. This was a momentous occasion when the Gate of Heaven itself was said to be open, and God's attention was especially directed toward the parturient: "The midwife keeps order among the women," Granqvist wrote. "They may not be noisy. They may not talk about their own sufferings. They may not quarrel or curse. If anyone does so she is reproved by the midwife. She exhorts them to remember the seriousness of the moment. The mother is in God's hands and she hovers between life and death. 'So pray,' she says, 'and do not curse! Angels go up and down to record what happens and what will happen!'" A continuous parade of angels and sympathetic neighbors: powerful support indeed!

Women in childbirth are vulnerable and in pain. This should naturally evoke empathy and compassion from external observers. This sense of compassion should be particularly compelling for women who have been in obstructed labor for three or four days. A woman who survives obstructed labor only to see her child stillborn and to suffer thereafter with an obstetric fistula should arouse the most tender of compassionate instincts in observers and promote a desire to help in some way. The intentions to alleviate pain and suffering that arise in such situations are the seedbed from which the practice of medicine blossoms in all cultural traditions. This compassionate instinct must be protected and nurtured—indeed, it must be institutionalized—so that it exerts a dominant influence in the value structure of healthcare institutions, particularly in obstetric institutions. We must continually be on guard against those— be they administrators and politicians or doctors and nurses—who "know the cost of everything and the value of nothing." The presence of compassion is deeply valued by all human beings. Health systems that provide compassionate care are respected, loved, and trusted by those whom they serve. The presence of compassion is a powerful force that should naturally motivate doctors, nurses, and midwives to overcome phase 3 delays.

A key issue in health systems management is how to develop an institutional culture that allows good practices to flourish. The environment should enable the provision of good medical care. As Godfrey Mbaruku demonstrated, there are often many barriers to overcome to provide compassionate care: lack of adequate skills, lack of adequate equipment, poor motivation, a sense of overwork, "burnout," specific personal issues, and so on. But Safiya should not have waited overnight in the hospital before she was evaluated. Professional standards require much more. Basic compassion demands prompt attention in such situations. Healthcare institutions that provide timely and compassionate care are also more effective because the patients who need care are more likely to utilize them, particularly in resource-poor countries.

Respect

Respect, like compassion, also originates in empathy. The English word "respect" derives from the Latin word *respectus*, which means "the action of looking around or back." It is related to the Latin *spectare*, meaning "to look or face in a specified direction." To respect means "to look again," to scrutinize more carefully, to see from a particular point of view. To respect someone means to see that person as the end to which viewing is directed; she is the focal point of regard, consideration, and notice. This particular characteristic of the word "respect" can also be used to convey deferential regard or esteem to the one who is thus respected.

How does respect arise from empathy? Both cognitive empathy (understanding) and affective empathy (feeling) are possible because we are able to recognize thoughts and feelings in others. Knowing how *we* think or feel in certain circumstances allows us, by a process of transference, to see others in the light of how we would see ourselves in similar circumstances. Smith's process of fellow feeling allows us to understand others through analogy with our own experience: "just like me" that person feels pain; "just like me" she wants to be happy and to avoid suffering; "just like me" she wants to be treated with consideration and respect; "just like me" she wants to matter, to be valued, to be the object of concern, to be treated as an end in herself, not just as a means to some other end or an instrument for someone to achieve her own purpose. To be respected means to be the focus of someone's attention, to be the object of his gaze rather than something that he looks beyond. The most successful physicians, religious leaders, and politicians all seem to have the ability to focus their attention on the individual they are with "in the present moment," concentrating fully on that person alone. Those who have experienced such deeply focused attention feel fully captured and absorbed in the moment, for they are deeply respected in the broadest sense of that word.

Conversely, to be disrespected means to be disregarded, not to be seen, to be looked past or overlooked entirely. At bottom, then, to be respected means to be worthy of consideration, to be the proper object of attention, to *matter*. As a patient needing medical attention—either a woman in labor or a woman living with a fistula years after her initial injury—to be respected means to have a voice, to be worthy of consideration, to be taken seriously as an individual, not merely to be the "work object" of a surgeon, a midwife, a doctor, or a nurse. Feeling oneself to be the proper object of caring is itself part of healing because this is one of the main pathways by which the multiple components of the internal self-healing system of the placebo phenomenon are activated. For compassion to be effective, it must be individualized and directed through respect.

The most fundamental principle of medicine is that the needs of the patient must come before all other considerations. This means that the practice of medicine, surgery, nursing, and midwifery must be actuated by an ethic of subservience and service. The individual needs of the doctor, midwife, or nurse—while important—should not come first. The only reason that patients go to a doctor is that they trust that the physician will work for their own best interests. It is trust that the obstetrician, midwife, or surgeon will put their best interests ahead of all other considerations that makes patients—who are often total strangers—expose their bodies, bare their fears, and reveal their most intimate secrets to a member of the medical community. It is only because they believe that their own best interests are the first priority that patients consent to inspection, examination, testing, surgery, and the like. "Disease" and "malady" are generalized concepts that doctors and nurses encounter only as they are manifested in the lives of individual patients. Although obstetrics and surgery have legitimate public health concerns, they can only be *practiced* one patient at a time: one obstructed labor with its unique circumstances or one fistula with its own particular individual characteristics. When this perspective is lost in clinical practice, the most important components of medical care are lost along with it. Healthcare systems that lose the perspective of respect are impersonal, unpopular, and ultimately ineffective because they lose the trust of the community and are underused as a result.

Safiya's Story, Continued

Safiya and her family bypassed the local health center on their journey to seek care because they thought that they would not be treated well there. They fared little better at the district hospital because the nurses were indifferent and the midwife treated her with contempt as a "bush-girl" unworthy of respect. Respect for patients requires prompt, competent attention to their medical needs. Their welfare depends upon it, and unnecessary delay may lead to serious complications. Safiya was ignored in labor for hours after she arrived at the hospital, and this contributed to the development of her injuries. When the urine leakage started after her delivery, Safiya was berated by the nurses for "making more work for them." She did not understand what was happening and felt guilty that she was constantly soiling the bed like a baby. This was shameful and embarrassing; it was psychologically wounding.

Worse, she was unable to walk. The entrapped fetal head had compressed the left side of her pelvis, injuring the lumbosacral nerve plexus. Safiya could not flex her left foot to walk properly, and she was very weak. She fell down when she tried to get out of bed. This made the nurses even angrier, since she knocked things over in the process. Her bed was always wet, and the bedding was not changed regularly. The nurses eventually put her on the floor so they wouldn't have to keep changing the bedding.

A few days after her delivery, Safiya was examined by a doctor. He told her that she had a fistula. She didn't know what that meant, but she was too shy to ask questions. He told her she should go home. There was nothing they could do for her. God willing, she would get better at home. That was it.

Fortunately, her obstetric palsy had gotten better. She could now stand up and walk with a stick for support. She managed to get transportation to a village near her own, riding in the back of a transport lorry that was carrying goods to a market. There were only a few other passengers. Safiya sat quietly by herself in a corner of the truck bed, her genitals wrapped as tightly as possible in old cloth to minimize the leakage and conceal the smell of urine.

When she reached the compound of Alhaji Arziki, she was greeted with indifference by Mairamu and the other members of the household. Her husband was polite but not very warm. The situation he had been looking forward to—a beautiful young wife having a fine baby boy—had turned to ashes. Such damaged goods were no cause for celebration. Safiya was sent to her hut, where she rested for hours at a time. Food and water were brought to her twice a day, but she kept mainly to herself. Her shame at having no urinary control was deep. She felt guilty but didn't really know why. What had she done to make God do this to her? She padded herself and washed often, but, in spite of her efforts, she often dribbled in the dust of the compound or soiled the floor of her hut.

Months went by with no improvement.

One day the cousin of a neighbor, who lived in a large city, came to greet Safiya. She had heard of Safiya's trouble and told her about a big hospital that might be able to help her. She said that if Safiya wanted to go, she would assist her in getting there. Alhaji Arziki gave his permission; he was rather glad to have Safiya go away for a while, and maybe, just maybe, she might be cured. So Safiya and her neighbor's cousin embarked on the journey, with only a few possessions and a little money.

The hospital was located on the outskirts of the city. Travel was difficult and took several days. It so happened that a charitable organization was giving money to the hospital to support fistula patients, so Safiya was admitted to the women's ward. The bed had no sheets, the floor was dirty and unwashed, the windows were small, and the ward was dark and overcrowded.

A few days later, Safiya was taken to the operating theater for an examination under anesthesia, which confirmed that she had a large vesico-vaginal fistula, but nothing else was done. None of the surgeons wanted to attempt the operation, and, in any case, the charity was paying a small amount of money every day for each fistula patient who was "under care." Safiya was now a cash cow: there was no incentive to actually do the surgery under these circumstances. The hospital was paid just because she was there. So, she languished, trapped in genito-urinary limbo, waiting, waiting. "Ha'kuri maganin duniya" (Patience is the world's medicine).

After four months of living on the hospital compound, Safiya was told she would have surgery from a visiting team of surgeons who came to the hospital once or twice a year. They would try to do as many operations as possible within two weeks, operating into the evening hours each day. Safiya happily waited her turn.

She was on the operating schedule for the last day of the surgical "camp." They took her to the operating room and injected her spine with anesthesia to numb her below the waist. Then they pulled her down to the end of the operating table and put her legs high up in stirrups. It felt funny; her legs were like lead. She could not move them at all, but it did not hurt. They covered her with sterile sheets. She had an intravenous infusion line in her left arm. The nurse talked to her during surgery.

The operation took a long, long time. When it was over, Safiya felt weak. One of the nurses told her she had lost a lot of blood. Her vagina was sore and she felt tremendous pressure. Safiya reached down. There was some kind of cloth packed into her vagina and a tube of some kind. She tugged on the tube and felt pressure in her bladder. There was urine in the tube and it was draining into a bucket on the floor—a catheter. She was told the catheter had to stay in place for two weeks so that her bladder would heal.

The next day the surgeons came by to see her. They took the vaginal packing out. Safiya felt better. Then the surgeons said goodbye. They were leaving and wished her well. They would be back in six months.

Over the next few days Safiya grew stronger and felt better. There was no leakage now—all of the urine drained into the catheter and out into the bucket on the floor. She was happy. Perhaps her problem was solved. The nurses paid less and less attention to her, especially now that the visiting surgeons had gone home.

On the third night after surgery, Safiya started to feel pain and pressure in her bladder. She had not felt this before. Something was wrong. The pressure got worse and worse. She sat up and looked over the side of the bed. The urine was no longer dripping out of the catheter, but there was blood in the urine in the bucket. She got out of bed and picked up the catheter and the bucket. It was dark. Other patients were sleeping. She could not find a nurse.

Then she slipped. The catheter and bucket fell out of her hands as she put them out in front of her to brace her fall. She fell flat on her belly. The pain was intense. There was urine everywhere. The bucket was tipped over. When she got up, she felt urine running out. She was leaking again.

The commotion aroused a sleeping nurse who grudgingly helped her back into bed. Safiya was sobbing. And wet.

Her catheter had become blocked and would not drain. Her bladder had filled with urine, stretching the line of sutures that had been used to bring the edges of the fistula together during the repair. Maybe the suture line was also infected. Maybe the sutures had been misplaced at the time of the repair. Maybe the scar tissue around the fistula had not been adequately dissected free so that it would not heal. Whatever the case, the repair had broken down. The fistula had reopened. She was back to square one.

A new catheter was finally inserted but even after three weeks of continuous bladder drainage, the injury did not heal. The fistula was open and leaked just as much urine as it had before her operation. Safiya was sent away from the hospital and told to return in six months.

Where to go? What to do?

She was now a long way from home. She was still wet. Her cowife was trouble: "Kishiya mai ban haushi." Her husband was unsympathetic. Her mother was dead. She had not seen her father for months and months. He didn't even know where she was.

Safiya drifted to the margins of society. She found a group of three women who also had fistulas living together on the edge of the city market. She joined them. They formed a small, desperate group of outcasts, doing what they could to hide their condition. They survived by begging, petty trading, doing odd jobs, whatever they could. Some of the more despairing women made money through sex acts. Life was precarious, difficult, and shameful, but Safiya continued to hope for deliverance someday.

Justice

Our basic sense of fairness—of justice—like compassion and respect, is also rooted in empathy. We all want to be treated fairly, and each of us knows the sting that comes from unfair treatment. This internal sense of basic justice and injustice is deeply rooted in our evolutionary past. There is substantial evidence that social species—such as chimpanzees, bonobos, and other primates—have an ingrained sense of fairness that helps regulate their behaviors with one another. Human societies have built upon this innate social instinct in constructing their moral codes.

In his celebrated book, A Theory of Justice, philosopher John Rawls attempted to determine the principles that would underlie a truly just society. Rawls defined "justice" simply as "fairness." He attempted to describe "a conception of justice that nullifies the accidents of natural endowment and the contingencies of social circumstances" to find a justice that would remove the inequalities of genetic heritage and social position. He distilled his theory of justice into two fundamental principles: (1) there should be "equality in the assignment of basic rights and duties"; and (2) "inequalities of wealth and authority are just only if they result in compensating benefits for everyone, and in particular for the least advantaged members of society."

But how could you reach agreement on these underlying principles? To answer this question Rawls developed an ingenious thought experiment utilizing what he called "the original position": the hypothetical beginnings of social organization when the rules had not yet been formulated. Rawls did not mean to suggest that this original position was an actual historical circumstance; rather, it was a way for him to examine the foundational principles of social organization through the lens of social contract theory. Let us imagine, Rawls hypothesized, how we could come up with these basic social rules in the society we were about to establish. What rules would we choose? For purposes of argument, Rawls presumed that everyone in these original circumstances was rational, equal to one other, and that they all had the same rights. In such circumstances, what rules would we choose to ensure society was fair to all? How could we devise rules of social regulation that would not give anyone an unfair advantage over others? Rawls suggested that the best way to do this would be to choose these fundamental principles of justice from behind "a veil of ignorance."

This veil of ignorance was a philosophical thought device Rawls explored to ensure that agreement could be reached on basic rules of fairness. It meant only that those who chose the foundational principles of social governance would not know what their own place would be in this society. The rule makers would not know their own social status or class position in the society that was about to emerge. They would not know their own physical characteristics, such as intelligence, sex, age, health, physical disabilities, or psychology; neither would they know anything about the specific nature of their society, such as its level of culture, its socioeconomic system, or its political standing in the world. They would know only "the general facts about human society," including, we may presume, the basic facts about human reproduction. Most importantly, those making these fundamental decisions about social organization behind the veil of ignorance would not know whether they would be male or female.

Rawls reasoned that, in these circumstances, none of the parties would have leverage with which to strike bargains with others. Since no one would know whether or not he or she would have some advantage over others, no one would want to choose principles of social organization that would put certain groups at a disadvantage from the beginning. If you did, you might end up being assigned to a disadvantageous group by chance. Rules chosen from behind the veil of ignorance would be fundamentally fair to all. There would be no built-in advantages or disadvantages. Everyone would start from an equal position. "The veil of ignorance," Rawls wrote, "makes possible a unanimous choice of a particular conception of justice."

It may seem a long reach from this Rawlsian worldview to the eradication of obstetric fistula, but a basic understanding of human biology makes clear that the physical burdens and medical risks of human reproduction fall entirely upon females. Women are humanity's childbearers. Women are the ones who risk death and disability from pregnancy, labor, and delivery. Women, not men, are at risk of developing obstructed labor during childbirth. It is women, not men, who will die or develop obstetric fistulas if their labors are obstructed. Maternal death statistics will never include men because pregnancy and childbirth are exclusively female activities. Given the facts of human biology, it follows from Rawls's "original position" argument that a just society in which no one knows whether he or she will be male or female, rich or poor, healthy or ill, will ensure that all pregnant women have high quality care in childbirth and ready access to comprehensive emergency obstetric services. The potential risks of "ending up female" would ensure that such medical services were available universally.

The choices imposed by the original position would also have to stipulate that all persons in society possess the right of personal autonomy. We all want the right to choose our destinies, insofar as this is possible. As embodied beings, we all want the right to determine what happens to our bodies. The right to control our bodily integrity includes the right to engage in consensual sexual relations as well as the right to refuse to do so. The right to control one's body includes the right to use contraception to prevent pregnancy and the right to permit the continuation of pregnancy should it occur—as well as the right to refuse to permit such continuation. Under these rules of basic fairness, the female body is not some "field" owned by a man, which he can "till" as he pleases. It is hers to control as a matter of fundamental personal and social justice. But should a woman consent to pregnancy, the basic principles of fairness adopted in the original position mandate that she receives effective antenatal care and skilled attendance at delivery, as well as access to emergency obstetric care, since the fact of her pregnancy puts her at risk for obstetric complications, which generally cannot usually be predicted in advance.

This is certainly true for obstructed labor. The best predictor of future reproductive performance is past obstetric history, but, even so, women who have delivered multiple times without difficulty can develop obstructed labor and a fistula in a subsequent pregnancy. Since all pregnant women are at risk of developing potentially catastrophic obstetric complications, no one, male or female, can be indifferent to this (particularly if they are determining the basic principles of social justice from behind a veil of ignorance).

From a practical point of view, providing comprehensive obstetric care to all women is straightforward and generally inexpensive (compared to other social costs). The technologies to overcome the most common causes of maternal death (hemorrhage, infection, hypertensive disorders of pregnancy, obstructed labor, and unsafe abortion) have been around for more than 75 years. It is clearly feasible to extend the lifesaving technologies that accomplished this in industrialized countries to all the women in the world, but only if the political will to do so exists.

This has yet to happen. Progress in solving these problems has been extraordinarily slow, largely because of the insidious combination of poverty and discrimination against women, both of which are pervasive among the bottom billion of the world's population. Many women are married against their will, become pregnant without their consent, carry their pregnancies without adequate medical evaluation, deliver under unsafe circumstances with insufficient social support in the hands of unskilled birth attendants, and either die from avoidable causes or become permanently injured by complications that could have been prevented with proper monitoring and timely intervention. Worse still, those women who do sustain a life-altering injury during childbirth (such as an obstetric fistula) frequently are unable to obtain curative surgery. This leads to unnecessary suffering, stigmatization, and marginalization from their families and society. Cases like Safiya's are not unusual.

In this respect, obstetric fistula is a neglected tropical disease (NTD). Traditionally, the neglected tropical diseases are a group of 13 parasitic infections with exotic names (ascariasis, dracunculiasis, hookworm infection, Chaga's disease, trypanosomiasis, Buruli ulcer, trachoma, schistosomiasis, trichuriasis, lymphatic filariasis, onchocerciasis, leishmaniasis, and leprosy) that are generally found only in the tropics. If these diseases are not treated, they cause disfigurement, severe disability, and stigmatization. Because these conditions affect the poor almost exclusively, there is no market to drive the commercial development of drugs to treat them. The World Health Organization and other groups have recently expanded the list of NTDs beyond the original 13 conditions, but the characteristics of the newly added diseases are similar: they are disfiguring, crippling, stigmatizing diseases of the poor that flourish among the bottom billion.

The term "neglected tropical diseases" is too narrow a term to encompass all of the pathologies that afflict this segment of the world's population. The very term "neglected tropical *diseases*" limits our view to *infectious* pathology, whereas in reality the suffering among the world's poor is very often due to noninfectious causes. Medical textbooks have shifted their focus to consider a broader range of disorders of form, function, and sensation rather than only derangements of tissues observable under the microscope. A better term that encompasses these other pathologies would be "neglected tropical *disorders*." This category would clearly include obstetric fistula, which is also a debilitating, stigmatizing medical condition more commonly found in conditions of tropical poverty. Like the other NTDs, fistula is directly linked to poverty, social instability, economic insecurity, and institutional mismanagement. This view returns our discussion to the concept of structural violence.

In chapter 5 structural violence was described as a concept used by social scientists to help explain the eccentric distribution of injuries and ill health in particular social groupings. In the words of James Gilligan, structural violence refers to "the increased rates of death and disability suffered by those who occupy the bottom rungs of society, as contrasted with the relatively lower death rates experienced by those who are above them. Those excess deaths (or at least a demonstrably large proportion of them) are a function of class structure; and that structure itself is a product of society's collective human choices, concerning how to distribute the collective wealth of society." Structural violence—the skewed patterns of illness and injury found particularly among the bottom segment of the population—is a manifestation of how healthcare resources are distributed in society. The distribution of healthcare resources reflects the values governing decisions about how to distribute those resources. How much should be spent, where should it be spent, and who should receive it?

Obstetric fistulas are a tangible manifestation of the unequal, unjust, and inadequate distribution of healthcare resources received by women generally (and childbearing women particularly) in poor countries. A healthcare system that is governed by values of compassion, respect, and justice will have extremely low numbers of obstetric fistulas. Prolonged obstructed labor will be rare because all pregnant women will have access to emergency obstetrical care when they need it. That women do not receive such care is a reflection of the values that have governed the distribution of healthcare resources in those countries. Poor men in poor countries have bad access to healthcare services; but for poor women in poor countries, their access is even worse, and the maladies to which they are subjected have no counterpart among males. There are no excuses for the persistence of these childbirth injuries.

The most effective technology for preventing obstetric fistula is usually Cesarean delivery, especially when it is carried out early. If Safiya's obstructed labor had been diagnosed early, she could have avoided a fistula and would have had a living child to raise. There are huge debates in the obstetrical literature about what is the "correct" rate of Cesarean section in any particular society, but the unquestionable fact remains that in those parts of the world where fistulas are most common, Cesarean section is not readily available, especially to the poor. In West Africa, for example, the observed rate of Cesarean delivery is about 1.3 percent, whereas the most conservative estimates of what would be needed to deal with life-threatening *maternal* conditions such as obstructed labor is at least 5.4 percent: a fourfold increase in Cesarean section is needed just to meet minimal maternal health needs, never mind those of the fetus. Conservative estimates from the World Health Organization in 1985 suggested optimal rates of Cesarean delivery around 15 percent, more than 10 times greater than those found in West Africa. Cesarean delivery is not expensive (certainly not compared to sports stadiums, military hardware, luxury cars, or presidential palaces), so why is it lacking for the women of the bottom billion? The poor generally (and poor women especially) do not have access to the levers of power in their societies. As a result, they remain vulnerable to life-changing injuries that could generally be avoided by the routine provision of competent medical care. Above all, they suffer from a lack of social justice.

Safiya's Story, Resumed

Safiya endured. She continued to believe that somewhere in this world, there was a place where her injuries could be treated. "Ikon Allah!" she thought. "If God so wills, I can find that place!" It was very difficult to live with her affliction, constantly trying to hide the leaking urine, relentlessly padding herself with old cloths every day, washing and drying, washing and drying. There were bigger, larger cities to the east: Kano, Katsina, Jos, even Maiduguri perhaps. She had never been to any of these places, but there had to be someone, somewhere, with the power and wisdom to help her. It took several months to acquire enough traveling money. Then once again she set out on her pilgrimage of hope.

She arrived in a large city where she heard of a clinic for women with *ciwon yoyo*, the "illness of dripping and leaking," which is what she knew she had, even if she didn't understand exactly why. Cautiously, she presented herself to the staff, who took her outside. They let her stay in the courtyard, where she had to scrounge for her own food as best she could. After a few days, she was brought inside for an examination. They told her she had a fistula. She still didn't really understand what this was or why it had happened to her. Only God knew. She only knew that she could not contain her urine and that life was miserable. They said they could help her.

The surgeon at the clinic was a tall, gruff, unsympathetic man. The patients whispered that he lacked *son mutane*, "humankindness." He treated the patients roughly, curtly. He didn't explain much. He spoke Hausa badly. To him the fistula women were only work objects, things to cut on, interesting cases. The government paid him good money. He cured some of the patients, and when this happened they were thrilled. Those who had bad outcomes he kept in the courtyard, where they waited their turn until he decided to have another try. Some stayed for many months. Where else could they go?

Safiya's surgery was scheduled. She asked whether she would get a "needle," an *allura*, a shot in the back to prevent pain, like she had at her first operation. No, she was told. You don't need that. It takes too much time and effort. All you need is patience. Be strong. Don't complain. Do as you are told. As a properly modest Hausa woman, she did as she was told.

It was not easy to have surgery without the needle in the back. It hurt. She had trouble keeping her legs apart, even after they were strapped into the stirrups and pulled aside. She cried out several times when the surgeon was rough while cutting or pulling. He spoke crossly to her, but she didn't understand what he said. It took a long time.

The pain and suffering of her second fistula repair operation would have been worth it all had it succeeded, but it didn't. Three days after her operation, the leaking started again. The surgeon was angry with her. The nurses wanted to know what she had done to make the operation fail. Safiya didn't know. She hadn't done anything, anything at all. Why would she do anything, she who had so much to gain or lose from the operation?

They sent her back to the courtyard to wait. Maybe in six months she could have another operation. Safiya was miserable. She sat under a thorny acacia tree in the rust-red dust of the courtyard, staring into the distance, wondering why this had happened to her.

Structural Violence and the Vulnerabilities of Poor Women

The root of the English word "vulnerable" is the Latin *vulnerabilis*, which means "wounding." To be vulnerable means to be susceptible to being wounded, and one's vulnerabilities are the special circumstances that increase such susceptibilities. Kenneth Kipnis has written thoughtfully about the kinds of vulnerabilities that patients face, especially those who are recruited to participate in medical research projects. There are many varieties of vulnerability, but in almost all societies vulnerabilities are heavily concentrated among the poor. Among the poor vulnerabilities are linked to one another, and their effects are synergistic, not merely additive. Together these vulnerabilities create a web from whose strands it is difficult to escape. This web of vulnerability is especially burdensome for poor women, who are the ones most likely to be wounded by obstructed labor and to develop an obstetric fistula thereafter. How would a healthcare system founded upon compassion, respect, and justice protect poor women who are the most likely to be injured because of their multiple vulnerabilities?

Kipnis has articulated seven categories of vulnerability: economic and allocational vulnerability, cognitive vulnerability, juridical vulnerability, the vulnerability of deference, social vulnerability, medical vulnerability, and infrastructural vulnerability. Consider how, in each case, Safiya was affected by these vulnerabilities. For her, each vulnerability compounded the next one. Cumulatively, they are overwhelming.

1. *Economic and allocational vulnerability*—Is the patient seriously lacking in important economic resources and social goods?

Where fistulas are common, access to Cesarean delivery is highly variable. The poor (who are those who will develop a fistula) have much less access to Cesarean section than do wealthier women. This occurs because the countries where fistulas are prevalent have not invested the time, money, and other resources needed to provide emergency obstetric care to the poor. Emergency obstetrical services tend to be concentrated in cities and to be accessible disproportionately by the wealthy. This is demonstrated graphically in figure 9.1, which shows the distribution of caesarean sections in 14 poor countries, each of which has a national Cesarean delivery rate of less than 2 percent. In each case, the poorest 20 percent of women have the least access to Cesarean section, and the wealthiest 20 percent have the greatest access, with increasing availability according to wealth for the middle 60 percent of the population. The same pattern is seen in countries with slightly better rates of access having Cesarean delivery rates between 2 percent and 4.9 percent (figure 9.2).

These differences also hold for urban/rural distinctions around the world. Urban areas have both higher concentrations of wealth and higher concentrations of healthcare facilities. This means that urban populations generally (and wealthy elites particularly) have better access to Cesarean section than do their rural counterparts. But, even in rural areas, it is the comparatively wealthy who have greater access to lifesaving surgical skills (figure 9.3).

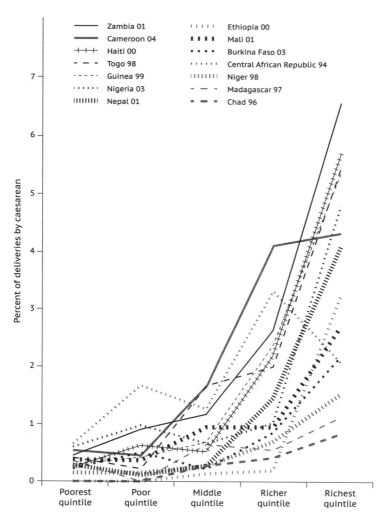

FIGURE 9.1. Cesarean section rates by wealth quintile in 14 countries with national Cesarean section rates of less than 2 percent. Notice how Cesarean section is most available to the wealthy. The numbers after the country names refer to the year in which data were collected. *Redrawn from C. Ronsmans, S. Holtz, and C. Stanton, "Socioeconomic Differentials in Caesarean Rates in developing Countries: A Retrospective Analysis,"* Lancet 368 (2006): 1518.

These differences in access to lifesaving emergency obstetric surgery are partially a matter of the geographic distribution of resources, but mainly they are a matter of poverty. It is almost impossible to overstate how devastating poverty is to women in obstructed labor who need Cesarean delivery. The same applies to poor women who

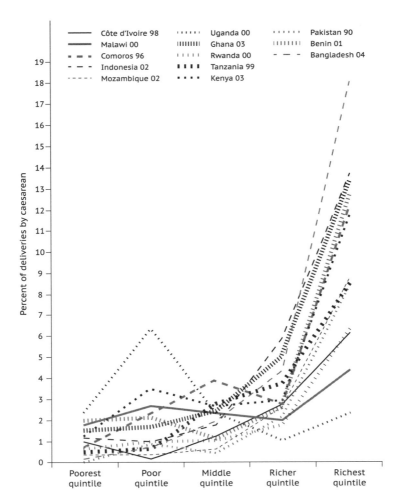

FIGURE 9.2. Caesarean section rates by wealth quintile in 13 countries with national cesarean section rates of between 2.0 percent and 4.9 percent. Notice how Cesarean section is most available to the wealthy. The numbers after the country names refer to the year in which data were collected. *Redrawn from C. Ronsmans, S. Holtz, and C. Stanton, "Socioeconomic Differentials in Caesarean Rates in developing Countries: A Retrospective Analysis," Lancet 368 (2006): 1519.*

already have an obstetric fistula and who are seeking surgical cure, the Safiyas of the world. User fees imposed to help recoup the cost of funding healthcare services is a huge barrier to the poor—especially under emergency conditions—but even if obstetric care (including Cesarean delivery) is ostensibly free, such "free" care is often overwhelmed by the hidden costs imposed on such patients in the form of travel expenses,

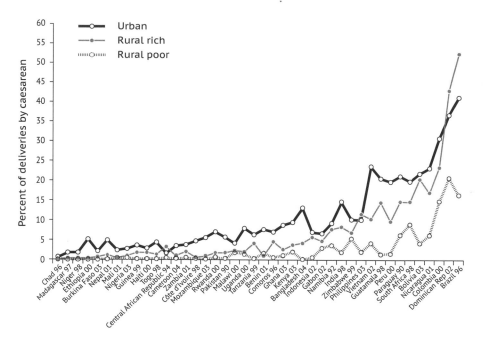

FIGURE 9.3. Cesarean section rates among urban, rural rich, and rural poor women from 42 countries. Notice how Cesarean section is most available to the wealthy. *Redrawn from C. Ronsmans, S. Holtz, and C. Stanton, "Socioeconomic Differentials in Caesarean Rates in developing Countries: A Retrospective Analysis,"* Lancet *368 (2006): 1522.*

admission fees, bribes, extortion, the costs of medications and surgical supplies, payment for food and laundry services, and other things. These uncovered expenses are often economically devastating to the poor. Indeed, fear of exploitation by health services workers is a major impediment to the prompt search for care. To have borne such costs only to receive substandard medical care and abusive personal treatment is simply intolerable.

To Western eyes, payment of $32 for a vaginal delivery or $118 for a Cesarean section seems trivial compared to the costs we associate with such services; however, for a Bangladeshi family with an average monthly income of less than $125, these expenditures are calamitous. A complicated Cesarean delivery for neglected obstructed labor followed by a postoperative wound infection and anemia requiring transfusion (none of which are unusual in such circumstances) turns a life-threatening medical condition into a financial catastrophe as well. One study on the hidden costs of "free" maternity care in Bangladesh found that 21 percent of families had to spend between half and all of their monthly income on obstetric costs after delivery, and that more than 25 percent of families had to spend up to eight times their monthly income covering healthcare costs. In such circumstances families must sell assets, abandon schooling, borrow cash from relatives or unscrupulous businessmen, and avoid other expenditures, the total effect of which is to plunge them deeper into poverty, from which they will never escape. No wonder they are reluctant to seek hospital care, even in emergencies. For some, death might be preferable to the economic destruction of their families.

Similar challenges face the woman who has an obstetric fistula. Rarely can she afford to pay the costs of treatment, and the lack of access to competent, caring fistula repair services means that many such women become trapped in an endless cycle of waiting, looking, hoping, and traveling from one hospital to another in search of relief. This takes an enormous toll on her family life and her finances, and is one of the major reasons that fistula victims become divorced or are largely abandoned by their husbands. Safiya's case, although a construction, is representative of the experiences of many of these women.

2. *Cognitive vulnerability*—Does the patient have the capacity to deliberate about and decide whether to receive the proposed care?

Cognitive vulnerability overlaps with several other categories described below, but in the first instance it refers to the question of whether the woman is capable of consenting to surgery. This is different for the patient currently suffering in obstructed labor than it is for the patient with an established fistula. In the first case she may be delirious with fever, unconscious from exhaustion or blood loss, and simply incapable of giving consent or participating in any deliberations because of her physical condition. But, beyond this, in many parts of Africa, the inability of a woman to deliver vaginally (irrespective of the cause) is equated with being a failure as a woman. Such cultural presuppositions of what is "proper" for a birthing woman to do may interfere with the ability to make a sound decision based on obstetric circumstances. Additionally, having adequate cognitive capacity to make a decision to undergo lifesaving Cesarean delivery means having someone explain clearly in the patient's native language the nature of her obstetric situation, why she is in that situation, and what must be done about it. This means that compassion, respect, and fairness must all be present—and often they are not. When patients become mere work objects, they are not respected, are not treated fairly, and are robbed of the compassion they deserve. Work objects become things that are disregarded, "looked beyond," disrespected. Full explanations and taking the time to make sure the patient understands are often neglected in these circumstances.

A woman who already has a fistula needs to have someone explain to her clearly, in her own language, what a fistula is, how it came about, and what the proposed surgical treatment involves. Patients must be given a fair understanding of the nature of the operation to be undertaken, what the likelihood is of success, and what complications might occur. Unfortunately, many patients at fistula centers are never told these things because they are seen as work objects for the surgeon, rather than beings to be respected in their own right. It is very useful to have fistula patients who have already undergone surgery explain the surgical process to newcomers. Understanding the risks and benefits is not only fair to the patient, but improved knowledge of her condition and an accurate understanding of what may occur afterward leads to improved patient satisfaction and better clinical outcomes.

3. *Juridical vulnerability*—Is the patient subject to the legal or social authority of others who may have an independent interest in her care?

In every country where fistulas are common, females are juridically vulnerable. As women, they have limited legal, moral, and social autonomy. Their reproductive capacity is viewed as something owned by males. Among the Hausa and other social groups, women cannot travel freely by themselves; they are expected to be under the control of a socially appropriate male: husband, father, brother. Such legal and social restrictions greatly hamper access to emergency obstetric care and to curative clinical services when injuries have occurred.

4. *The vulnerability of deference*—Are there patterns of deferential behavior present that may hide an unwillingness to participate or comply?

Almost everywhere the poor are intimidated in the presence of authority, be it social, political, legal, religious, or economic authority. Lacking power, lacking education, lacking wealth, lacking standing, the poor have learned that deference is usually (in most circumstances) less risky than active engagement. A poor, uneducated woman facing a difficult clinical situation—prolonged labor or an obstetric fistula, for example—may not express her worries or concerns, particularly if she must confront a powerful educated authority figure in doing so. Imagine an illiterate woman from a remote rural area trying to navigate a hospital bureaucracy where everyone in a position of power or authority is of a different ethnicity, educated, gowned with institutional status, and of unsympathetic demeanor. Her concerns are unlikely to be voiced, and therefore to be heard or addressed. Most likely her concerns will remain unmet. *Kunya*, the culturally sanctioned Hausa idea of deferential female modesty and submission is an ideal example of how this deference compounds women's vulnerability.

5. *Social vulnerability*—Does the patient belong to a socially undervalued group?

By being poor, a woman already belongs to a socially undervalued group in many societies, but this disvalue can be increased exponentially by rural residence, by ethnicity, by membership in a religious minority, by lack of appropriate marital status, by lack of education, or by her clinical circumstances. Fistula patients in particular are often disvalued—both by themselves (having a deep sense of personal shame at their condition) and by society at large, which fails to understand the mechanism by which their injuries have occurred, often misattributing them to transgression on the part of the afflicted woman rather than to faulty obstetrical mechanics. If hygiene is a problem (as it often is), a physical unattractiveness further worsens the woman's plight.

6. *Medical vulnerability*—Does the patient have a serious medical condition for which there are no satisfactory remedies?

Obstructed labor has a satisfactory remedy: Cesarean section, but for that remedy to produce a satisfactory outcome, it must be delivered as soon as the diagnosis is made. Once a fistula has developed, the available remedies are less satisfactory. If the injury involves extensive tissue destruction, surgical repair of the fistula may not even be possible, but there is no way to know this until the patient has been examined by a competent fistula surgeon. In most countries where fistulas are prevalent there is a shortage of surgeons qualified to undertake fistula repair (especially for complex or difficult cases), yet because the condition of the afflicted women is so miserable—the unremitting stream of urine or feces producing a daily struggle to maintain basic cleanliness and an even more difficult struggle to maintain their human dignity—fistula patients are often desperate for relief, making them potential prey for those who promise care that they cannot deliver but who profit nonetheless from the financial support they receive from the government or outside agencies. In many instances fistula patients are simply "warehoused" by these organizations, using these women to raise money while they wait—sometimes for years—for help that never arrives. Exploitation of this kind is intolerable.

7. *Infrastructural vulnerability*—Are the necessary resources available to provide the care that is needed? Considering the total context (political, economic, social, and organizational) does the institution have the integrity and stability to provide an acceptable level of care?

This is the real heart of the matter. When all is said and done, the bottom-line question is whether medical institutions can deliver appropriate care in an acceptable manner. By definition, the women of the bottom billion live in a world of social and infrastructural vulnerability. The poor are generally the last to receive needed social and medical resources because they are remote from those who make the decisions about how such resources are allocated. Being remote from the levers of power, they have little influence by which they can improve their lives. The institutions that serve the poor (if they exist at all) in countries where fistulas are prevalent are typically hamstrung by inadequate physical facilities, by insufficient numbers of staff (who are often poorly trained and even more poorly motivated), by inadequate and inconsistent supply chains, and by lack of effective administrative supervision and organizational support. It is the lack of dependable, effective medical infrastructure that creates the fistula problem in the first place, and the same lack of infrastructure also makes the care of birth-injured women so difficult thereafter.

A healthcare system that operated according to principles of compassion, respect, and justice would ensure that all women receive a "fair deal" with respect to their pregnancies: safe and effective obstetric care, tailored to their specific needs, provided by competent personnel, and in a timely, respectful, and affordable manner. Chapter 8 discussed this as the problem of overcoming the third delay in the receipt of emergency obstetric care. Timely, respectful, competent, and affordable care for women in obstructed labor is a matter of making healthcare institutions in poor countries functional and accountable.

Obstructed labor is a life-threatening condition. If timely care is not received, the outcome can be fatal for the pregnant woman, as it often is for her fetus. If she survives her ordeal only to develop a fistula, a woman is unlikely to die immediately, but the life she lives thereafter is difficult and often worsens over time. Most hospitals at the first referral level in the world's poor countries do not offer fistula repair services. Even hospitals that provide comprehensive emergency obstetric care generally do not perform obstetric fistula surgery, and even if they do, often they do not perform it well. Fistula operations are frequently challenging, requiring meticulous attention to detail both during surgery and afterward. Belonging overwhelmingly to the bottom billion as they do, patients with fistulas cannot afford to pay much—if anything—for surgery. Because the operations require considerable skill, because the condition is stigmatizing and the patients are poor, because the nursing demands are significant, and because the rate of operative failure in inexperienced hands is high, few institutions want to care for these women. They are seen as a burden, not as an asset. As the story of Safiya demonstrates, the quest for cure often becomes an all-consuming task for a woman with a fistula, involving far-ranging travel, prolonged time away from home and family, increasing financial and marital strain, and protracted personal suffering. Under such conditions, how can these women get a just deal?

The argument has already been made that under reasonable first principles of justice, all women should have access to timely, competent obstetric care. Simply from the fact of their being female, women's lives and health are at risk by the biology of human reproduction. Because the treatment of most causes of maternal mortality and childbirth injury are now well understood and (theoretically) easy and inexpensive to provide, universal access to comprehensive emergency obstetric care is a woman's right, a basic human right. The same argument can be made with respect to women with an obstetric fistula. Because effective treatments are available and because the cost of care is low in terms of the long-term disability that is avoided, proper care for obstetric fistulas is also a woman's right, a basic human right. Simply because a woman is poor and female, she should not have to endure such misery.

A just deal for women suffering with an obstetric fistula means providing compassionate, respectful, care in a fair manner. A just deal for women with fistula is grounded in the recognition of their basic human rights. A just deal for these women can be summarized, succinctly, as a Bill of Rights for women who have an obstetric fistula.

A Bill of Rights for the Obstetric Fistula Patient

- Every woman with an obstetric fistula has the right to be treated with compassion, dignity, and respect, irrespective of her socioeconomic status.

- Every woman with an obstetric fistula has a right to privacy. She has the right to refuse to be interviewed, photographed, or displayed in any fashion without her express consent. Receiving care at any institution where patients with fistulas are treated should not be contingent on interviews, photographs, or displays that are not relevant to a woman's immediate clinical care.
- Every woman with an obstetric fistula has the right to have the nature of her condition—its causes, prognosis, and possible treatments—explained to her fully and completely in a language she can understand. She has the right to ask questions about these subjects and to participate actively in deliberations about her care.
- Every woman with an obstetric fistula has the right to food, clothing, and shelter sufficient to sustain her basic needs while receiving care for her condition.
- Every woman with an obstetric fistula has the right to self-determination. She has the right to be free from coercion, proselytizing, or exposure to any form of undue influence when making decisions about how, when, where, or whether she is to undergo treatment.
- Every woman with an obstetric fistula has the right to refuse treatment, to refuse to participate in research studies, and to leave an obstetric fistula treatment center whenever she chooses to do so, without penalty or retribution.
- Every woman with an obstetric fistula has the right to receive competent care from qualified doctors, nurses, social workers, and therapists during the course of her treatment. The receipt of competent care is an integral part of a just deal. The obligations to avoid harming patients (non-maleficence) and to serve their best interests (beneficence) are fundamental ethical obligations of doctors and nurses.

Because fistula treatment services are often funded largely from external donations in the countries where these injuries are prevalent, external funders have an obligation to ensure that these rights are respected at the institutions they support. Regular human rights reviews and the presence of an on-site ombudsman to deal with complaints of unjust treatment should be part of such external aid packages.

A Code of Ethics for the Fistula Surgeon

If a bill of rights encapsulates the basic expectations that a fistula patient should have when she is evaluated and then treated, its mirror image is a code of ethics for the fistula surgeon. The fistula patient should be an active participant in her care. She should provide accurate information about her medical history and should consent to treatment only after thorough counseling and thoughtful consideration of the issues involved. She should ask questions when she does not understand what is happening or what is required of her, and she should comply with the medical instructions she is given to maximize the chances of a good outcome after surgery. Fistula surgeons have substantial obligations to the patients who have entrusted themselves to their care. Surgeons must respect the basic rights of these birth-injured women while striving always to create a favorable environment in which the delivery of excellent clinical care can flourish.

Dr. Reginald Hamlin, who along with his wife, Dr. Catherine Hamlin, founded the Addis Ababa Fistula Hospital more than 40 years ago, used to speak of the problems posed by "fistula tourism." This was the term he coined to describe the phenomenon of surgeons from affluent countries dropping in to resource-poor parts of the world to try their hands at fistula repair and then buzzing off back home again afterward. Because fistulas from obstructed labor are almost unknown in advanced industrialized societies due to the smooth functioning of their obstetrical services, obstetric fistulas became an exotic medical curiosity. For some, doing a fistula repair in a poor country became a "trophy" they could brag about to their surgical friends back home.

It doesn't take deep thought to uncover the potential problems associated with this. Unlike the vesico-vaginal fistulas that sometimes occur after a hysterectomy (which are the result of a discrete injury to otherwise normal tissues during a surgical procedure), the obstetric fistula is a "field injury" involving widespread tissue necrosis as the result of prolonged impacted labor. This often involves extensive tissue loss and substantial scarring in patients who may already be malnourished and suffering from medical comorbidities seldom seen in Europe or the United States. The surgical challenges presented by such patients are unique, and the conditions under which their injuries must be repaired are often challenging to those accustomed to the comparative luxuries of Western surgical practice. When entering difficult clinical environments to provide surgical care, surgeons must always be cognizant of the practical and ethical challenges presented by such cases. They must strive to make sure the patient receives a just deal, remembering that the normal rules of medical ethics still apply, even in remote tropical locations. A Code of Ethics for the Fistula Surgeon summarizes the basic ethical obligations involved in the care of these women. Both the visiting surgeon and the local practitioner must always put the best interests of their patients ahead of all other considerations, remembering to treat patients with compassion and respect, to provide benefit, to avoid harm, and to treat them fairly while providing competent care.

- The fistula surgeon shall be dedicated above all else to providing the best possible care permitted by the resources available and the local circumstances in which care is rendered. The welfare of the obstetric fistula patient must be the overriding concern in all medical judgments made during her care, and the fistula surgeon shall not participate in any activity that is not in her best interests. Lack of resources is never a justification for the abandonment of basic ethical principles in patient care.

- The surgeon must treat all fistula patients with respect, dignity, compassion, and honesty, safeguarding their confidentiality while recognizing that they are uniquely vulnerable to exploitation due to the circumstances in which their injuries have arisen. The ethical fistula surgeon recognizes the right of fistula sufferers to participate in decisions regarding their treatment and will not engage in any treatment or research upon them without their consent. The fistula surgeon will further strive to support decision-making processes that are free from bias or coercion.

- The highest duty of surgeons is acceptance of direct personal responsibility for the care of patients on whom they have operated. Once fistula surgeons have accepted a patient for care, she must not be neglected. Fistula surgeons must ensure that all patients under their care receive an appropriate preoperative evaluation, undergo competent treatment, and have access to adequate, ongoing postoperative care, particularly in the critical period immediately following surgery. The pre- and postoperative care of fistula patients is the surgeon's direct responsibility, unless such duties are specifically delegated to another competent practitioner who can provide the same level of care as the operating surgeon, including repeat operation should it prove necessary.

- Fistula surgeons must restrict their practice to that which they are competent to deliver by education, training, experience, and available resources. Fistula surgeons should not hesitate to refer patients needing a higher level of care than they can provide to surgeons and healthcare facilities with appropriate advanced expertise. Fistula surgeons should strive to provide adequate and effective training for other less experienced surgeons who are committed to learning the art of fistula repair and practicing among these vulnerable patients, and they should inculcate in these trainees a respect for and a commitment to the high ethical ideals enshrined in this code.

- Fistula surgeons must practice a method of healing founded on science and should strive to improve their clinical skills through the regular review of objective data on treatment outcomes. This process is enhanced when surgical objectives and outcome criteria are explicitly defined in advance and data are collected prospectively. The fistula surgeon should strive to engage in regular critical self-scrutiny. When surgical innovation departs in a significant way from the standard of accepted practice, such innovation should be evaluated at an early stage through a formal well-constructed research protocol to determine its risks and benefits. All such research should be approved and supervised by an appropriate ethical board. Where such boards do not exist, it is imperative that mechanisms to ensure critical oversight of innovation are put into place. Not only should surgeons engage in critical self-scrutiny themselves, but they must also be open to objective external scrutiny from the wider community of fistula surgeons in the true spirit of scientific inquiry. Fistula surgeons should advocate, promote, maintain, and uphold the highest ethical standards for the care of women with obstetric fistulas, wherever this condition exists in the world.

- Fistula surgeons must never take advantage of a patient, nor allow anyone else to take advantage of a patient in any way that might subject her to physical, emotional, economic, or sexual abuse.

- Fistula surgeons must neither pay nor receive a commission for the referral of patients. They must exercise good stewardship over the financial resources entrusted to them for the care of women with obstetric fistulas and should not involve themselves in fistula-related endeavors for the purpose of personal financial gain.

- Fistula surgeons must uphold the dignity and honor of their profession, safeguarding both themselves and the public against surgeons deficient in moral character or professional competence; surgeons should also obey the laws of the country in which they practice. Fistula surgeons should respect and cooperate with other surgeons, physicians, nurses, and healthcare workers, always safeguarding the best interests of patients in so doing. Behavior that diminishes a fistula surgeon's capability to practice must be avoided. If such behavior occurs, it must be addressed immediately, and prompt remedial action must be undertaken. Fistula surgeons should not practice while impaired by alcohol or drugs, or by other physical or mental disabilities.

- Fistula surgeons must acknowledge the fundamental social inequalities that promote the development of obstetric fistulas and must help eradicate these injustices. Fistula surgeons should actively support programs that seek to prevent fistulas. Fistula surgeons should work to remove barriers that hinder access to emergency obstetric care. Fistula surgeons should strive to ensure that all women afflicted with fistulas receive adequate and appropriate care regardless of their age, marital status, ethnicity, race, cultural traditions, religion, political affiliation, economic status, level of education, concurrent disease, or other disabilities. Fistula surgeons should support programs that help women who currently suffer from or who have been afflicted with this condition in the past reintegrate successfully into their societies. Fistula surgeons' social responsibility should extend to the prevention of recurrent fistulas in women who have been cured of their injuries by promoting access to effective prenatal and intrapartum care should they become pregnant in the future.

Under what circumstances will fistula patients receive the best care? Where will fistula patients have their rights respected while receiving care from surgeons who strive to live up to their ethical obligations? The complex nature of their injuries, the technical surgical difficulties commonly associated with repair, and the complicated social, economic, and psychological ramifications of their life circumstances all argue that the care of obstetric fistula patients should be concentrated in centers that spe-

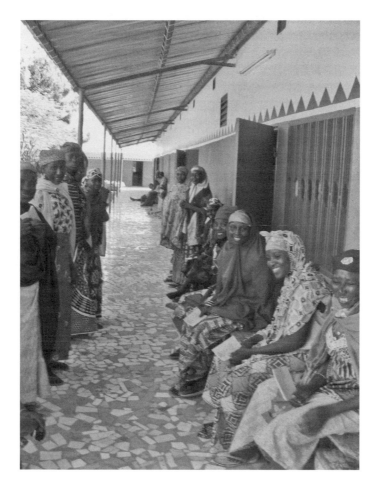

FIGURE 9.4. Women with obstetric fistulas waiting to be seen at the Danja Fistula Center in Niger. *Photo by the author.*

cialize in such cases, rather than scattered throughout the surgical wards of general hospitals. When the mission of an institution is focused specifically on the needs of these women, it is much more likely that they will be treated with compassion, respect, and justice.

Safiya's Story Concluded

Random pieces of information, observations, opinions, and rumors circulate haphazardly and unpredictably in all societies. This grapevine of unofficial communication exists to greater or lesser degrees among all social groups, and fistula patients are no exception. As Safiya sat in the courtyard, hungry, depressed, sorrowful, and wet, she started to hear about a place called Danja. It was said that Danja was a place where fistulas were fixed. A few women had left the center where Safiya was living and had actually been to Danja. They told her that they had been treated with respect there. Danja was full of *son mutane*, humankindness. Many patients were actually cured. The whole experience was different. That was why they had come back to tell others. The recommendations were good. Safiya resolved to go.

Danja lay to the north. In fact, it turned out that Danja was not even in Nigeria—it was over the border in Niger, a country that had been colonized by the French, not the British as had been the case in Nigeria. But the border was porous and there was a good all-weather road leading out of Katsina. Once she saved enough money for travel, Safiya managed to take public transport across the border. She was nervous about being so far away, but everybody spoke Hausa just like she did. She blended in.

The Danja Fistula Center lies along the road between Katsina and Maradi. It sits on the campus of the Centre de Santé et de Leprologie, a leprosy hospital (the only one in Niger) established by Christian missionaries in the 1950s. This "Christian business" bothered Safiya a bit. She didn't know any Christians. She was Muslim, but nobody in Danja objected. There seemed to be plenty of Muslims around. She asked several people for help after she arrived, and they took her to the clinic in a new hospital building. The staff told her the clinic was not open today, but they did not turn her away or deposit her in the courtyard to wait. Rather, they took her across an open field to a hostel, where she met dozens of women who also had fistulas. It was a whole village of fistula women, dozens and dozens of them, with their own huts and everything. She was given a mat and a place to sleep. She was shown where to wash (there was water, running water!) and where the latrines were. Best of all, she was greeted warmly by the matron of the fistula village and was given food. That night, the hunger went away.

Two days later Safiya was taken to the clinic for an examination. The doctor was kind and rather quiet. He smiled at her when he spoke. Eventually, she smiled back at him, too. He spoke Hausa and explained to her what had happened during her labor. He was gentle when he examined her and explained what he was doing as he did it. They put a catheter in her bladder and filled it with blue water. It ran out through the fistula so that he could see where all the leakage came from. He explained that her fistula was still rather large, that there was a lot of scar tissue from her obstructed labor, and that she had had two failed operations, but he was hopeful that something could be done. If she wished, they could do the operation next week. Safiya's heart leaped in her chest.

The day before surgery, Safiya was taken up to the ward. It was a big, light airy room. The beds were lined up neatly. They all had sheets! The floor was clean (it was mopped several times each day). The nurses helped her wash thoroughly and clean herself up. The beds all had absorbent pads on them with a waterproof backing. Everything was carefully explained to her.

The next morning they started an intravenous line in her arm and took her to the operating theater. The anesthetist was very nice. He was from Danja village. His family had worked at the hospital for years and years. He smiled and joked and made her feel at ease. The surgeon came and greeted her and reviewed her hospital notes. The anesthetist gave her an injection in her back. Soon her legs were numb and heavy. They put her in the stirrups, washed her genitals with iodine, and put the sterile drapes on her. She could hear what was going on, but couldn't see what was happening. She did not feel any pain.

The operation took several hours. When it was over, the surgeon came up and took her hand. He smiled at her. "Mun gama da aiki," he said to her in Hausa. "Our work is done." She smiled back.

They took her to the ward and put her in bed. Her catheter was carefully adjusted. She was told to notify the nurses immediately if it ever stopped draining. There was blood in the catheter at first, but it soon cleared up. In a few hours the feeling came back into her legs. She sat up. She was a little sore. She felt the vaginal packing up inside her.

The next day the surgeon came to see her. He asked her how she felt. He asked her whether she had any leakage. She said no. He took the packing out and looked at her catheter. It was draining nicely. "Yau da gobe za ki warke," he said. "You'll get better day by day. The catheter must stay in for a few days more." He saw her every day and spoke kindly to her each time.

On the tenth day after surgery, he took the catheter out. Safiya was nervous. The nurses gave her water to drink. In a couple of hours, her bladder felt full. She told the nurses. She was very nervous now, but there was no leakage.

The nurses said, "Go pee."

Go pee! What wonderful words! Safiya hadn't peed in nearly three years! All of her urine had been leaking out through the fistula, continuously, day and night, with every motion, every time she moved, 24 hours a day, every day of the week. Her bladder never filled, so she never had to pee; she couldn't pee even if she had wanted to. Go pee indeed!

Safiya went to the latrine, hitched up the body cloth that covered her lower half and squatted over the hole in the tiled floor. Did she even remember how to pee? What was going to happen? And then, at first slowly and then more forcefully, it started. A stream of urine came out—not through her vagina like it had for months and months, dripping and dribbling down her legs and onto the floor—but urine shooting out through her urethra straight into the hole in the floor of the latrine where it splashed and spattered and actually made noise! She could pee again! She stood up and felt herself. No more urine came out.

She stepped out of the latrine and said to herself, "I can pee! I can actually pee!"

A grin burst forth from her face as she ran into the ward. She opened the door and shouted "I can pee!" She laughed as the rest of the patients on the ward clapped, cheered, and began the celebratory ululations that mark the presence of joy in Hausa festivities. Safiya could pee again.

The nurses had her lie down in the bed. They wheeled a small ultrasound machine over to the bedside. They squirted some cold gel onto her abdomen behind her pubic bone and placed the transducer there. They pressed a button. The machine whirred and clicked. The nurses looked at the screen and said, "You have emptied your bladder! Congratulations!"

For the next three days Safiya exulted in her urinary physiology. She went to the latrine every two hours and grinned each time the urine came out. She was no longer leaking. And she could pee!

Every week or so a "graduation ceremony" was held on the ward for the patients who were leaving after their fistulas were repaired. The nurses brought in new dresses for each patient who was going home to help mark the start of her new life. Drums appeared on the ward. The surgeon with the quiet smile came by to say hello. The patients danced in their new dresses and the surgeon danced with them.

Safiya. "Dawn." The start of a new day, a new beginning, a new life.

The Danja Fistula Center in Niger

I know the Danja Fistula Center well, because my wife, Helen, and I worked hard for many years helping to create it and fund it. We were supported in this project by family and friends, collaborating with many generous donors and many wonderful, dedicated people from all over the world who shared a vision of what could be done for the victims of obstructed labor in West Africa. The Danja Fistula Center was built in Niger by the Worldwide Fistula Fund, a not-for-profit US charity based in Chicago, Illinois. The center was built and operates in collaboration with SIM (Serving in Mission), a Christian missionary organization that has carried out charitable and educational work across Niger since 1924. The Danja Fistula Center is a specialist hospital, dedicated to meeting the medical, surgical, mental, social, spiritual, and rehabilitative needs of women with obstetric fistulas and other childbirth injuries. Services are provided free of charge to patients, irrespective of their ethnicity, religion, or socioeconomic status. All are welcome, and many Safiyas arrive each week.

The Danja Fistula Center is rooted in the values of compassion, respect, and justice. These roots are long and deep. They stretch nearly 3,000 miles to Addis Ababa, Ethiopia, where a remarkable couple named Reginald and Catherine Hamlin first encountered the fistula problem more than 50 years ago and felt compelled to make it their life's work. The Danja Fistula Center is an attempt to replicate their vision in another part of the world. The utterly compelling story of how that vision developed and finally was realized is the subject of the next chapter.

CHAPTER 10

The Vision of Hamlin Fistula

Helen and I descended the steps behind the fistula ward onto the lawn in the center of a stunning tropical garden, bursting with white and lavender petals, the blooms of red and orange flowers, and dense green foliage backlit by a clear blue Ethiopian sky. Turning left, we descended the hillside along a sidewalk that undulated through the greenery until we reached the wrought-iron fence halfway down the slope. Unlatching the gate, we worked our way down the steep stone staircase through another magnificent garden until we reached the modest mud-brick house with the sheet-metal roof at the bottom of the hill. We were greeted by Birru, Catherine's handyman and gardener for more than 50 years, who waved us onto the veranda where we knocked on the door. It opened and there was Catherine Hamlin, bright and lively, a cane for balance in one hand, the other extended in greeting. After smiles and hugs, she ushered us into the sitting room, where tea was prepared and waiting, old friends greeted with unwavering hospitality.

The little house is modestly furnished. It is typical of a 1950s home in Britain or Australia, perfectly reflective of the era in which Catherine and her late husband, Reg, arrived in Ethiopia. They were both obstetrician-gynecologists who came to serve the people of Ethiopia. They planned initially to stay only a few years, but they never left; rather, they invested their lives in caring for the women of this fascinating country in northeastern Africa.

We chatted about her health, the weather, family and friends, fundraising, and the challenges associated with charitable work. Mamitu Gashe smiled at us as she carried in the cookies, lemon cake, sugar, and milk. Gazing out the front window, we could see the edge of the river running by the bottom of the hill, flattening out into a small lake, the hillside covered with flocks of sacred ibis resting in the afternoon sun.

Catherine and Reginald Hamlin Come to Ethiopia

The Addis Ababa Fistula Hospital is a tranquil oasis set on a steep hillside in the middle of the chaos that is Addis Ababa, the capital city of Ethiopia. The hospital represents the life's work and continuing legacy of a remarkable couple, the Drs. Hamlin, Catherine and Reg, and their quest to heal the wounds (both physical and spiritual) of poor women with childbirth injuries. It is the oldest, largest and most successful fistula hospital in the world, and it has made a tremendous impact on this ancient country. As Richard Hamlin remarked on the occasion of his mother's ninetieth birthday, "Catherine Hamlin has one son but 35,000 daughters" (figure 10.1).

Catherine Nicolson was a 1946 graduate of the University of Sydney medical school who became a resident in obstetrics and gynecology at the Crown Street Women's Hospital. The only female resident, she soon caught the eye of the hospital's medical superintendent, Dr. Reginald Hamlin. They gradually discovered that they liked each other (a lot), and they were married in 1950.

There were strong traditions of Christian missionary service in both of their families, which made them aspire to something more than ordinary medical careers. Motivated by a sense of Christian compassion and rather wearied by Australian medical politics, in 1958 they answered an advertisement placed in a prominent medical jour-

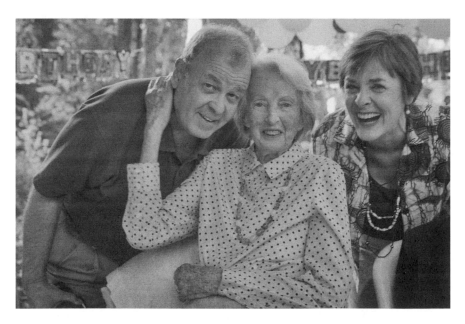

FIGURE 10.1. Lewis and Helen Wall with Catherine Hamlin on the occasion of her ninetieth birthday, Addis Ababa, Ethiopia. *Photo copyright Joni Kabana, used by permission.*

nal, the *Lancet*, by the government of Ethiopia. The government was seeking to hire obstetrician-gynecologists to establish a midwifery school at the Princess Tsehai Hospital in Addis Ababa. Princess Tsehai was the third daughter and fourth child of Emperor Haile Selassie. A remarkable young woman, she had trained in nursing in London during her father's forced exile from Ethiopia during the Italian occupation of the country in the late 1930s, and she returned home as the first fully qualified Ethiopian nurse when he was restored to the throne. She was determined to set up a hospital. Unfortunately, she herself died in childbirth from an uncontrolled hemorrhage in Welega Province in 1942. The hospital she longed to create was established in her memory in 1951.

The Hamlins had an inauspicious arrival to Ethiopia in 1959. The cable announcing their arrival had not been received (it appeared two weeks later), and when they landed in Addis Ababa by airplane from the French colony of Djibouti on the African coast after a turbulent, stomach-churning flight, no one was there to meet them. They trudged into town on foot with their six-year-old son, Richard, in tow and eventually located the hospital.

Their unexpected arrival caused considerable consternation, but the welcome they received was warm nevertheless. They made do in improvised housing, the first in a lifelong series of improvisations necessitated by their circumstances. They were soon heavily immersed in clinical work, seeing complications of childbirth they had scarcely imagined were even possible based on their professional experience in Australia. Catherine still vividly remembers the words spoken to them shortly after their arrival by Dr. Margaret Fitzherbert, one of the hospital's gynecologists, who said, "The fistula patients will break your heart."

The First Fistula Cases

The first fistula case to come to their attention arrived only a few days after they themselves did. She was a 17-year-old girl who had been in obstructed labor for five days out in the countryside. Her child was stillborn, and she had developed a massive fistula as a result of her ordeal. Reg and Catherine were stunned by the damage they saw but still considered themselves to be too "green" and too uncertain about how to approach a clinical problem of this magnitude. They referred her to a German gynecologist working at another hospital who had some experience in fistula surgery.

But the fistula patients kept appearing; obstetric fistula was not a "one-off" clinical oddity in Ethiopia. It was a major medical problem that was not being addressed by anyone. Fistula was clearly a condition about which the Hamlins would have to educate themselves, and rather quickly. Telephone service in Ethiopia was poor, and the Internet would not exist for another 30 years, so Catherine and Reg started writing letters, corresponding with the handful of world experts on obstetric fistula: Naguib Mahfouz in Egypt, Chassar Moir in Britain, and Heinrich Martius in Germany (who had developed a novel tissue flap for use in vaginal reconstructive surgery). In reply to their letters, these men sent them articles and books, which Reg and Catherine began digesting. Catherine got a copy of J. Marion Sims's autobiography, *The Story of My Life*, from England and sat up late into the night reading about his struggles to repair fistulas and to set up the world's first fistula hospital in New York. After absorbing all they could from these sources—and faced with a steady stream of patients with heartbreaking injuries who appealed to them for help—Reg and Catherine began to operate.

They chose a relatively straightforward case for their first attempted repair: a young woman from a rural area with a small fistula. As Catherine recounted in her autobiography, *The Hospital by the River*, "She was a brave little soul, trusting and calm. She had no idea that her case was such a landmark for us." Reg performed the operation with Catherine's assistance. They closed the injury, placed a catheter to drain the bladder, and waited anxiously for the outcome. Two weeks later when the catheter was removed, her bladder had healed. The fistula was closed. The patient was dry and voided normally. The joy produced by this operation and the gratitude expressed by this young woman to the Hamlins upon her departure from the hospital made a deep impression on them. They immediately carried out two more operations, both of which were successful. Soon Reg had done 22 operations as the primary surgeon, with only one failure, and then Catherine started operating.

Reg and Catherine continued their normal duties, but as word spread of their success in repairing fistulas, the stream of patients with these injuries started to increase. Some would travel for weeks on foot from remote areas to get to Addis Ababa. They were poor women from rural areas. They arrived destitute, begging for help, with no place to stay. So Reg and Catherine personally began paying their hospital admission fees and scrounged for places to house them. They had six beds available for their use, but far more fistula patients than that. The number of fistula patients began to strain the hospital's resources.

Although desperate for help, a woman with a fistula is not generally a surgical emergency, and scheduled fistula repairs were frequently bumped from the operating schedule by emergency cases who needed urgent life-saving treatment. Many women with fistulas were told by the gate attendants that there were no beds available, but they waited anyway. Reg would find them, feed them, and sequester them around the hospital wherever he could, sometimes in storerooms and stairwells (a practice that created some problems of its own).

Eventually the number of patients became so large and so noticeable that Reg was called to the Ministry of Health to explain the fistula "epidemic" that seemed to have hit Addis Ababa. He explained to the government that this had been going on for decades because of the poor medical services in rural areas, but now for the first time someone was trying to do something about it, and the women were responding. As they later wrote in the *Ethiopian Medical Journal*, "It is not surprising, therefore, that almost every day a young woman with a vesico-vaginal fistula arrives at the Princess Tsehai Memorial Hospital from the provinces seeking a cure. To meet only one of these sad patients and to listen to the history she gives, is to be profoundly moved."

Fistula Pilgrims

Reg referred to these woman as "fistula pilgrims." In medieval times, a pilgrimage was a long arduous journey to a sacred place such as Santiago de Compostela, Jerusalem, or Canterbury, done as an act of religious devotion, often in search of healing or a cure. The analogy was apt; and in caring for these fistula pilgrims, Reg and Catherine found the meaning of their lives and the cause to which they would devote themselves.

Their description of the existential situation of the patients they met with these childbirth injuries is eloquent:

> In vast areas of the world . . . [i]n South East Asia, in Burma, in India, in parts of Central America, South America and Africa, 50 million women will bring forth their children this year in sorrow, as in ancient Biblical times, and exposed to grave dangers. In consequence, today as ever in the past, uncounted hundreds of thousands of young mothers annually suffer childbirth injuries: injuries which reduce them to the ultimate state of human wretchedness.

> Consider these young women. Belonging generally to the age group 15–23 years, and thus at the very beginning of their reproductive lives, they are more to be pitied even than the blind, for the blind can sometimes work and marry. Their desolation descends below that of the lepers, who though scarred, crippled and shunned, may still marry and find useful work to do. The blind, the crippled and the lepers, with lesions obvious to the eye and therefore appealing to the heart, are all remembered and cared for by great charitable bodies, national and international.

> Constantly in pain, incontinent of urine or faeces, bearing a heavy burden of sadness in discovering their child stillborn, ashamed of a rank personal offensiveness, abandoned therefore by their husbands, outcasts of society, unemployable except in the fields, they live, they exist, without friends and without hope.

> Because their injuries are pudendal, affecting those parts of the body which must be hidden from view and which a woman may not in modesty easily speak, they endure their injuries in silent shame. No charitable organization becomes aware of them. Their misery is utter, lonely, and complete.

These women sustained their injuries because of lack of timely access to emergency obstetric care. They exemplified all of the delays that lead to obstetric tragedy discussed in chapters 6, 7, and 8. Ethiopia is a rugged country with an incomplete road system and difficult communications, even today. Although much has improved in the past 20 years, 85 percent of the people still live in rural areas. In the

1960s the medical, educational, transportation, and administrative infrastructure of the country was woefully inadequate.

As a result of these infrastructural deficiencies, the Hamlins often faced a cavalcade of daunting obstetric complications that would never have occurred in a modern industrialized country with an efficiently functioning system of maternal healthcare.

A woman arrived after eight days in labor, with the dead baby's head delivered (and now starting to decay) but the body stuck in her birth canal. She died from infection a few hours after her delivery.

Another woman arrived in shock after several days in labor, also with her dead baby's head protruding. Her belly was tender and grossly distended, suggesting a ruptured uterus from prolonged obstructed labor. In surgery, the diagnosis of uterine rupture was indeed confirmed, but the abdominal cavity was filled with a tangle of limbs. She had been carrying twins. For some reason, Reg couldn't do the delivery. He couldn't get the dead babies out. Then he discovered the unimaginable reason why: this was a case of conjoined ("Siamese") twins, which could never have been delivered through the vagina. That was why the uterus had ruptured, but now he couldn't get them out even by Cesarean section. They were immovably jammed into the pelvis. The twins were already dead, so delivery was finally accomplished by decapitating the twin stuck in the vagina to relieve the obstruction, then extracting the remnants of their conjoined bodies through the uterine incision. The uterus was so damaged that it had to be removed as well to save the woman's life. Fortunately, she survived.

Another patient arrived declaring she had been pregnant for 18 months but had not yet delivered her baby. She had an enlarged abdomen, and the clinical suspicion was that she probably had a large ovarian tumor. But the patient was actually right. At operation she turned out to have an abdominal pregnancy: a rare condition in which implantation of the fertilized egg takes place outside the uterus and the placenta embeds itself into an adjoining structure, usually the bowel. Such pregnancies can actually become quite advanced, but the pregnancy will always die without good medical care and Cesarean delivery because, lying as it does outside of the uterus, there is no way that a vaginal delivery can occur. Many women who develop an abdominal pregnancy also die, particularly when this occurs in a remote African setting. In this case the pregnancy had died and subsequently became calcified, creating a stone-like fetal mummy in the woman's abdomen (known medically as a "lithopedion"). It was removed successfully.

An adolescent girl was brought in one day, horribly wounded. To Catherine it looked like she had been the victim of a shark attack—an impossibility in rural Ethiopia—but the actual story turned out to be just as surreal as a shark attack would have been. The girl had been in labor at home in her hut, when it unexpectedly caught fire. Her relatives hurriedly hauled her out of the burning *tukul* and placed her under a tree while they attempted to put out the fire. They were distracted from this task only when they heard her screams and rushed to her assistance. She had already delivered by herself, and it was not labor pains that were causing her to scream. Astonishingly, after giving birth she had been attacked by a hyena that had been lurking in the vicinity. The hyena first killed her baby and then turned on the horrified girl, severely mauling her buttocks and thighs. With excellent clinical care, she survived.

The fistula patients continued to arrive, but there was no place to put them. Reg and Catherine raised enough money to build a small 10-bed hostel in which patients could stay while awaiting surgery and for their aftercare, but this was not enough. They built another hostel. Then they built a third one, but still there was not enough bed space. These patients really needed their own hospital. The Ethiopian government was not convinced and did not embrace the idea. If Reg and Catherine wanted a fistula hospital, they would have to build it on their own.

The Idea for a Specialist Fistula Hospital

With able salesmanship, they secured the patronage of Princess Tenagnework for their project and slowly set about locating an appropriate parcel of land on which to build a hospital. Throughout Africa land tenure issues are convoluted, complex, and often intractable. Finding land and getting clear title to it is not easy. Disputes concerning ownership may last for generations, constantly moving into and out of court. While out riding on horseback (a favorite pastime) one day, Catherine found a piece of bare land running down a steep hillside to a river, just below a shirt factory. The land was owned by the Armenian community. After considerable discussions, Reg and Catherine managed to purchase two parcels of land for what would eventually become the Addis Ababa Fistula Hospital. They established a charitable trust to oversee the work, obtained serendipitous funding from the United States and Australia to begin the work, and (most importantly) received permission (which they needed, as foreigners) from Emperor Haile Selassie to purchase the land.

Ethiopia is a proud country (never colonized) with its own deep bureaucratic tradition and ways of doing things. It took four years from the acquisition of the land to construction of the hospital. Reg and Catherine designed it themselves, with specific goals in mind. It was to have a large open ward of 40 beds (to encourage social interaction and a communal spirit). It was constructed with large windows down the long sides of the ward, with open doorways to encourage light and cross-ventilation (a rather important characteristic in a hospital for fistula patients). The operating room was large enough to hold three operating tables, and it had plenty of space for all of the subsidiary rooms needed to run such an enterprise (sterilization room for instruments, offices, changing rooms, storage for supplies, etc.). The operating theater opened onto the ward, so the patients could see everyone coming and going. A large open veranda was constructed along the whole length of the ward, to provide shelter from inclement weather as well as a convenient social gathering place for patients.

The enormous effort it took to put this project together occurred at a very difficult time in the history of modern Ethiopia. The early 1970s was a period of poor rainfall and subsequent crop failure throughout the country. Slowly, inexorably, famine began to grip the country, particularly in the Wollo and Tigray regions of the north. Because of the poor communication infrastructure and central government indifference toward rural areas, word of the developing catastrophe was slow to reach the capital. When it did, it was not taken seriously. Many of the educated elite of the country (especially the young) were becoming increasingly hostile to Emperor Haile Selassie's heavy-handed, undemocratic rule and the feudal social system that supported him. Furthermore, the country was bogged down in an unpopular war with the one-time Italian colony and sometime Ethiopian province of Eritrea.

Political unrest was growing in the cities, on university campuses, and in the military, when in 1973, British television journalist Jonathan Dimbleby came to Ethiopia to investigate the reports of famine that were filtering out of the country. His ITV documentary film, *The Unknown Famine*, aired in Britain, showing heartbreaking images of starving people. It claimed that more than 200,000 people had died so far. This film shocked the world's conscience and accelerated the rapidly growing discontent within the country. It did not help matters when a copy of the film was produced juxtaposing images of starving peasants to those of the emperor and his friends feasting in a lavish setting. Retitled *The Hidden Hunger*, the film was shown around the clock on Ethiopian television the day the military staged its coup. The country was further destabilized by soaring oil prices in the aftermath of the 1973 international oil crisis, a general strike, and several army mutinies.

Rise of the Derg

The 82-year-old Emperor Haile Selassie was deposed by the military on September 12, 1974, and driven away from his palace crammed into the back of a Volkswagen Beetle. The government was taken over by an army group known as the Armed Forces Coordinating Committee. In Amharic, the principal language of Ethiopia, a committee is called a *derg*, and so the new government became known as the Derg. What started out as possibly a hopeful stumble toward more democratic government quickly turned into a nightmare. The Derg itself was quickly taken over by radical communist elements, who imposed a military dictatorship on the country. Soon afterward, the killing of prominent citizens and former government officials began. On November 23, 1974, more than 60 former nobles and officials (including the patriarch of the Ethiopian Orthodox Church) were executed in a mass murder. The country began a slow, bloody, downward spiral toward totalitarian dictatorship and genocide.

This was not a propitious time to be opening a new hospital for poor women with childbirth injuries, but the obstetric problems would not go away. Under the worsening circumstances within Ethiopia, it was far more likely that the problem would get worse. Reg and Catherine persevered. Wary about garnering any publicity at all in the rapidly deteriorating political climate, they held a private "opening ceremony" in their own home, snipping a ribbon inelegantly strung between two chairs, and declared their hospital open. It was May 24, 1975.

Because Princess Tsehai Hospital was close to the airport, the Derg took it over for military purposes and sent all of the patients and staff to Black Lion Hospital in the middle of Addis Ababa. This was a blow to Catherine and Reg, because their hospital was located close to Princess Tsehai. They had hoped to be able to use the laboratory and x-ray facilities there for their fistula patients, but this was not to be. Their new hospital was busy but understaffed and undersupplied. Electric power was irregular, and they had no generator. Bandages had to be washed by hand, sterilized, and then reused. There was no anesthesiologist, so when patients needed an anesthetic, Reg and Catherine had to give a spinal injection themselves, then rush around to the other end of the operating table, position the patient, and do the surgery. Eventually the Derg gave them permission to take two nurses from a government hospital (reuniting them with old friends) to help with their work. The rest of the nursing staff—the nursing aides who did most of the hands-on nursing care—were former fistula patients whom the Hamlins trained themselves. This led to an astonishingly high level of empathy among the staff, since almost everyone working on the wards had experienced a fistula herself. They knew what it meant, for they had lain in a similar bed themselves, facing similar fears and worrying about the same deep existential questions all of these women face about their futures.

On August 28, 1975, the Derg announced that Emperor Haile Selassie had died the previous day, ostensibly from "respiratory complications" following prostate surgery. Nobody actually believed this. The commonly accepted story is that the emperor was smothered in his own bed with a pillow at the hands of Mengistu Haile Mariam, the leader of the Derg.

Whatever the truth concerning the emperor's death, Mengistu took full advantage of his passing, emerging in its aftermath as the sole dictator of Ethiopia. He proved to be a ruthless totalitarian ruler, aligning himself with the Soviet Union, which provided him with substantial military and economic aid. He became a major African ally in the geopolitics of the Cold War. Mengistu proved to be an able student of Soviet political theory and practice. To consolidate his power, he launched a brutal crackdown on all opposition groups that would have made even Joseph Stalin proud. Eventually he slaughtered more than 500,000 people. Ethiopia was now ruled by the Red Terror.

The political situation in Ethiopia only worsened the already appalling medical conditions in rural areas. The numbers of fistula pilgrims continued to increase. As Catherine wrote in her memoirs, "Our poor neglected fistula patients still came flocking to our door in rags and smelling of urine, hoping that we could give them a new life. People asked me why we did not leave. How could we turn our backs on so much need?"

Reg and Catherine simply set to work, kept their heads down, avoided controversy, and tended to their patients. The Derg were not much interested in poor women with childbirth injuries, and, for the most part, they left the Hamlins alone.

"Professional Beggars"

Running your own hospital in a poor African country without adequate staff, supplies, or money was more than a full-time job. Reg was often up by five o'clock in the morning, writing letters to foreign foundations and dignitaries in search of funding and supplies. Money arrived sporadically from many sources, often unexpectedly, but keeping the hospital going was a constant hand-to-mouth struggle. The clinical load increased as more and more fistula pilgrims arrived. Catherine and Reg operated on Mondays, Wednesdays, and Fridays. In between, they saw new patients in the outpatient clinic and prepared the operating room for the next round of surgeries.

When they were able to leave Ethiopia to go abroad, their holiday time was often spent looking for funding. Catherine and Reg were engaged in a constant round of meetings and speeches. They spoke to many churches about their work, which was motivated by deep Christian compassion for these injured Ethiopian women who suffered from nothing other than faulty obstetrical mechanics. The Hamlins were faithful members of St. Matthew's Anglican Church in Addis Ababa (which, because the congregation was almost entirely composed of expatriates, was largely ignored by the Derg). A favorite story involves a meeting that Reg had on one of these trips abroad with the vicar of a church where he was about to speak. Reg said to him, "You do understand, vicar, that I'm a gynecologist who deals with childbirth injuries. I won't be able to explain to your congregation what I do without using the word 'vagina.'" The vicar looked at him thoughtfully for a moment and then said, "Good! Maybe they'll pay attention for a change!"

Mamitu

Of the thousands of stories surrounding the Addis Ababa Fistula Hospital, that of Mamitu Gashe is one of the most remarkable. Mamitu was born in a remote rural area in the province of Shoa in central Ethiopia, a land of remarkably rugged terrain. Her father was a farmer. She had five sisters and four brothers, but no schooling. As was customary in this part of the world, Mamitu's future marriage was arranged by her family while she was still a child, and she was wed at the age of 14. Two years later, she became pregnant.

When the time came for her delivery, her labor was obstructed. She sat, squatting, on the floor of her hut, trying to push the baby out for four long days. No attempt was made to get to a hospital because, quite simply, there were no hospitals to get to. Mamitu had a "natural" labor—and a "natural" complication. When her child was finally delivered, it was stillborn. The baby had died during labor, and after death had softened until it could slip past the obstruction in her pelvis into the outside world.

Mamitu was exhausted by this ordeal and lay in her hut for three weeks trying to recover. She had sustained massive injuries to her bladder, rectum, and vagina during labor, and she now was leaking both urine and stool from combined vesico-vaginal and recto-vaginal fistulas. Because one of her sisters had moved to Addis Ababa, the family thought they might be able to find help for her there. Her brothers and an uncle built a stretcher using two wooden poles and some goatskins, and they set out on foot in search of medical help. They carried Mamitu, feverish and semiconscious, from their village down the mountainside until they reached the town of Debre Sina. It took three days to make the journey. At Debre Sina they managed to catch a bus to Addis Ababa, a distance of 200 kilometers.

Once they reached Addis Ababa, they didn't know where to take her. Eventually, she was brought to the Princess Tsehai Hospital, where she met the Drs. Hamlin. Mamitu was very weak and very ill, and it took many weeks before she was strong enough to undergo surgery. Her injuries were breathtaking, involving the whole of the lower urinary tract and the rectum. Multiple reconstructive operations were undertaken in an attempt to restore normal functioning anatomy. As Catherine later wrote, "Mamitu stood these operations with courage and the optimism of youth." But it was eventually clear that the damage was so extensive that things could never be fully restored to normal. What was to be done with Mamitu?

Mamitu was unschooled, but she was clearly highly intelligent. She had a pleasing personality. Catherine described her as having "a soft and tender heart and winsome ways," so the Hamlins decided to put her to work as a nursing aide. She soon mastered the routine tasks on the fistula ward. It was also quite obvious that Mamitu was especially fond of Reg. Before her injuries, Mamitu had been very close to her father, and Reg now filled that place in her life. He began taking her from the ward to the outpatient clinic, where she worked as his assistant. By now Mamitu had learned passable English, and she started to serve as his interpreter while interviewing patients. This arrangement worked out so well that Reg soon began taking her to the operating theater, where she began assisting him in surgery. At first she only cut sutures and handed him instruments when they were needed, but she was a quick study, and soon she understood the natural flow of fistula repair operations. There was so much work to be done—often with three operations in progress simultaneously—that Reg started letting Mamitu close the vaginal incision herself after the bladder repair had been completed, while he moved on to place the spinal anesthetic and start the next case across the room.

Gradually, with increasing experience and rapidly improving skill, Mamitu began operating by herself under Reg and Catherine's supervision. Finally she began operating independently. Eventually Mamitu became the principal instructor for new surgeons arriving in Addis Ababa to learn the craft of fistula surgery. In 1989, when

Dr. Reginald Hamlin was awarded the Gold Medal of the Royal College of Surgeons for his work in fistula surgery, Catherine and Mamitu shared the award with him. Mamitu had become a gold-medal-winning surgeon without ever having been to medical school.

Surviving the Red Terror

Throughout this period, things in Ethiopia had been growing progressively worse. Mengistu's communist government was a disaster for the country, and opposition to his rule had grown progressively more intense since 1974. In 1977 Ethiopia was invaded by Somalia in a bold attempt by that country to annex the Somali-speaking parts of Ethiopia. With massive assistance from its Soviet bloc allies, the Mengistu government was able to defeat the Somalia forces and repel the invasion, but the war with Eritrea (which had been started by Haile Selassie's attempted annexation of the country) continued. Mengistu's attempts at land reform were hobbled by corruption and mismanagement. His brutal political repression solidified the opposition of the people (particularly the peasant farmers) to the government. Hundreds of thousands fled the country. Within Ethiopia itself, armed opposition groups arose, particularly in the north, where the Tigray People's Liberation Front was becoming both a powerful political as well as an effective military force. Headed by a former medical student named Meles Zenawi from the northern town of Adwa (the site of the battle where Ethiopian patriots had handed the Italian imperialist army a humiliating defeat in 1896) the Tigray People's Liberation Front was beginning a war of attrition against the Derg that would last 17 years.

In the mid-1980s Ethiopia was again struck by famine, which caused additional turmoil and suffering within the country. The Mengistu government was destabilized further by the structural weaknesses that began to appear in the communist bloc at this time. Foreign aid to his regime declined as the Soviet Union began lurching toward dissolution. By this time numerous other "People's Liberation Fronts" had emerged throughout Ethiopia to fight the communist government. Eventually these disparate groups joined together to create the Ethiopian People's Revolutionary Democratic Front, a very effective guerilla military force. By the late 1980s much of the countryside had fallen under its control, and its military forces were beginning to move on the capital, Addis Ababa. The casualties they inflicted were notable; many of Mengistu's soldiers were killed or wounded.

One day Reg was down at their house working on some administrative details, when a convoy of buses arrived at the hospital, full of wounded government soldiers. Catherine was on the fistula ward at the time and ran to the house to alert Reg. The military was taking over their hospital. Reg ran up to the ward to meet the officer in charge. He calmly gave him a guided tour, showing him that all the beds were full and there was no more room for patients. As the major looked around, Reg continued to explain to him that the hospital was a specialist institution for women with childbirth injuries. He doubted they had any such patients among his wounded troops. Oh, and by the way, the hospital didn't really have much of a lab or even a blood bank—and there was no x-ray equipment to use in diagnosing fractures or other injuries. Disgusted by the shoddy facilities (for military purposes) they had been shown, the soldiers left, moving down the road to a leprosy hospital that was better equipped for their needs. Reg's cool head, calm demeanor, and quick mind had saved their life's work.

The defeats of Mengistu's army piled up as the rebel forces advanced. In May 1989, while Mengistu was out of the country on a state visit to East Germany, several military officers attempted to stage a coup. Mengistu quickly flew back to Ethiopia to crush the attempt to oust him, but the tide of events was now running the other direction. Two years later, in May 1991, the Ethiopian People's Revolutionary Democratic Front forces had the capital surrounded. As they were tightening their stranglehold on the city, Mengistu and his family fled the country. He was granted asylum in Zimbabwe by his fellow dictator Robert Mugabe. The long civil war to free Ethiopia from grip of a bloodthirsty tyrant was over; now the healing could begin.

The change in government gradually brought new life to the capital and a new freedom to the economy. Over the years since then, many Ethiopians among the diaspora who fled the country under Mengistu's bloody rule have returned home, releasing and reinvigorating the country's entrepreneurial spirit. Those working at the hospital breathed a large, deep, collective sigh of relief and took up their work with renewed enthusiasm. There was indeed a rebirth of freedom under the new, noncommunist government (now headed by Meles Zenawi), but huge challenges remained. The state of maternal health in Ethiopia was slow to improve. There were still thousands of women with obstetric fistulas to reach and no clear prospect of stemming the influx of new cases every year.

Transitions

After returning to Ethiopia from a family holiday to Kenya for some much-needed rest and relaxation in 1991, Reg Hamlin noticed a lump on the inner surface of his right thigh. A visiting surgeon who examined him thought he had developed a large hematoma—a blood clot—inside the muscle. Perhaps he had fallen over or run into something? Reg couldn't remember any such incident. The swelling didn't subside, so he went to see an orthopedic surgeon at Black Lion Hospital for another opinion. An attempt at a needle biopsy of the mass was unsuccessful, so the surgeon recommended an operation under spinal anesthesia to excise the mass. The mass was encapsulated and removed successfully, but the pathology report revealed bad news. The tumor was a fibrosarcoma, a cancer of the connective tissue, in the thigh. Everyone hoped that the excision of the mass would lead to a cure, but the tumor recurred within a few months. This was a bad sign.

No further treatment for a condition like this was available in Ethiopia, so Reg and Catherine went to Britain for expert consultation. What they were told was grim. Surgery might be curative, but if so it would involve a radical and debilitating operation: amputation of the entire right lower extremity at the hip joint, a so-called hindquarter amputation. Reg was 82 years old and not robust. An operation like this would be daunting even for a young man in excellent health. They discussed it and together decided against surgery. The only alternative treatment was radiation therapy, but fibrosarcomas are not generally very radiosensitive. The prognosis was not hopeful. Reg and Catherine stayed on in Britain for several weeks while he received radiation treatment. They stayed in the London home of the British ambassador to Ethiopia and hoped for the best. Radiation completed, they returned to Addis Ababa.

Reg was exhausted by his therapeutic ordeal in Britain. He was unable to resume his clinical duties after returning to Ethiopia. A film crew from the BBC arrived and spent a month at the hospital, filming a documentary called *Walking Back to Happiness*. Reg appeared in the film, enthusiastic and engaged—but obviously not well. He and Catherine both knew that his time was running out. As he began to weaken, Mamitu stopped her hospital duties and became his full-time nurse. Catherine began doing more and more; a transition was occurring. By July, Reg was clearly fading. He was now completely bedridden. In the early hours of August 5, 1993, he died peacefully at home with Catherine by his side, on the grounds of the hospital to which he had devoted most of his life. After a funeral service at St. Matthew's Anglican Church, he was buried in the British War Graves Cemetery in Addis Ababa. His tombstone was inscribed with the words "I know that my redeemer liveth," from Handel's *Messiah*.

Reg's death accelerated the changes that were occurring at the fistula hospital. Catherine had to assume new administrative and fund-raising duties while simultaneously dealing with her grief. Her commitment to the institution they had founded together never wavered, but the tasks that she had to shoulder were not easy. The fistula pilgrims continued to come; the workload increased. There were continual staffing challenges. It was difficult to train and retain Ethiopian surgeons for fistula work since they could make considerably more money in private practice. Most of the doctors they had trained left after a few years for financial reasons. It proved difficult to find suitable expatriates who would take on fistula surgery in Ethiopia as a career. The hospital had an unsuccessful experience with a missionary surgeon released from his organization. A retired professor of surgery left because of administrative and personality issues. In spite of the challenges, Catherine persevered, and the hospital grew and prospered.

The hospital was redesigned and reconstructed in the 1990s. The hodgepodge of buildings that had grown up over the years was replaced with a more coherent master plan. An on-site well was drilled to supply a continuous source of clean, fresh potable water—an absolute necessity for an institution of this kind. Although the need for continuous fundraising never abated, regular donors began to appear, including World

Vision (United States and Canada), Rotary International, the British charity Ethiopiaid, and the Australian government. Reg and Catherine had developed a large international network of friends over the years, many of whom remained inspired by and loyally engaged with their work. Over time a network of charitable trusts developed throughout the industrialized world to support the programs at the fistula hospital: Australia, New Zealand, the United Kingdom, Germany, the Netherlands, Sweden, Switzerland, the United States, and a fledgling organization in Japan.

While visiting the United States to receive an award for her lifetime's work from the American College of Surgeons, Catherine Hamlin appeared on television as a guest on *The Oprah Winfrey Show* in January 2005. Her appearance was an eye-opening experience for millions of viewers, who had never dreamed that childbirth injuries of the kind she described were even possible, much less that they occurred with such alarming regularity to tens of thousands of poor women around the world each year. Catherine's passionate advocacy for her cause generated millions of dollars in donations for her work and catapulted the Addis Ababa Fistula Hospital to new international prominence. Oprah herself wrote a generous six-figure check in support.

Results

In 2010 the hospital published an analysis of nearly 15,000 fistula cases in a Swedish medical journal, *Acta Obstetricia et Gynecologica*. It was a review of patients seen between 1974 and 2006 based on a standardized, structured, intake questionnaire, supplemented by additional information from 434 patients who were seen in 2007–2008. This paper gives a very clear picture of the women who developed obstetric fistulas in Ethiopia and of the treatment they received at the Addis Ababa Fistula Hospital.

- 57 percent of the patients developed their obstetric fistula during their first pregnancy.
- In these first pregnancies, over 50 percent of women were still in labor, undelivered, after three days; in 31 percent they were still in labor after four days.
- 43 percent developed their obstetric fistula in their second or later pregnancy.
- 35 percent of patients were under the age of 20 when they developed their fistula.
- 77 percent were illiterate.
- 36 percent were divorced or separated as a result of their fistula.
- Only 26 percent were accompanied to the hospital by their husbands.
- 77 percent had had no antenatal care during the pregnancy in which their fistula occurred.
- 92 percent had a stillborn baby at the delivery that caused the fistula.
- Over 99 percent had a urinary-vaginal fistula (mainly vesico-vaginal fistulas).

- Only 0.3 percent of patients had an isolated recto-vaginal fistula.
- 13 percent of patients had a combined vesico-vaginal and recto-vaginal fistula.
- The fistula was closed successfully in 93 percent of the cases, but—
- In 19 percent of the cases where the fistula was closed successfully, there was a "continence gap," meaning the fistula was closed but urine loss through the urethra persisted for a variety of reasons, including severe damage to the urethra, bladder emptying difficulties, and uncontrollable spams of the bladder muscles. To get such women dry after surgery was an ongoing treatment challenge.

Women who developed a fistula tended to be short (152 cm in height) compared to the national average of 157 centimeters for women of reproductive age (short maternal height is roughly correlated with decreased pelvic capacity, predisposing short women to obstructed labor). The average age at marriage was 17 years. Since adult pelvic capacity is not reached until several years after menarche, a young age at marriage (when followed by a pregnancy) also predisposes young girls to difficult labor. There are few life opportunities for rural Ethiopian women other than marriage, so it is not surprising that many marry young, soon after their first menstrual periods. Almost a quarter of the fistula patients had been married before the age of 15. Interestingly, among those women with fistulas for whom the sex of the baby was known when their fistula occurred, 77 percent reported having a stillborn male child. This is most likely explained by the fact that male babies tend to have heavier birth weights than females, and large babies predispose a woman to obstructed labor.

The young women who developed obstructed labor in their first pregnancies had longer labors, more extensive damage to their pelvic tissues, and a higher rate of recto-vaginal fistulas, indicating more severe tissue compression during labor. They also had a greater likelihood of being separated from or divorced by their husbands, and far less likelihood of being accompanied to the fistula hospital by their spouses. This probably reflects the lack of other children at home from the marriage and correspondingly less investment in the marital relationship by their spouses.

These data also illuminate the many challenges faced by those who are attempting to combat the fistula problem in Ethiopia. The women come from rural areas, where attendance by a trained midwife during childbirth is rare. It is difficult to move laboring women from rural villages to hospitals because of the rugged terrain and the distances involved. The number of hospitals to which these women can be brought is still far too small (but improving). Under these circumstances, fistula prevention is difficult simply because it is difficult to get timely help. As a result, many patients have a neglected labor that lasts for days, resulting in extensive injuries: more than a third of all patients in this series had a fistula greater than 4 centimeters in width, and 15 percent had a vagina that was severely scarred or totally obliterated from the damage that had occurred. What was to be done with the women whose fistulas could not be repaired because there was no normal tissue left to work with? What was to be done for women whose fistulas were closed successfully but who still remained incontinent for other, unclear, reasons?

Some patient stories were heart wrenching. The problems encountered by poor women in poor countries who seek help for these afflictions are incomprehensible to citizens of the affluent world. Reg once encountered a girl who arrived at the hospital bearing a grubby old envelope with an almost illegible referral letter tucked inside. The letter had been written by a missionary down along the Kenya-Ethiopian border, asking them to treat her fistula—but the letter was seven years old! When asked where she had been all this time, the girl replied that she had been hanging around the bus station begging, trying to raise the pitifully small fare (about three dollars) required to get her to Addis Ababa.

Intractable Fistulas and Desta Mender

One of the more pressing problems was how to deal with patients who had unsuccessful surgery, those whose fistulas could not be closed in spite of the very best efforts made on their behalf. The number of such patients was small—only about 7 percent of the total—but their circumstances were often precarious. The injuries they had suffered were severe; sometimes there was not even enough normal tissue remaining to close the hole that had formed in the bladder. In other cases there was so much scar tissue that nothing could be mobilized to even make the attempt at closure. Women with these sorts of injuries were going to remain severely incontinent for the rest of their lives. Having endured several surgeries without success, with no place to go and families not particularly interested in receiving them home again, they stayed in and around the hospital, lingering on the edge of despair, hoping that something, anything, might yet be done for them. How could this challenge be met?

The simplest surgical solution to this problem appeared to be urinary diversion. In the normally functioning urinary tract, the urine produced by the kidneys is transported through the ureters (two long thin muscular tubes) into the bladder where it is stored until urination takes place. A fistula creates a hole in the bladder so that it cannot store urine. If fistula repair surgery is successful, the hole in the urinary "bucket" (the bladder) is plugged, and most of the time all is well. If the hole cannot be fixed, if the "bucket" is too damaged to be salvageable, the problem is how to manage the continuous stream of urine that flows into the damaged bladder through the ureters. One solution is to divert the urine to another location.

The simplest diversionary surgery is called an "ileal conduit." In creating an ileal conduit, the surgeon removes 6 to 8 inches of the lower end of the small intestine (the ileum) and sews the two ends of the ileum back together so that the small intestine maintains its normal continuity. A hole (called a "stoma" or a "urostomy") is made through the abdominal wall and the piece of ileum is sewn into it as a tube. The surgeon then mobilizes the two ureters, cuts them loose from their attachment to the bladder, and reimplants them into the other end of the repositioned ileal segment, which now acts like a hose pipe. In this rearranged anatomy, the urine flows through the ureters, into the ileal segment (which forms a conduit to the skin surface, hence the name), and out through the stoma in the abdominal wall. Thus diverted, the urinary stream no longer goes into the bladder; therefore, the bladder no longer leaks.

But this does not solve the problem of urinary control. If the patient is going to be continent, the urine flowing out of the abdominal stoma must be contained. This is done by affixing a stoma bag over the urostomy to collect the urine. The bag is emptied periodically. The stoma bag functions as an external, artificial bladder, and the patient voids by emptying the urostomy bag.

Technically, this is rather simple; psychosocially, however, it is often quite difficult. Without access to a reliable supply of stoma bags, this operation only moves the fistula from the pelvis to the abdominal wall. Some patients find this new arrangement more stigmatizing than the original fistula. At least with a fistula the urine is coming from approximately "where it is supposed to come," whereas no normal person passes urine through her abdominal wall. An ileal conduit is a surgical creation, and as such it may develop surgical complications. The new "bladder" produces mucus (which the original bladder did not do), and this may become a problem. Patients with an ileal conduit require specialized nursing care, uninterrupted access to stoma bags, and monitoring for potential long-term complications of the surgery. Patients with an ileal conduit are never really free to go back to remote rural villages and live as they did before the fistula occurred. If you create an ileal conduit in a patient, you "own" her for life. The surgery creates a permanent dependency in the attempt to solve the problem presented by the obstetric fistula. This presents challenges of an entirely new kind.

Thus was born the idea for Desta Mender, the "Village of Joy," as a refuge for patients with intractable injuries and those who needed urinary diversion to become dry. Catherine's youngest brother, Jock Nicholson, was the driving force behind the creation of Desta Mender and helped facilitate its construction. Much of the cost was paid for by an AusAID grant from the Australian government. A series of two-bedroom houses were constructed for the patients, and soon the number of residents at Desta Mender climbed to more than 100. A rehabilitation and job-skills training program was created as the staff began to grapple with the practical problems of managing such a large cohort of urologically disabled women. Within a few years, it was obvious that changes were needed.

Although Desta Mender is in an idyllic location, many women living there felt isolated and alone, cut off from community ties and urban excitements. Although the intentions underlying its creation were honorable and compassionate, over time, institutionalizing these women seemed less and less like the correct approach to their problems. As a result, Desta Mender was gradually transformed from a long-term nursing facility into a rehabilitation institute, with a mission to give birth-injured women improved life skills so that they could make a transition from institutional to semi-independent or even fully independent living.

Desta Mender has now developed into a skills management institute located in the suburbs of Addis Ababa. It has vegetable gardens, an orchard, and even a combination restaurant and conference center run by the women of Desta Mender called the Juniper Café. Women are now making the transition from rehabilitation patient to vocational student to independent businesswoman. Not only do residents run the Juniper Café as a profit-making enterprise, but former residents of Desta Mender are moving into the surrounding community to start their own businesses including a dairy farm, a jewelry business, and a café.

More importantly, however, the Desta Mender experience has helped the organization understand the importance of individualized patient assessment linked to tailored rehabilitation and job-skills training. Under the direction of Beletshachew Tadesse, the on-site director of Desta Mender, each patient who is admitted to the Fistula Hospital in Addis Ababa undergoes an individual assessment of her physical and socioeconomic situation and gets a rehabilitation plan specifically crafted for her own needs. Some women require extensive help in surmounting the daunting barriers which have arisen to their resumption of a normal life; other women have fewer, more easily managed, physical and psychosocial needs.

Both at Desta Mender and at the main hospital in Addis Ababa, there are comprehensive programs of physical and occupational therapy to help birth-injured women regain their physical capacity to resume normal activities of daily living. In about 15 percent of fistula cases, for example, the prolonged pressure of the fetal head trapped against the pelvic sidewall injures the nerves that control motor function to the leg and foot. This creates a lower extremity neuropathy called "foot drop" in which the injured woman can no longer dorsiflex her foot to step over physical obstacles in her path. When this happens the foot becomes little more than a floppy appendage, dragging the ground, knocking against rocks and roots, often injuring the skin and toes. Women with foot drop must walk with a stick or staff for support and usually assume an awkward high-stepping gait, if they can walk at all. Recovery from this injury is possible, but it requires regular, supervised therapeutic exercise (and prosthetic devices to support the foot) to be successful. If the woman is unlucky enough to have injured the nerves on both sides of her pelvis, she may develop bilateral foot drop and be unable to walk at all. With time and skilled care, most women can recover from this injury; but if they are bedridden in a hut in a rural village (constantly lying in a pool of urine, or worse), they will develop contractures of their lower limbs that disable them for life—all because they could not get timely obstetric care for a labor gone awry.

After a presentation on obstetric fistula that I made at a medical conference several years ago (at which I presented the high rates of divorce and separation that are commonly found among fistula patients), a member of the audience asked me whether the women who were still married had smaller fistulas than those who were separated or divorced. "No," I replied. "They just have better husbands." To a large extent, this really is true. Some women (often women who have living children from previous pregnancies) arrive for care accompanied by a devoted husband and other family members. Such women are likely to require shorter and less intensive rehabilitation than will the adolescent patient who became a fistula victim in her first pregnancy, has been abandoned by her husband, and who has seen her only recently formed adult social world shattered by one horrific obstetric experience. The key to effective social services for the fistula patient is individualized care, provided with compassion, respect, and justice.

Regionalized Care

The haunting memory of the fistula patient who sat begging for bus fare along the Kenya border for seven years before she could get transportation to Addis Ababa was a stark and constant reminder of the inaccessibility of curative surgical services for fistula patients throughout Ethiopia, much of which is rugged, mountainous, and poorly served by transportation links. For example, the city of Mekelle in the Tigray region of northern Ethiopia is 300 miles from Addis Ababa "as the crow flies." It takes just over an hour by air to make the trip on Ethiopian Airlines, and there are four flights per day—but no fistula patient could navigate the complexities of purchasing an airline ticket and the social barriers to boarding the plane, even if she could afford the ticket. The trip by road is 470 miles, and it takes two days to drive. The most common way that fistula patients are transported to health centers in rural areas when they are in labor is by stretcher, carried by supportive relatives and neighbors, just as Mamitu was carried down from the mountains herself. Was there a way to move fistula surgery closer to the women who needed it, rather than expecting them to make their way somehow to the capital city?

The answer was decentralization of fistula services, with the creation of regional fistula centers around Ethiopia. Starting in 2003, the Hamlin organization began an aggressive program of outreach involving the development of regional hospitals, staffed by expert fistula surgeons who had trained at the main hospital in Addis Ababa. The first regional hospital was built in Barhir Dar near the shores of Lake Tana in northwestern Ethiopia. Within a few years, four other centers followed: Mekelle in the far north, Yirga 'Alem in the south, Metu in the west, and Harar in the east. Each center is a small replica of the Addis Ababa Fistula Hospital, complete with a ward of about 20 beds, an operating theater, dedicated nursing staff, and rehabilitative services. Each hospital is located close to a large government general hospital so that non-fistula-related medical problems can be referred appropriately, and ancillary services (such as laboratory testing, radiology, etc.) can be shared. The regional centers have been enormously important in moving fistula care closer to the women in rural areas. Patients with difficult problems (such as those requiring urinary diversion or complex diagnostic evaluation) are still referred to Addis Ababa for specialized care. The Hamlin organization performs roughly 2,500 surgical operations each year; about half are performed in Addis Ababa, and about half are performed at the five regional fistula centers.

Preventing Fistulas: The Hamlin College of Midwifery

But even with expanded access to surgical repair, it would still be better to prevent fistulas in the first place than to repair them after the fact. As has been emphasized throughout this book, the fistula problem results from the combination of obstructed labor and obstructed access to emergency obstetric care. The problem will not be solved until access to skilled delivery services improves in areas where fistulas are common.

The original reason that Reg and Catherine Hamlin moved to Ethiopia in 1959 was to establish a midwifery school at Princess Tsehai Hospital. Political turmoil, the press of clinical duties, and their compassionate embrace of the crowds of suffering fistula patients they found in Ethiopia (who were ignored by everyone else) all contributed to sidetracking the development of an effective midwifery training program. In 2007, Hamlin Fistula was able to return to its historic roots in midwifery education with the creation of the Hamlin College of Midwives, nestled in the beautiful Desta Mender campus outside Addis Ababa.

Midwives are the front line in the prevention of obstetric fistula and the reduction of maternal morbidity and mortality in countries like Ethiopia. A qualified midwife should be able to handle routine deliveries safely; to provide education to patients, families, and communities about potential complications of pregnancy and what to do when those complications arise; to diagnose abnormalities in labor; to prevent complications from worsening after they appear; and to facilitate the prompt referral of complex emergencies that require advanced obstetric care. Most importantly, a midwife should be a valued public figure within her community: known, respected, approachable, and trusted. The Hamlin College produces midwives with these characteristics.

The population of Ethiopia is more than 90 million people, and there are roughly 4.5 million pregnancies in the country each year. At the present rate of growth, the population will expand to 138 million by 2030. According to the 2014 report on the state of the world's midwifery produced by the United Nations, there are fewer than 7,000 midwives in Ethiopia to handle this workload. By simple arithmetic alone, it is obvious that the obstetric needs of Ethiopian women are woefully underserved: obstetric fistulas still persist, uterine rupture from obstructed labor is common, and the maternal mortality ratio in Ethiopia is estimated to be as high as 567 maternal deaths per 100,000 live births, with a lifetime risk of a woman's dying in childbirth of 1 in

64. (Consider this in the context of comparable statistics for the United States, Britain, or Australia, which have maternal mortality ratios of 14, 9, and 6 respectively, with lifetime risks of maternal mortality between 1 in 3,800 and 1 in 8,700). Because 85 percent of the population still lives in rural areas, the need to place midwives in these locations is critical to improve maternal health.

Placing midwives in rural areas is not enough. They must have solid clinical training and work within a supportive environment that allows them to practice effectively. Unfortunately, there are huge barriers in Ethiopia to achieving effective midwifery care for all women. Most governmental midwifery training programs are classroom based, focus on the rote learning of textbook material, lack testing for clinical competence, and provide inadequate practical clinical experience to their students. In some cases graduates of midwifery training programs have been certified without ever having delivered a baby by themselves.

The Hamlin College of Midwifery was created in 2007 to shatter the unsatisfactory paradigm for midwifery education that existed in Ethiopia. It was designed to produce excellent clinicians who have a clearly defined professional career pathway with incentives to keep them working in rural areas where they are most needed. This is how it works.

First and foremost, the curriculum is designed to high academic standards. It involves four years of training after completion of secondary education. The training is in English and is based on the standard midwifery texts and curricula used in western Europe and other industrialized nations, modified for the Ethiopian environment. The curriculum is built to international standards and is competency based; that is, the graduates must demonstrate proficiency in the practical skills of midwifery before they can graduate. Supervised one-on-one clinical training is carried out throughout the course of study. Each midwifery student has attended a minimum of 50 deliveries by the time she graduates, usually more, and some have handled case-loads three times this size.

The midwifery students are carefully recruited from rural communities, to which they will return as practicing midwives after graduation. After their training has been completed, Hamlin midwives are posted to work at a government clinic within the catchment area of one of the regional Hamlin fistula centers. The new midwives are sent out in pairs so that each will have a colleague to consult and to share the workload. They also receive regular supervisory visits from a clinical midwifery mentor to monitor their progress and to help them solve problems. They are given suitable housing, decent pay, and the opportunity to invest in a retirement plan. Additionally, their clinics are linked to the regional fistula centers and the partnering government hospitals by an ambulance service so that patients who need more advanced care can be transferred swiftly and reliably. The midwives run antenatal clinics, provide family planning services, perform routine mother-baby care, and do deliveries in their local health center.

Hamlin midwives are wildly popular in the communities they serve. In some locations to which they have been posted, institutional deliveries at their health centers have increased sixfold since their arrival. The Hamlin College of Midwives graduated its first class in 2010, and there are currently 27 Hamlin-supported midwifery clinics throughout Ethiopia. Maternal mortality in Hamlin midwifery clinics is remarkably low compared to the rest of the country. Between 2011 and 2015 there were only 9 maternal deaths out of 23,744 deliveries, a maternal mortality ratio of only 38 deaths per 100,000 deliveries. But Hamlin produces only 15–25 midwifery graduates per year. How does this impact the country as a whole?

The success of Hamlin graduates is striking, especially compared with the performance of most government-run midwifery training programs. It is hoped that Hamlin-trained midwives will be recruited for increasingly senior positions within the health services, where they can serve as role models and supervisors for more junior midwives. The Hamlin model works because it produces graduates with demonstrated high levels of clinical competence who fit well into their communities. The midwifery clinics are integrated into local health service networks, facilitating timely referral of patients. In addition, the Hamlin model consistently demonstrates the values of compassion, respect, and justice (part of which is providing high-quality care) in the services it provides for the women of Ethiopia. Because Hamlin patients know that they are valued and because they receive high-quality clinical care whether they are first-time mothers in labor or multiparous women who have experienced a catastrophic birth injury and need reconstructive surgery, they give their trust to these institutions. Effective clinical services are the key to reducing maternal mortality and morbidity, including obstetric fistula; but being known for their commitment to compassion, respect, and justice is the key to having such services *utilized* by the women who need them.

This raises the problem of what to do when a fistula patient becomes pregnant after repair of her injury. The fistula develops as a result of faulty obstetrical mechanics a baby that is too big or that is positioned in such a way that it will not fit through the birth canal during labor. Often this is a recurrent problem. A woman with a small pelvis who develops a fistula may still very well have a pelvis that is too small for easy delivery in a subsequent pregnancy. Leaving a woman with this history in a rural village to have another pregnancy under the same circumstances is unwise and risks a catastrophic outcome. We know from long experience that the subsequent reproductive history of such women is poor; often they have another stillbirth, a ruptured uterus, or a recurrent fistula if their labors are unattended. Women who develop a fistula (particularly those who do so during their first pregnancies) often desperately want to have another, living, child. No one wants to experience the agony of obstructed labor, another stillbirth, and possibly a recurrent fistula.

Patients who undergo successful fistula repair are discharged from the hospital in Addis Ababa or from one of the regional fistula centers with a new dress and the advice to return in the eighth month of a subsequent pregnancy so that they can be delivered by Cesarean section before they go into labor. In the past few years, the Hamlin fistula hospitals have begun providing obstetric care to former fistula patients who have again become pregnant. In March 2013, Dr. Fekade Ayenachew, the medical director of the Addis Ababa Fistula Hospital, performed the first on-site Cesarean delivery of a fistula patient. Careful follow-up like this for fistula patients will further improve reproductive outcomes and lessen the likelihood of recurrent fistulas. It also provides an opportunity for patient and community education about the risks of obstructed labor and the need for better obstetric services.

Beyond the Eradication of Fistula

Since the fall of the Derg and the restoration of a freer society, Ethiopia has experienced remarkable economic progress. Gross domestic product has increased in Ethiopia by nearly 11 percent per year over the past decade. Although still a relatively poor nation, Ethiopia is poised to become a "middle-income country" within the next ten years. The hope is that this increasing prosperity will be widely shared by the population, especially by its women, and that this will be reflected in improvements in maternal and child health. The government of Ethiopia has declared its intention to eradicate obstetric fistula by 2020. Although this is an extremely ambitious goal, achieving it is not beyond the bounds of possibility. Undoubtedly there will be isolated pockets in remote areas where fistulas will continue to occur, but in many areas home deliveries attended by untrained lay midwives or relatives of the pregnant woman are already declining. These traditional home births are being replaced by deliveries in health centers where laboring women are attended by skilled professionals (like Hamlin midwives). For example, in Tigray, in the far north of Ethiopia, the percentage of deliveries occurring in health facilities is now over 60 percent and continuing to rise. The Hamlin Fistula Center in Mekelle (the main catchment facility for women with fistulas in this region) is beginning to see a decline in the number fistula cases, and rigorous outreach programs to rural areas are discovering fewer and fewer women with these injuries. This is very encouraging.

But reproductive life for Ethiopian women remains difficult, particularly in rural areas. Motherhood and childbearing remain the focus of Ethiopian women's lives: 44 percent of the population is under the age of 14. According to data compiled in the *CIA World Factbook*, the rate of population growth in Ethiopia is high (2.9 percent per year), with 37.3 births per 1,000 population and a contraceptive prevalence rate of only 29 percent. A woman's average age at first birth is less than 20, and she can expect to bear more than five children in the course of her reproductive life. Only 41 percent of Ethiopian women are literate, and most will go to school for six years or less. Because most women live in rural areas, they are heavily engaged in agriculture and the heavy physical labor that rural life entails: hauling firewood, hauling water, tilling the fields by hand, lifting heavy burdens, such as clearing rocks from the fields. The combination of high fertility, multiple births, marginal nutrition, heavy agricultural labor, and high rates of obstructed labor produce other problems: behind the tragedy of obstetric fistula another looming medical problem is coming into view: utero-vaginal prolapse.

The word "prolapse," when used with respect to a bodily organ, means "to slip out of place, to fall downward and outward," usually protruding outside the body. Like obstetric fistula, prolapse of the genital organs is another sex-specific malady that afflicts women almost exclusively. The anatomy that allows a full-term fetus to pass through the birth canal in the middle of the pelvis and to exit the vagina also creates weaknesses of support for the surrounding pelvic organs: the uterus, vagina, and bladder. The male pelvis is closed except for a small urethral opening through the penis that allows the passage of urine and semen, and for the anus, which allows defecation to occur; but in the female not only are the bladder, urethra, and rectum weakly supported anatomically; this anatomic support is frequently damaged during delivery of a child, especially if labor is obstructed. Much of this damage occurs to the muscles that normally hold the genital opening (genital hiatus) closed. Over time, injury to the pelvic nerves, connective tissue, muscular supports, and ligaments causes the bladder, vagina, and uterus to sag out of position. When heavy physical labor is added to this, the supports give way, and the uterus and surrounding tissues bulge out through the vagina. At first, this may only be a nuisance, with occasional discomfort; but when it becomes more advanced, the entire uterus may fall outside the body, causing pain, ulcers to the vaginal tissues, obstruction of urination or defecation, and an inability to have sexual relations—serious problems indeed.

It is now apparent that vast numbers of women in Ethiopia have untreated pelvic organ prolapse. A recent survey of more than 23,000 women in 113 villages in three rural zones in Ethiopia carried out by Hamlin Fistula found a fistula prevalence of 6 cases per 10,000 women of reproductive age, but only 2 *untreated* fistula cases per 10,000 women. The combination of decades of outreach to provide fistula surgery and the increasing numbers of women undergoing institutional as opposed to home delivery have started to reduce the number of fistula sufferers in Ethiopia. In contrast, 1 percent of the female population (100 per 10,000 women of reproductive age) suffer from symptomatic pelvic organ prolapse. In absolute terms, the authors estimate that there are now only 5,000 untreated fistula cases throughout Ethiopia, but at least 200,000 cases of utero-vaginal prolapse. It is still incredibly difficult to be a woman in the bottom billion of the world's population.

These data present a clear challenge to the Hamlin organization. With an estimated 5,000 untreated fistulas scattered throughout Ethiopia, there is still plenty of surgical repair work to be done, but the decreasing number of cases also means that institutions dedicated solely to fistula care will slowly become less relevant to women's healthcare needs as the patterns of disease and injury change. To meet this challenge—and also to train the generations of doctors who will guide Ethiopian gynecology in the future—Hamlin Fistula has joined an ambitious partnership with Mekelle University in northern Ethiopia and the Worldwide Fistula Fund to create the first fellowship training program in urogynecology and reconstructive pelvic surgery in Ethiopia. The three-year program is open to graduates of Ethiopian residency programs in obstetrics and gynecology and will train them not only to become expert fistula surgeons but also to master the techniques of pelvic organ prolapse repair and the complex procedures in reconstructive urology (such as continent urinary diversion and ureteral reimplantation surgery) that are generally outside the scope of the clinical practice of gynecologists in the industrialized world. The program is approved by the federal Ministry of Education and accredited by Mekelle University, through which the graduates will receive a subspecialty certificate in urogynecology. It is an official Ethiopian program, designed for Ethiopian needs.

Hamlin Fistula has blossomed into something its founders never would have imagined possible when they started their work more than 50 years ago. When they first encountered these urinary pilgrims, a vesico-vaginal fistula from obstructed labor was an injury that hardly ever occurred among women in affluent countries. In Australia and New Zealand, in Britain, in Canada and in the United States, the vesico-vaginal fistula from obstructed labor was an exotic curiosity of medical history, not a grim reality of reproductive life. Ethiopia slapped Reginald and Catherine awake both professionally and spiritually and pushed them into an unexpected venture to which they devoted their lives. From seeds tentatively sown in the rocky ground of the Princess Tsehai Gynecology Department, starting with a few beds in the general gynecology ward (with patients hiding under stairwells and camped out on the hospital grounds), Hamlin Fistula has grown to encompass a tertiary care specialist fistula hospital, five regional medical centers, a rehabilitation complex, and a school of midwifery. The impact of Hamlin Fistula on healthcare in Ethiopia has been profound. It has kept a spotlight on the reproductive health needs of women who otherwise would have been neglected. While emphasizing the importance of individualized care, the institution has nonetheless managed to tackle the intertwined problems of fistula prevention, surgical cure, and physical and psychosocial rehabilitation. The Addis Ababa Fistula Hospital has trained fistula surgeons from all over the world who now work to alleviate the suffering of women with these preventable childbirth injuries from Senegal to Afghanistan and beyond. In so doing Hamlin Fistula has consistently emphasized the importance of tending to the needs of the whole woman—not simply repairing the hole in her bladder. It is no wonder that Catherine Hamlin has twice been nominated for the Nobel Peace Prize.

The success of Hamlin Fistula in Ethiopia has been due to its unfaltering guidance by an ethical vision that demands that women are treated with compassion, respect, and justice. Recognizing that the roots of the fistula problem lie in the inequalities of the country's social and economic structure (which mean that poor rural women suffer disproportionately both because they are women and because they are poor), Hamlin Fistula has been able to provide world-class curative surgical care, to emphasize the dignity and importance of each woman no matter where she is from, and to work toward raising the quality and accessibility of midwifery care within the country, so that ultimately no woman should have to give birth without adequate medical assistance. Although the complete transformation of the position of women in Ethiopia—or any other country—is the responsibility of that country's government, visionary activists like Reg and Catherine Hamlin can wield a disproportionate influence in the debates over women's health, women's rights, and women's lives. Such conversations—in which the voices of dedicated activists are loudly heard—can transform the world and lead to the ultimate eradication of obstetric fistula from the human experience.

Lessons Learned and the Way Forward

Pregnancy and childbirth are not diseases. They are normal physiological processes by which the human species is perpetuated; but like all biological events, they often run imperfectly. They are prone to failure and they are vulnerable to innumerable maladies. From basic subcellular components all the way to the complex integrated physiology necessary to sustain life, biological systems are faulty, fragile, subject to disease, and prone to misadventure. Tragedy results when things go wrong. The biological burden of human reproduction falls upon females who carry and bear our young. Females are subject to these (potentially fatal) risks by genetic chance alone. The genetic lottery that randomly allocates the presence or absence of a Y chromosome to a father's gametes determines which of his offspring will be female, and thus at risk for possible reproductive misadventure and injury later in her life. Childbirth injury happens to women through no fault of their own. They are the victims of reproductive biology gone awry.

The anatomical changes in the human pelvis necessitated by upright, bipedal locomotion collided with progressively increasing brain size over millions of years of hominin evolution to produce the human obstetrical dilemma: how to get babies with big brains and big bodies through a relatively narrow pelvis whose shape is convoluted and whose planes are misaligned. As a result of these biological constraints, the mechanics of human childbirth are slow, painful, complex, and difficult as the fetus is moved through the birth canal by the contracting uterus during parturition. In about 5 percent of cases labor becomes obstructed. From the standpoint of biology, this is just part of the natural history of childbirth. Many organisms die in the process of reproducing; humans too.

When obstructed labor is not treated promptly and properly but instead lingers for days, it may result in catastrophic, life-changing injuries such as a vesico-vaginal fistula. Obstetric fistula formation is also part of the natural history of childbirth, as Queen Henhenit and others have learned to their sorrow. These childbirth injuries render miserable the lives of the women who are afflicted by them. Although medicine, science, and technology have eliminated these problems among their affluent sisters in industrialized countries, even today avoidable childbirth injuries like fistula cause immeasurable suffering for millions of poor women among the bottom billion of the world's population.

Obstetric fistulas have been surgically curable for over 150 years. For well over 75 years the major causes of maternal mortality—hemorrhage, infection, pregnancy-induced hypertensive disorders like preeclampsia and eclampsia, obstructed labor, and complications of unsafe abortion—have been treatable using low-technology, easily implementable solutions: blood transfusion, drugs to make the uterus contract after delivery, antibiotics, surgical curettage of retained placental tissue left behind in the uterus after birth, medications to lower blood pressure and prevent seizures, instrumental vaginal delivery, and Cesarean section. When these technologies became available to all child-bearing women in industrialized countries during the twentieth century, maternal mortality plummeted to previously unimaginable low levels. In the process, obstetric fistulas vanished as a public health problem in these countries. This has not yet happened among the world's poorest childbearers, and it is inexcusable.

With the scientific knowledge and medical technology that now exist, all women everywhere have an inalienable right to safe childbirth. They have this right because they are individuals worthy in themselves, not merely because they are the reproductive machinery of human societies, not merely because they are fields to be "tilled" by men in order to produce a "harvest" of children. The technologies to accomplish safe motherhood—and the economic resources to do so—exist, but they have not been distributed effectively, justly, or systematically to all of the women of the world. The unequal distribution of healthcare resources is especially notable among the world's poorest women, who continue to die and to sustain crippling childbirth injuries unfairly and unnecessarily. This is a clear and spectacular instance of gendered structural violence. This must change.

From a practical political standpoint, this change must begin by convincing men of the stake that they themselves have in women's reproductive health. All men have mothers, most have wives, some have sisters and daughters. No man wishes to see harm come to the women he loves, much less reproductive harm that ends in crippling injuries or death. Men and women all want flourishing families and offspring who are successful themselves.

All too often human reproductive biology is regarded as embarrassing, private, not to be spoken of, or a gendered domain that—because women are the childbearers—is regarded as only the business of women. When these conditions exist (especially in strongly patriarchal societies) men are likely to regard women's reproductive affairs as unseemly, disgusting, or unworthy of (or improper for) their attention. Not only is this attitude wrong, it is stupid. Both sexes have huge stakes in women's reproductive health, both at the personal, familial level as well as at the level of society. There is abundant evidence that societies thrive when girls and women are healthy and well educated. Not only do educated women make better wives and mothers who are better able to take care of their families, but in an increasingly globalized world economy, no society can afford to waste half of its available brainpower if it hopes to be competitive. The education of girls and women helps delay childbearing until a more suitable biological age. It leads to increased use of health facilities and improves both the maternal and neonatal outcomes of pregnancy. High rates of maternal death and the continuing prevalence of obstetric fistulas are markers of inequality and injustice in those corners of the world where gender equity does not yet exist.

The eradication of obstetric fistula is simple, in the sense that it is straightforward, not necessarily in the sense that it will be easy to accomplish. The process of eradicating obstetric fistula must begin by making sure that every woman in the world delivers her children in the presence of a skilled birth attendant who can summon emergency care when complications arise. Such deliveries must be accomplished in an atmosphere of compassion, respect, and justice (which includes technical competence as one of its fundamental components) if the healthcare system is to be valued and is to produce the desired results. People no matter where they live must hold their governments accountable for creating health systems that provide such services and for creating the communication and transportation infrastructures that tie its component parts together in an effective manner. The medical, nursing, and midwifery professions must likewise be held accountable for providing competent, respectful, ethical care to all pregnant women. These professionals must serve as advocates for childbearing women to ensure that effective policies and programs are put in place to eliminate fistulas and to reduce maternal mortality.

Competent, compassionate, respectful care must also be provided to those unfortunate women who have developed obstetric fistulas as complications of human reproductive physiology gone awry. This care is a basic human right and should not be contingent upon a woman's economic resources. The technical clinical challenges presented by fistula patients strongly suggests that their care is best provided in specialized fistula centers like the Addis Ababa Fistula Hospital in Ethiopia or the Danja Fistula Center in Niger, where the focus of every activity is on healing the physical and the psychosocial injuries these women have sustained. The injuries suffered by the women of the bottom billion is a direct manifestation of the structural violence that has been directed toward them by the societies in which they live. To recover from their injuries they must find a place within a therapeutic community that welcomes them and helps them heal. Recognition that they all belong to a "sisterhood of suffering" as a result of their shared experiences in childbirth is a powerful bond. Within that bond lie opportunities to provide economic rehabilitation and life-skills training in addition to medical and surgical intervention. These women often need such help if they are to rebuild social lives that have been sundered by catastrophic childbirth injuries.

The sisterhood of suffering among fistula patients is very real. Recall again the Hausa song "Fitsari 'Dan Duniya" that was analyzed in chapter 5. The full impact of this song cannot be appreciated without seeing it performed. Picture a church on a hospital compound, filled with 150 or 200 women, many of them fistula patients themselves. Drums are thundering out an interwoven series of polyphonic rhythms. Many of the congregants have recently had surgery and are carefully carrying small plastic basins into which the open ends of their catheters are draining (the luxury of disposable closed urinary drainage systems is often beyond the budget of many African hospitals). Other women, yet to have their operations, simply dribble onto the floor. It doesn't matter. All are welcome—this is their community, their sisterhood. The leader calls out the verses, and the congregants respond, loudly and enthusiastically. The air is split with the ululations of celebration, interspersed with rhythmic clapping. The lines of dancers form in the aisles at the front of the church and weave through the congregation. The building is awash in unfettered exuberance at the joy of deliverance or in the expectation that it soon will come.

To have danced with the fistula patients is to be submerged in a unique community of caring, which is bound together by an almost indescribable knowledge of the nature of suffering. To have danced with the fistula patients is to recall why you went into medicine in the first place and to mourn what we in the West have lost, in spite of our advanced healthcare, affluent economies, and technical expertise. To have danced with the fistula patients drives home the importance of compassion, respect, and justice, and to realize that with these three things, the world may yet be transformed.

ACKNOWLEDGMENTS

It is hard to know just where to begin to acknowledge the many people who have somehow contributed to this book, which has been in gestation for more than 20 years. I have accumulated many personal debts in that period of time.

I entered medical school (still trying to write my doctoral dissertation) after completing nearly two years of anthropological field research in northern Nigeria, and for a decade thereafter I was totally immersed in rigorous clinical training. I appeared to be headed in a totally different direction. My late, great friend Dr. Tom Elkins (a.k.a. "The Big Guy") opened the door for me to create a career which combined anthropology and medicine, when as the new chair, he recruited me to the Department of Obstetrics and Gynecology at the Louisiana State University Medical Center in New Orleans with a mandate to work in West Africa and to develop one of the first US fellowship programs in urogynecology. We both got much more than we had bargained for in New Orleans. The story of our time there together is far stranger than fiction; it could easily be the stuff of novels and screenplays (someday, perhaps). Tom's premature death at the age of 48 was a terrible tragedy that deprived the world of a wonderful, compassionate, visionary medical leader with a strong sense of ethics and the courage to stand up against corruption and injustice. I miss him.

Dr. Jane Bertrand and Dr. Barnett Cline welcomed me into the School of Public Health and Tropical Medicine at Tulane University (International Health and Development, and Tropical Medicine, respectively) and expanded my horizons considerably.

Dr. Doug Brown and I have discussed issues in medical ethics generally, and the topics discussed in this book specifically, over many years and in many places, ranging from O'Reilly's Tavern in New Orleans, to kitchen tables, and our own back yards.

Dr. Catherine Hamlin of the Addis Ababa Fistula Hospital has been a continuing inspiration for as long as I have known her. I hope this book does justice to her vision and her work.

I have had an ongoing conversation for many years about obstetric fistula with Nick Kristof, intrepid champion of the "bottom billion" at the *New York Times*. He has done more to bring the fistula issue to the world's attention than almost anyone I can think of, and, without his support, the Danja Fistula Center would never have been possible. The pen is truly mightier than the sword.

Greg and Melissa Fleming provided substantial personal and financial support to help make the Danja Fistula Center a reality.

Lynn and Mike Coatney have been generous supporters of this work and good friends for decades. My debts to them are almost incalculable.

At Washington University in St. Louis, I owe debts of thanks and friendship to Dr. Jim Schreiber and Dr. Dave Mutch, who recruited me to join the Department of Obstetrics and Gynecology. Dr. George Macones allowed my international career to flourish and provided both permission to go and generous financial support for my stay as a Fulbright Scholar at Mekelle University in northern Ethiopia.

On the Danforth campus of Washington University, I owe an enormous amount to Dr. Richard Smith, who as chair of the Department of Anthropology, took a gamble on allowing me to teach a course that I proposed to him called "Anthropology of Human Birth," and to Dr. T. R. Kidder, his successor in that role, who embraced me warmly as a full-time member of the faculty. David and Paulina Conner created the Selina Okin Kim Conner Professorship in Arts and Sciences through a generous endowment to the university, and Chancellor Mark Wrighton stunned me by naming me as the first holder of that chair. I am deeply grateful to all of them. Writing this book would not have been possible without their support.

Egyptologists Dr. Joyce Tyldesley of Manchester, England, and Dr. Chrystal Goud-souzian, of Memphis, Tennessee, reviewed my treatment of Queen Henhenit and made many helpful suggestions. Any Egyptological defects that remain are my own responsibility.

Kelley Squazzo and Robin Coleman guided this book through Johns Hopkins University Press with care and attention. Carrie Watterson's meticulous copyediting made this book much better than the original manuscript that I turned in. I am deeply grateful to all of them for their assistance.

Drs. Steve and Jan Arrowsmith have been the source of many courtesies and kindnesses on multiple fistula-related trips to various African countries. Steve in particular has taught me an enormous amount about fistula surgery.

In Niger, I owe debts of thanks of Steve Schmidt, Chad and Amanda Winsor, Bert and Elaine Haaga, Bunmi Oluloto, Dr. Itengre Ouedraogo and his wife Rasmata, the intrepid pilots of SIMAir, and all of the service and support personnel at SIM-Niger.

In Ghana I have benefited greatly from my long friendships with Drs. Demi and Anyetei Lassey, Dr. Kwabena Danso, Dr. Henry Opare-Addoh, Dr. E. Y. Kwawukume, Dr. Ali Samba, Dr. Cecil Klufio, and Prof. J. B. Wilson. I owe much to the late Dr. J. O. Martey, who did so much to help build residency education in obstetrics and gynecology in Ghana. The late Dr. T. S. Ghosh, Ghana's pioneer fistula surgeon, gave me valuable instruction early in my career.

My debts in Nigeria run deep as well. With respect to maternal health and obstetric fistulas, I am indebted to Professor Kelsey Harrison, Dr. Nimi Briggs, Dr. Carolyn Kirschner, and especially to *babban abokina*, Dr. Jonathan Karshima.

I also have to thank Dr. Abo Hassan Abo, the late Dr. John Kelly, Dr. Andrew Browning, Dr. Frank Asiimwe, and Alice Emasu for numerous enlightening conversations regarding obstetric fistula at various times and places in Africa, the United States, and Europe.

To acknowledge all my debts to Ethiopian friends and colleagues would require a book in itself. I especially thank Dr. Melaku Abreha, Dr. Yibrah Berhe, Eyoel Berhan, Dr. Loko Abraham, Shewaye Belay, Dr. Kindeya Gebrihiwot, Dr. Angesom Kebede, Dr. Samson Mulugeta, Dr. Hagos Gidey, Dr. Zerihun Abebe, Dr. Yazezew Kebede, Dr. Amanuel Haile, Dr. Fekade Ayenachew, Beletchatschew Tedesse, Dean Zelalem Belete, Martin and Harriet Andrews, Alison Shigo, and, most especially, "our Ethiopian family": Freweini Mebrahtu, Sami, Gideon, and Mariam.

I have enjoyed much camaraderie and useful work with colleagues involved with the Worldwide Fistula Fund. I acknowledge especially Benson Smith (who has been a trouper since the organization's founding), John Adams, Dr. Nancy Muller, Dr. Chris Payne, Dr. Rahel Nardos, Dr. Tracy Spitznagle, Michael Wittek, Soja Orlowski, Casey Shipman, and especially Wendy Weiser. Jeanette Bax-Kurtz has been a loyal and powerful stabilizing influence behind the scenes in many different capacities, with many different projects, over several decades.

Within the Hamlin Fistula organization (worldwide), I offer thanks to the many loyal supporters of the Hamlin fistula hospitals in Ethiopia. I especially thank Julie Rosenberg for service above and beyond the call of duty. In the United States I owe special thanks to Joe Kinahan, Steve Sockolov, Katie Baggley, and Dr. Senait Fisseha for their service to the organization.

Eugene New has been drawing medical illustrations for me for many years, including some in this book. Sophia Brown redrew the figures on maternal death rates and Cesarean section from the sources cited.

Numerous people have read and commented upon various parts of this book in several drafts. In some cases, they have given me diametrically opposed suggestions! The book is much better as a result of their observations, but any defects that remain are my own responsibility. For their services I would like to thank (in alphabetical order): Dr. Fekade Ayenachew, Dean Zelalem Belete, Drs. Lars and Sarah Breimer, David Conner, Dr. Peter English, Melissa Fleming, Robin Hart, Dr. Ali Heller, Malcolm Hewitt, Mary Lehoczky, Natasha Myers, Lord Naren Patel, Dr. Peter Petros, Julie Rosenberg, Dr. Todd Savitt, Dr. Tracy Spitznagle, Sara Veltkamp, Helen Wall, Jimmy Wall, Julie White, and Dr. Jeff Wilkinson.

The deepest and most important acknowledgements are to family. In his autobiography, *Out of My Life and Thought*, theologian-physician-humanitarian Albert Schweitzer remarked of his childhood that "it struck me as incomprehensible that I should be allowed to lead such a happy life, while I saw so many people around me wrestling with care and suffering." Anyone who studies anthropology will immediately recognize that much of what we are is determined by where and to whom we are born. My brother, Terry, and I "won life's lottery" by having most fortunate births.

Our parents, Evelyn and Leonard Wall, were members of what Tom Brokaw called the "Greatest Generation," those who suffered through the Great Depression and fought (and won) the Second World War. They were hardworking, perseverant, humble, kind, honest, generous, and extraordinarily loving people.

My mother, Evelyn, was a dynamic, engaging, fun-loving, and deeply empathetic woman. She was passionate about the cause of obstetric fistula and raised (as well as personally donated) tens of thousands of dollars toward its treatment and eradication. If compassion alone were enough to eradicate obstetric fistula, my mother could have done it by herself.

My father, Dr. Leonard A. Wall, repeatedly emphasized to me as a child that the most important thing in life was to be born wanted and loved. Never for a minute did I doubt that this was true in my case. Dad went into obstetrics and gynecology as the result of his horrific experiences fighting in World War II (part of which was spent as a prisoner of war). He wanted to be a force in helping bring new life into the world— and he was. He was also dedicated to the cause of obstetric fistula. Among the most memorable of my life experiences were our travels together in Ghana, Nigeria, and Ethiopia to investigate aspects of the fistula problem when he was in his 80s. He accompanied me on my first visit to Addis Ababa in 1995 and became good friends with Dr. Catherine Hamlin, with whom he had much in common. More than anything, it was his example that made me decide (rather late) to become a doctor and (to my shock and his quiet amusement) ultimately to pursue a career in obstetrics and gynecology, in spite of my previous vociferous, lifelong disavowals of any such inclination. He rose from rural poverty in the Oklahoma Dust Bowl to become a leading member of the medical community in Kansas City, the "obstetrician's obstetrician," supremely competent, hardworking, reliable, caring, and utterly devoted to his patients. This book is dedicated to his memory.

My brother, Terry, who also became a physician (but not an obstetrician), has devoted much time, effort, and money to the cause of obstetric fistula, serving (as did our father) on the board of directors of the Worldwide Fistula Fund. I value his integrity, his dedication, his counsel, his generosity, his love, and his friendship.

My wife, Helen, is my greatest friend and most loyal supporter. I cannot begin to describe the many contributions she has made both to my life and to the fistula cause. She has devoted many hundreds of hours to fistula-related fundraising, bookkeeping, and administrative tasks, serving on the Worldwide Fistula Fund board while traveling with me to places most people would find difficult and unpleasant at best. She has "kept the home-fires burning" throughout my medical career, especially when our sons—Jimmy and Thom—were young. One indication of the impact that my overseas travels was having on family life occurred one morning when the boys were still in elementary school. One of them looked up at breakfast and asked Helen, rather quizzically, "Mom, is Dad in Africa again?" To which she replied, "No, Dear. He's in the bathroom. He'll be out in a minute."

My final and most important debt is to the hundreds of women suffering from obstetric fistulas whom I have met over the years. The purpose of this book is to help the world hear their stories and to end this terrible scourge. It's about time.

The Controversy concerning Sims's Experimental Surgeries on Slaves

In the second edition of his monograph on vesico-vaginal fistula published in 1968, the British obstetrician-gynecologist J. Chassar Moir wrote of "the skill—almost legerdemain—of Sims and Emmet" and noted that in spite of modern advances in surgical lighting, anesthesia, and antisepsis, "Sims's position, Sims's speculum, and Sims's silver wire could achieve the seemingly impossible a century ago, and they can do so now." He concluded his positive assessment of Sims and his surgical procedures for vesico-vaginal fistula repair by writing the following:

> The treatment of vesico-vaginal fistula has a fascination of its own. No branch of surgery calls for greater resource, never is patience so sorely tried, and never is success more dependent on the exercise of constant care both during operation and, even more perhaps, during the anxious days of convalescence. But never is reward greater. Nothing can equal the gratitude of the woman who, wearied from constant pain, depressed by an ever-growing sense of the humiliating nature of her infirmity, and desperate with the realization that her very presence is an offence to others, finds suddenly that she is restored to full health and able to resume a rightful place in the family—who finds, as it were, that life has been given anew and that she has again become a citizen of the world. To J. Marion Sims, more than to any man, is due the honour for this transformation. And if in these days a moment can be spared for sentimental reverie, look again, I beg, at the curious speculum and, gazing through the confused reflections from its bright curves, catch a fleeting glimpse of an old hut in Alabama and seven negro women who suffered, and endured, and had rich reward.

In 1976, this generally positive (perhaps even laudatory) view of Sims started to change with the publication of a peculiar book by G. J. Barker Benfield entitled *The Horrors of the Half-Known Life: Male Attitudes towards Women and Sexuality in Nineteenth-Century America.* Sims was one of the central figures in this book, where he was portrayed as a ruthless, domineering misogynist who cynically—and cruelly—exploited helpless females (slaves and otherwise) to advance his personal medical career. A product of the social turbulence of America in the 1960s and 1970s, when venerable institutions of all kinds were being reevaluated or attacked, when both the feminist movement and the civil rights movement were becoming important social forces and opposition to the Vietnam War was calling traditional values and political processes into questions, the book resonated with certain aspects of the popular zeitgeist.

But *The Horrors of the Half-Known Life* was a book of abysmally bad scholarship. It was uniformly demolished in professional academic journals by historians and social scientists alike. Sociologist Michael Gordon summed up his reaction to Barker-Benfield's book by writing, "From a sociological perspective this is, in most respects, a rather unsatisfactory book. . . . [T]he author relies almost exclusively on the interpretation of literary material, and his interpretation is strongly informed by a rather fundamental brand of psychoanalytic thinking. To make matters worse, the writing is rather turgid and various sections of the book are not well integrated." In *Reviews of American History*, Anita Clair Fellman and Michael Fellman observed:

> The engine driving this book is a strange and bitter vision of fundamental male hatred of women. Women are merely projectees, nonexistent in any other manner than as the victims of raging, misogynist, self-loathing men. Destroyed generally in male fantasy, women are literally tortured and mutilated by men's representatives, male doctors. . . . Fantasy and reality blur in this book in a seemingly intentional manner. Nevertheless, the intellectual argument is muddled and presented in somewhat conflicting versions, and the prose is often vague and frequently royal purple. . . . Barker-Benfield frequently chooses the most extreme and implicitly sadistic reading possible. Thus the real purpose of Sims's surgery was vaginal warfare; surgery was the legitimized version of rape. . . . Sims is portrayed generally as a sadist, operating inhumanly and maniacally first on poor women, "the supply of human material" dredged up for him first from southern slave quarters, and then from northern, urban slums. Later he mutilated rich women, because he also resented them. By extension, doctors had no sincere desire to help women in distress, nor even essentially ambivalent motives. They only wished to inflict pain and to use women's bodies as a means of male conquest and success. . . . *The Horrors* is written utterly without reservation, humor, or irony; it ends up being a caricature in the name of psychohistory.

The most damning review of Barker-Benfield's book, however, appeared in the country's most prestigious medical history journal, the *Bulletin of the History of Medicine*, by respected medical historian Regina Morantz. She began her lengthy review of *The Horrors of the Half-Known Life* by questioning what "serious historians" were to make of it, calling it "a persistently annoying work—often ahistorical, frequently speculative, and only occasionally sensitive to the traditional principles of historical inquiry." In the following three and a half pages, she proceeded systematically to eviscerate the book as the product of inept, if not downright incompetent, historical research. She accused Barker-Benfield of engaging in "ingenious distortions of the past." "Apparently freed by his own a priori reasoning to pick and choose among the various bits of evidence," she wrote, "he remains undaunted by factors like chronology, data, statistics and methodology." "It is, in fact, in his treatment of the American medical profession, symbolized for Benfield by the rise of surgical gynecology, that the author makes his most fantastic forays into the art of historical fiction. Although Benfield grudgingly admits that the emergence of modern gynecology 'in some sense . . . may be construed to have advanced medicine,' he prefers to see the development of the specialty as a conspiracy against women by hostile, insecure men." His methodology is shoddy: "Benfield's generalizations about the medical profession are based upon a highly selective and idiosyncratic examination of the careers of just two men—J. Marion Sims and Augustus Kinsley Gardiner. Even allowing for the book's limited cast of characters, however, Benfield's Sims is a grotesque, imprisoned in a world of sexual fantasy. His interest in gynecology is portrayed as an outgrowth of both his hostility toward women and his ferociously competitive instincts." Only negative thoughts about Sims are allowed within the book: "Sims is pictured as incapable of purer or more complex motives." The basic problem with the book, however, is simply this: "Benfield is ignorant of the history of medical therapeutics." The book is work of amateur psychoanalysis based on superficial research and in many places it is nothing more than a speculative critique of Sims's autobiography. "Unfortunately," Morantz writes, "Benfield's cast of characters are not flesh and blood actors in the past. Their behavior is solely a function of their gender. They respond, not as doctors, lawyers, ministers, fathers, politicians, but exclusively and mechanistically as anxious males. Women, too, are merely figments of the male imagination. They exist solely to shape men's perceptions of reality."

With a stake driven so resolutely through its heart, one would think that the book would have died a quiet death, bleeding out its purple prose on dusty library shelves, remainder bins, and the back rooms of seedy secondhand bookshops. *The Horrors of the Half-Known Life*, however, has turned out to be a prime example of what Princeton economist and New York Times columnist Paul Krugman called "zombie ideas": "ideas that keep being killed by evidence, but nonetheless shamble relentlessly forward, essentially because they suit a political agenda." Barker-Benfield's view of J. Marion Sims as a sort of "antebellum Joseph Mengele" torturing helpless female slaves is a zombie idea. Sims has become a particular kind of "meme."

The concept of the "meme" was coined by evolutionary biologist Richard Dawkins in his book *The Selfish Gene*. He used it to refer to a self-replicating unit of cultural transmission—seen as analogous to a gene in the field of genetics. A meme, by definition, is a bit, not a whole. It is a piece of intellectual flotsam or jetsam, swirling through the currents of popular thought. It is a "factoid," not a fact, used in popular bricolage to buttress a worldview, rather than something that has resulted from critical historical research. Its main characteristic is "truthiness," not truth.

"Truthiness" is a concept popularized by the comedian Stephen Colbert, which (according to the American Dialect Society) means "the quality of preferring concepts or facts one wishes to be true, rather than concepts or facts known to be true." This approach to historical events—making them what one wishes them to have been, rather than what they actually were—is part of the phenomenon that historian Herbert Butterfield called the Whig interpretation of history: "the study of the past with direct and perpetual reference to the present."

This pernicious approach to history extracts events from their historical context and judges them solely from the perspective of the present. This inevitably involves abridgement, simplification, distortion, and quite often—as is certainly true in the case of how Sims has been presented by these authors—the deliberate falsification of historical facts to make the narrative confirm to a predetermined judgment. As Butterfield noted, "For the compilation of trenchant history there is nothing like being content with half the truth." A common feature of these writers is that, while they are intent on passing moral judgments on past events, "it is really something in the present that the historian is most anxious about."

That "something" in the present may be a truly righteous cause—such as the exploitation of workers, the degradation of women, poverty, racial injustice, lack of access to decent medical care, and such like—but hammering past events into a predetermined mold to produce the story you want to hear only recapitulates the conclusion you reached before starting out. As Butterfield wrote, "If we look for things in the course of history only because we have found them already in the world of today . . . the upshot of all our history is only to send us back finally to the place where we began, and to ratify whatever conceptions we originally had in regard to our own times." While it is indeed possible to mount the steed of moral outrage and to ride it all the way to a national book award (as Harriet Washington has done with her book *Medical Apartheid: The Dark History of Medical Experimentation on Black Americans from Colonial Times to the Present*)—the end result is still bad history. When the past is seen only in the light of incandescent indignation about present circumstances, that light distorts the past rather than illuminates it.

Sims's early surgical attempts to cure the vesico-vaginal fistula must be understood within their proper historical context. To locate Sims's surgeries within that context the historian must understand the nature of the injury itself (the end product of a prolonged obstructed labor), the clinical context of the patients with this condition (the real-life experience of a woman with a vesico-vaginal fistula), the medico-historical context (the lived realities of clinical practice in the 1840s, including a familiarity with the medical literature and practice of the time), the ethical context (the generally accepted principles of early nineteenth-century medical ethics), and the legal framework in which his operations were carried out (including the legal status of slaves). None of Sims's modern critics comes close to meeting these basic prerequisites in their analysis of his early surgical operations. To do this properly would require an entire monograph; however, at least nine fundamental flaws in the revisionist approach to Sims can be outlined briefly. Many of these operate as unquestioned fundamental assumptions to their approach, which lead to skewed results because they begin from flawed starting points.

1. Sims's modern critics lack clinical experience in obstetrics and gynecology generally, and they are particularly lacking in experience with vesico-vaginal fistula repair. The vast majority of Sims's critics are nonclinicians who are unfamiliar with obstructed labor and who do not understand the awful damage it does. They are likewise unfamiliar with the surgical challenges these patients present. They look with incredulity at the repeated failed operations these women underwent without understanding the reasons for the failures and the determination—common among fistula sufferers worldwide—to try one more time to escape the hell into which their injuries had thrust them. They focus on Sims's personal surgical failures while ignoring the fact that such failures were the norm at that time. They also ignore how common such failures are today, particularly in the low-technology settings found in Africa and Asia, where these injuries are prevalent. Careful review of the nineteenth-century surgical literature reveals numerous patients who underwent multiple attempts at surgical repair of their fistulas by numerous surgeons. Sims was by no means alone; he simply was more perseverant than most, which is one of the main reasons he was ultimately successful.

2. The lack of familiarity with obstetric fistulas leads Sims's modern critics to consistently downplay the suffering that drove these women to seek surgery. Their desperation is ignored; instead, vesico-vaginal fistula is presented as a "trivial" complaint, unworthy of surgical attention. This ignorance concerning the suffering produced by an obstetric fistula is almost always paired with the tendency to exaggerate the pain involved in fistula surgery.

3. The lack of experience in gynecologic surgery manifested by Sims's modern critics means that these authors have no realistic understanding of how painful a fistula operation would actually be, compared with other surgical operations as they were performed in the

1840s. This is not by any means to suggest that fistula surgery undertaken without anesthesia was painless, but the operations were relatively short, the motivation of the patients was very high, and, in terms of anatomy, the vagina is poorly innervated and is therefore much less sensitive to pain than the external genitalia, which is richly innervated. It is a commonplace observation in gynecological surgery that transvaginal operations are far less painful than transabdominal or intra-abdominal surgeries. Most of the pain experienced during fistula operations occurs from manipulation of the bladder, rather than from incising or suturing the overlying vagina. For that reason (as well as fear of infection and concerns about poor healing), nineteenth-century surgeons tried to avoid cutting or suturing the bladder itself during these early operations. The overlying vagina was incised, or "saucerized," and sutures were placed through the *vaginal* layer, which upon being tied down, would pull the edges of the bladder and the rest of the fistula into apposition. Many nineteenth-century authors remarked on how little pain was experienced by patients during cauterization of the fistula or even during attempted surgical closure of the fistula. Even Sir James Young Simpson, the discoverer of chloroform anesthesia and an ardent proponent of anesthesia for women during labor, did not believe that anesthesia was needed during most fistula repair operations. Indeed, at least one fistula surgeon working in Africa today has advocated routine fistula repair without anesthesia as more convenient and less troublesome for patients. (This is an assertion that I strongly contest. In any case, to do this today when safe spinal anesthesia is easy to provide and anesthetic protocols are well developed is a far different matter than employing anesthesia as soon as it had been discovered, when almost nothing was understood about its safety, its potential abuses, and its possible long-term effects.)

4. Modern critics of Sims uncritically adopt a presentist view of anesthesia when looking at the late 1840s. The modern critics being comfortably accustomed to the achievements of modern medicine (and blissfully unaware, it seems, of the disasters and abuses that propelled medicine to its current position in the twenty-first century), they immediately assume that "newer is necessarily better," and, once anesthesia was discovered, everyone should have "shouted hurrah!" and embraced it enthusiastically, uncritically, and immediately. This viewpoint ignores the deeply conservative nature of preanesthetic surgical practice, the stunning lack of major advances in therapeutics up to the middle of the nineteenth century, and legitimate concerns by prudent practitioners about the proper use of these powerful pharmacological agents. What uses of anesthesia were ethical? Was it worth the risk of possible anesthetic death to overcome pain that was generally regarded as "bearable" based on past experience? For many different reasons, it took almost thirty years before the use of anesthetics was fully embraced by the surgical community.

Sims began his fistula operations nearly two years before the discovery of ether anesthesia, using the accepted surgical processes in place at that time. He was a prudent practitioner by the standards of his time. Sims, like many other surgeons, saw no necessary benefit to change in these particular circumstances, and he was not alone. As historian Martin Pernick has written, "Our twentieth-century sensibilities recoil at the thought that sane, responsible physicians could ever have opposed the use of anesthetics. Today, the concept of operating on a fully sentient patient conjures up only hellish images of concentration camp doctors. Yet in mid-nineteenth-century America, humane, conscientious, highly reputable practitioners and ordinary lay people held many misgivings about the new discovery.

Neither sadists nor fools, these critics alleged a variety of rational drawbacks to the use of anesthesia." In fact, among those most opposed to the introduction of anesthesia were military surgeons, who, while caring for horrific battlefield injuries during the Mexican-American War refused to use ether because they thought it would weaken the constitution of soldiers, prolong their recovery from surgery, and make them unfit for service. It turned out that they were wrong, but this opinion was commonly held and was considered prudent surgical practice at the time.

While criticizing Sims for surgical innovation, Sims's critics seem united in the view that he should have started using anesthesia immediately after its discovery. Blinded by the glare of twenty-first-century anesthetic achievements, they are completely oblivious to the ethical issues posed by the introduction of anesthetic agents in the late 1840s. These powerful drugs were not evaluated systematically for safety and effectiveness before they became widely used; rather, they were introduced in a series of utterly uncontrolled experiments by individual physicians and surgeons without any standards or formal consent procedures—they very things Sims is now attacked for doing with his fistula operations.

From our modern perspective, for example, the way chloroform was introduced into clinical practice in 1847 simply beggars belief. James Young Simpson, having heard of the anesthetic properties of ether, was convinced that he could find a better anesthetic agent. He personally started experimenting by inhaling virtually every volatile chemical liquid he could lay his hands on. His "experimental procedure" consisted of organizing early morning or late afternoon "sniffing bouts" around his dining room table, aided by his colleagues Matthew Duncan and George Keith. The three would pour whatever volatile substance they had on hand into a saucer or glass, inhale the vapors and record their impressions of its effects. It was, as Simpson's biographer Morrice McCrae wrote, "a procedure that was foolhardy and even potentially lethal."

On November 4, 1847, the hardy trio of Simpson, Duncan, and Keith, accompanied by Simpson's wife Jessie and her sister Wilhelmina, along with Jessie's brother-in-law Captain Petrie and his daughter Agnes, participated in a chloroform-snorting party to see what the effects might be. George Keith went first and became impressively snockered. Delighted with what they had observed with Keith, Matthew Duncan and Simpson immediately inhaled the stuff. They became high almost immediately, being both elated and exuberantly garrulous before crashing to the floor, senseless. When Simpson awoke from his chloroform-induced stupor, he saw Matthew Duncan lying under a chair, snoring, and George Keith under the dinner table lying on his back, kicking the tabletop from below. When they had more or less recovered from their first inhalation, they snorted the stuff again and drew the ladies into their frolics as well. Simpson reportedly chased his sister-in-law, Wilhelmina, around the house with a tumbler full of chloroform trying to get her high, while she squealed and ran away from him. This continued until 3 a.m., when the chloroform finally ran out. Within a few days, Simpson was using the drug in practice, and he was even giving it to women in labor within a week.

Chloroform anesthesia thus was the product of an orgy of uncontrolled recreational drug use by members of the Edinburgh medical community. Imagine what the reaction of the modern critics would have been had Sims done something similar to his enslaved fistula patients—and imagine if the outcome had been unfavorable or even fatal in such a case. The ethical issues are just as compelling with respect to the introduction of anesthesia as they are to surgical procedures, yet the modern critics blithely ignore them on the assumption that modern anesthesiology sprang to life full-blown, safe and effective at its discovery. Nothing could be further from the truth. The early anesthetists faced enormous ethical issues and controversies in trying to find the best way forward. This history is simply excised from the story of Sims.

5. Sims's modern critics also uniformly fail to distinguish between therapeutic and nontherapeutic medical experimentation. They describe Sims's "surgical experiments on slaves" in language calculated to bring to mind the Nazi medical experiments on concentration camp inmates during the 1930s and 1940s. This is both inaccurate and blatantly unfair: the Nazi experiments were straightforward atrocities involving the senseless and sadistic abuse of helpless victims who were subjected to scientifically worthless procedures that had no possibility of benefitting them.

In more benign circumstances, nontherapeutic experimentation involves research that may contribute to medical knowledge but that will not provide any benefit to the research subjects who participate in the experiment. An example would be a person who agrees to participate in studying the metabolism of a new drug early in its development. She is given the drug voluntarily and then provides blood and urine samples every few hours to measure the blood levels and excretion of the drug that occurs after administration of a specific dose. The information is potentially valuable, but the study subject is unlikely to gain therapeutic benefit from a pharmacological study of this kind.

In a therapeutic experiment, however, the circumstances are very different. Here the study subject potentially has much to gain from participating. A classic example would be a woman with metastatic cancer in whom all previous therapies have failed. She is offered a chance to take an experimental drug to see whether she responds. In return for her participation in the drug trial, she is offered the chance of clinical benefit, perhaps even cure. This is a far different set of circumstances, and many people in such a situation jump at the chance to participate. This was, in fact, the situation for Sims's fistula patients. There was no known cure for their dehumanizing, stigmatizing obstetric fistula. If they agreed to participate, the possibility existed that they would be cured. They took a therapeutic gamble, and, in this case, eventually they won. This is very different from the way Sims is usually portrayed, but it appears to be gradually emerging as the ethically correct point of view. (See the discussion by historian Robert Baker in his comprehensive review of American medical ethics, *Before Bioethics: A History of American Medical Ethics from the Colonial Period to the Bioethics Revolution*, for example.)

6. In similar fashion, Sims's current critics typically use a late twentieth- or early twenty-first-century view of medical ethics to evaluate his early fistula surgeries. Unsurprisingly, he fails to measure up when evaluated with a modern yardstick. This is the historical fallacy of anachronism. Sims is condemned (to borrow a phrase from Herbert Butterfield) "for not being sufficiently original in [his] thoughts to rise above the rules and standards of [his] own day." How many of us would be comfortable being criticized for failing to live up to the ethical standards of the twenty-third century? We have no way of knowing what those standards might be, and therefore we cannot possibly adjust our behavior to accord with them. The best we can do *now* is to strive to reach the highest level of ethical behavior that seems possible from our present perspective. A few moral visionaries may succeed in surpassing present standards, but that is a very high bar indeed to require for the average man or woman.

Consequently, all that can be gained from using twenty-first-century standards to judge nineteenth-century behavior is, perhaps, a little more insight into our twenty-first-century standards and the difficulty of applying them.

The proper standards by which to judge Sims are the ethical standards of his own time. To evaluate Sims in this way would require the modern critic to engage in actual historical research to elucidate the then-existing ethical framework upon which to construct such a critique. None of them have done so. In the mid-1840s the prevailing standard of medical ethics was that "a doctor should act like a gentleman." Although Sims was involved in numerous controversies during his professional career, none of the charges raised against him by contemporary critics include any of the ethical lapses alleged by the modern reviewers. To date, I have not found anyone during his lifetime who accused him of being unethical by operating on slaves in the manner in which he did. Such critiques may have been made, but if so, they were not widespread and remain poorly accessible if they exist at all.

7. A common point of view with respect to Sims is to declare that the slave system was unjust and unethical, and because Sims was part of the system of slave medicine, his entire practice was unethical by default. While there is no question that the American system of racial slavery was a moral atrocity, if one adopts a universally condemnatory viewpoint like this, there is little point in proceeding with further historical research of any kind. The really illuminating historical questions are those that involve trying to understand how individuals caught up in a highly flawed economic system like plantation slavery navigated their day-to-day ethical behavior. How did a doctor make practical decisions when it came to working with slaves and slave owners? Given the fact that one lived and practiced in a slave-owning economic system, how did one act ethically? How could and how well did Sims address his patients' needs under these circumstances?

I am sure we would all cheer if Sims had become a resolute opponent of the slave system, working within to destroy it while simultaneously caring for these victimized fistula sufferers—but if Sims been an active opponent of slavery, he wouldn't have had a medical practice at all. He would have been a pauper and an outcast, shunned by white society as a whole. More likely still, had he been an active opponent of slavery living and working in Alabama in 1845, he probably would have been killed. He certainly wouldn't have become the respected and successful physician and surgeon that he was in his local community. Sims may not have been a moral giant who rose above the rules and standards of his day, but who of us are? Most of us go along to get along, doing the best we can as we see fit. Few, if any, modern surgeons would take a stand so radically at odds with the prevailing social norms of their communities and still expect to have a clinical practice. In this Sims was no different than the rest of us. If we condemn him for not being a moral genius who could see past the times in which he was living, we need to understand that almost all of us will fall short of that exacting standard as well.

8. It is common for modern critics to argue that because slaves were slaves, they couldn't consent to undergo experimental surgery. From a legal point of view, this is true. By definition, slaves were not autonomous human beings; rather, they were "a species of property." Legal consent had to be obtained from the owners of the slaves for them to receive treatment. But to use this clever turn on "consent" as an argument to condemn Sims raises other, even more awkward, questions. If it is unethical to treat those who cannot consent, and if slaves are unable to give consent, then it is unethical to provide *any* medical care to

slaves because they cannot consent to treatment. Are the modern critics really suggesting that slaves should *never* have received *any* medical or surgical treatment, no matter what their condition, because they could not consent? This is an ethically ludicrous position.

Although it is true that slaves could not give *legal* consent, slaves could certainly give *practical* consent, agreeing in their capacity as rational beings to accept treatment when they were ill or injured. Sometimes they were bitterly opposed to a proposed treatment, but sometimes they were enthusiastic participants in such care if they had the expectation of gaining relief from unbearable conditions in so doing. Long personal experience with obstetric fistula patients suggests that these women would have been *eager* to have their burden relieved. Even if they could not legally consent to surgery themselves, nonetheless they were "all in" with Sims to find a cure for their malady. Rather than being the unwilling victims of sadistic experiments, they were active participants in Sims's attempts to solve the problem of fistula closure. Reconstructive surgery—putting something back together so that it works again—is more difficult than extirpative surgery—removing something, cutting something off, or taking something out. Extirpative surgery (such as the amputation of a limb) can often be carried out quickly, sometimes brutally. Carefully trying to put the edges back together so that a fistula is closed is delicate, painstaking work that requires the cooperation of the patient—just like Sims's operation for congenital double harelip. If the patients actively resisted, closure would have been impossible. Had the patients actively resisted, this actually would have been a compelling reason for Sims to use anesthesia, which he did not do—because he did not need it when operating on cooperative patients. Particularly in the preanesthetic era (which is when Sims began his operations), surgery was very much a "team effort," requiring speed and dexterity on the part of the surgeon coupled with cooperation, fortitude, patience, and resolve on the part of patients.

9. The easiest charge against Sims to refute is the "race card": the accusation that he performed surgery without anesthesia on slave patients but then used anesthesia on white patients who couldn't bear the operations without it. Sims operated on white women without anesthesia on a regular basis, even after ether had been discovered. The operations at the Woman's Hospital in New York, where the patients were overwhelmingly (but not exclusively) white, were carried out without the use of anesthetics for a decade or more after the hospital opened. As Sims's associate and cosurgeon Thomas Addis Emmet noted many years later, "Anaesthesia did not come into use, at least in the Woman's Hospital except for special cases such as ovariotomies, until about the close of our Civil War"—20 years after the discovery of ether. The reason for this was therapeutic conservatism: a legitimate ethical concern that anesthesia should be used on patients only when absolutely necessary, not exposing them to excess risk. Living as we do in an era when anesthesia is ubiquitous and very (but not totally) safe, this is difficult to understand, but that is also why good history is difficult to write.

GLOSSARY

albumin. A common protein circulating in the blood needed to maintain "osmotic pressure" so that fluid does not leak out of the vascular system into surrounding tissues.

altriciality. The property of an individual's being born or hatched in an immature and helpless condition that requires significant (usually parental) care for a time until it is independent. Its opposite is "precocial." The term originated in ornithology with reference to altricial birds, which are incapable of moving about on their own after hatching, as opposed to precocial birds, which can move around after emerging from the egg.

amniotic fluid. The fluid that surrounds the fetus within the amniotic membranes. In British obstetrics, this fluid is also called the "amniotic liquor."

anterior. In anatomy, this means toward the front (ventral surface) of the body, as opposed to the back (posterior, dorsal) surface of the body.

anthropometry. The measurement of the human body.

antiseptic technique. Similar to aseptic technique. Antiseptic technique was a method of surgery developed by Sir Joseph Lister in the late nineteenth century. Initially it involved using antiseptic fluids such as carbolic acid, to clean instruments used in surgery and the hands of members of the surgical team, and so on. Lister also used an intraoperative spray of carbolic acid (an antiseptic) to decrease surgical infections. The development of the steam autoclave allowed for much more efficient sterilization of the materials used in surgery, including gowns, drapes, and so forth. Antiseptic technique was replaced by aseptic technique as more efficient. Aseptic technique is what is used in surgery today.

aseptic technique. A procedure (such as a surgical operation) that is performed under sterile conditions. This means that microbes are excluded from the operative field. This is done by carefully sterilizing all drapes, instruments, sutures, and so forth used in the procedure and by all participants in the operation using sterilized gowns, gloves, and so on. The need for aseptic technique in surgery was not recognized until the development of the germ theory of disease in the nineteenth century. Aseptic technique was preceded by antiseptic technique.

atony. Lack of tone, particularly with reference to a muscle. In the obstetric context, it refers to a lack of uterine contractility. After delivery, failure of the uterus to contract properly is a major cause of postpartum hemorrhage, which may lead recently delivered women to bleed to death, particularly in parts of the world where emergency obstetric care is not readily accessible.

barrier nursing. Refers to the use of proper infection control techniques in nursing care to avoid contamination.

beneficence. The ethical obligation to do good; that is, the obligation to put the best interests of the patient ahead of all other considerations and to act accordingly. See also *non-maleficence*.

bipedalism. The ability to walk about on two legs. Obligate bipedalism (which pertains to humans) means that this is the normal and expected means of locomotion.

birth canal. The bony pelvis. The fetus must traverse the birth canal during labor. Obstructions to birth are commonly due to abnormalities of the bony pelvis.

breech. An antiquarian term referring to the buttocks. In obstetrics, it refers to the fetal buttocks, generally in the context of a delivery in which the fetus presents buttocks-first in the birth canal, instead of in the normal head-first position. There are numerous variants of breech presentation, depending on whether or not the fetal legs are flexed or extended. Because the largest part of the fetus is the head, breech deliveries can be complex and traumatic. See also *malpresentation* and *presentation*.

case fatality rate. Is a cause-specific measure of mortality. It refers to the percentage of individuals with a condition (such as Ebola fever or malaria) who die of that condition over a specified period. For example, the case fatality rate for hysterectomy is the percentage of women having a hysterectomy who die as the result of complications of that surgical operation within a specific time (for example, six weeks or three months or one year) after surgery. Many people erroneously use the term "mortality rate" when what they really want to refer to is the case fatality rate for a particular condition. The mortality rate is a population-wide statistic, sometimes broken down by sex, referring to total deaths (or sometimes disease-specific deaths) over the course of a period, such as a year, in the total population, including people not exposed to the condition.

cephalo-pelvic disproportion. A mismatch between the size of the fetal head and the birth canal through which it must pass, resulting in difficult labor. See also *feto-pelvic disproportion*.

chorioamnionitis. The medical term for infection of the amniotic membranes and fluid. See also *sepsis*.

cicatrix. The scar or seam remaining after the healing of a wound.

comorbidity. See *morbidity*.

contracted pelvis. A condition in which the diameters of the pelvis are abnormally small, making delivery difficult.

craniotomy. Refers to puncturing or opening the skull. In obstetric use, it refers to opening the fetal skull to remove the brain, "lessening the head," to allow vaginal delivery in cases of obstructed labor. Usually the fetus is already dead from prolonged labor when this is done; in some cases, however, a living fetus is sacrificed in an attempt to save the life of its mother.

curettage. Scraping of the lining of the uterus with a surgical instrument called a curette. Curettage is a reliable way of removing retained tissue after delivery. Retained tissue (placental fragments and pieces of the amniotic membranes) often lead to serious infection and must be removed as part of the treatment of such infections.

cystitis. Infection or inflammation of the bladder.

decubitus ulcer. A bedsore, caused by the prolonged pressure of the body compressing the soft tissues of the back and buttocks if such pressure is not relieved by regular turning and movement in bed.

direct maternal death. See *maternal mortality.*

dose-response curve. A simple x-y graph showing the relationship between the amount of "exposure" (the dose, of a drug or a pollutant, for example) to its effects (the biological "response" that occurs in the affected organism).

dystocia. Difficult birth.

eclampsia. See *preeclampsia.*

encephalization. Increasing brain size over evolutionary time. One of the characteristics of hominin evolution.

endomyometritis. Medical term for infection of the lining of the uterus (endometrium) and the underlying muscle (myometrium).

episiotomy. An incision made in the posterior vagina and perineal body at the time of delivery to open a larger space for delivery of the baby.

feto-pelvic disproportion. A mismatch between the size of the fetus and the birth canal so that labor is difficult. Feto-pelvic disproportion is usually synonymous with cephalo-pelvic disproportion, because the head is usually the largest portion of the fetus. In some cases, however, other parts of the fetus may be larger than the fetal head (e.g., fetal abdominal distension in cases of pathological swelling of the fetus called "fetal hydrops," etc.). See also *cephalo-pelvic disproportion.*

fimbria. An anatomical term referring to a "series of threads or thread-like projections, a fringe." The Fallopian tubes have a fimbriated end, the projections of which help them to capture an egg that is ovulated from the ovary and bring it inside the tube, where it is fertilized.

fistula. An abnormal communication between two body cavities or organs that normally are not connected. Fistulas are usually described using the two cavities or organs involved; thus, *vesico-vaginal fistula* refers to a passageway between the bladder and the vagina, *recto-vaginal fistula* refers to an abnormal opening between the rectum and the vagina, *uretero-vaginal fistula* refers to a connection between the ureter (which carries urine from the kidney to the bladder) and the vagina, and so on. An *obstetric fistula* is a fistula that develops from obstetric causes, most commonly from prolonged obstructed labor.

foot drop. A condition in which a patient is unable to dorsiflex the foot (flex the foot upward) due to an injury to the nerve that innervates the muscles involved. This injury can occur at the level of the peroneal nerve itself or higher up along the side of the pelvis in the lumbosacral nerve plexus. This may occur because of prolonged squatting and pushing, trying unsuccessfully to deliver a baby, or because of obstructions to labor high in the birth canal. The old term for this is "obstetric palsy."

fundus. Refers to the upper portion or dome of the uterus or bladder.

genital hiatus. The female genital opening. Technically, the genital hiatus is defined/measured as the space between the middle of the urethral opening to the line of the hymen on the back of the vagina (technically, from the external urethral meatus to the posterior midline hymen), measured in centimeters.

genito-urinary. Referring to the genital tract and the urinary tract together. Most obstetric fistulas are genito-urinary fistulas, usually involving the bladder and the vagina. Other combinations are possible.

grand multipara. See *parity*.

hematoma. A localized collection of blood outside of blood vessels, such as blood pooling within a large bruise or blood collecting within a surgical incision.

hominid. The group consisting of all modern and extinct great apes, which includes modern humans, chimpanzees, bonobos, gorillas, orangutans, and all of their immediate evolutionary ancestors. See also *hominin*.

hominin. A term used in human evolutionary biology to refer to the group that consists of modern humans (*Homo sapiens*), extinct human species (such as Neanderthals), and all of our immediate evolutionary ancestors (including members of the genera *Homo* (such as *Homo erectus* and *Homo habilis*), *Australopithecus* (such as "Lucy," *Australopithecus afarensis*), *Paranthropus*, and *Ardipithecus*. See also *hominid*.

impaction. The condition of being wedged in and fixed in position; said of the situation of the fetal head in the pelvis in obstructed labor.

incidence. The number of new cases of a specified disease or condition during a defined period. This is usually expressed as the incidence rate or number of cases per 1,000 or 100,000 population per year. See also *prevalence*.

index pregnancy. A term referring to the pregnancy in which the fistula occurred.

indirect maternal death. See *maternal mortality*.

indurated. Hardened and thickened, as by the formation of scar tissue.

infarction. The obstruction of blood flow to tissues or organs, usually resulting in their death. A myocardial infarction, for example, is a heart attack; the blood to the heart has been obstructed, with death of the affected tissues, sometimes (but not always) sufficient to kill the entire organism.

intraoperative. Occurring during the performance of a surgical operation.

ischemia. Lack of adequate blood supply. See also *necrosis*.

labor. The process by which contractions of the uterus expel the fetus from the uterus through the cervix and vagina into the outside world. Labor is traditionally divided into three stages. The first stage is from the onset of regular uterine contractions through complete effacement (thinning) and dilation (opening) of the cervix. The first stage is complete when the cervix is fully effaced and dilated to 10 centimeters. The second stage of labor is from complete effacement and dilation of the cervix until the fetus is expelled. The third stage of labor lasts from the expulsion of the fetus through expulsion of the placenta (afterbirth).

lie. The fetal lie is the orientation of the long axis of the fetus in relationship to the long axis of the mother. Most of the time, the lie is longitudinal. In the worst case, the lie is transverse, meaning that the fetus is lying sideways in the uterus. Such cases cannot be delivered vaginally and if a cesarean section does not occur, there is a substantial risk of uterine rupture. See also *malpresentation* and *presentation*.

lithotrite. A surgical instrument used for crushing urinary stones.

lochia. The normal vaginal discharge that occurs after birth, including blood, mucus, fragments of tissue, and so on. If an intrauterine infection occurs, the lochia will be infected and foul smelling, with the presence of pus and large numbers of bacteria.

lumbosacral nerve plexus. The interlacing network of nerves emerging from the lumbar and sacral portions of the spinal cord in the pelvis, from which the peripheral nerves to the lower extremities originate.

malpresentation. The presentation of the fetus refers to that portion of the fetus that lies lowest in the birth canal. Normally, the fetal head is the presenting (lowest) part, in which case the *presentation* is referred to as a vertex presentation or a cephalic presentation. In some cases, however, other parts of the fetus may present first: such as the *breech* (legs or buttocks), the face or chin, and so on. In rare cases the fetus may present sideways (a transverse *lie*), with an arm or shoulder presenting. These cases are extremely difficult to manage without cesarean section.

maternal morbidity. Nonfatal obstetric injury or disability, as opposed to maternal mortality. A vesico-vaginal fistula is one form of maternal morbidity. See also *maternal mortality*.

maternal mortality. A maternal death is the death of a woman while pregnant or within six weeks of the termination of a pregnancy (irrespective of the duration or site of the pregnancy), from any cause related to or aggravated by pregnancy (but not from accidental or incidental causes). It is usually measured using the maternal mortality ratio, which is the number of maternal deaths per 100,000 live births. The maternal mortality rate is different from the maternal mortality ratio. These are often confused with one another. The maternal mortality rate is the number of maternal deaths per 100,000 women of reproductive age, usually between the ages of 15 and 45. Calculating the maternal mortality rate requires accurate total population statistics, which are generally lacking in most developing countries. This is why live births are generally used as a proxy, since newborn babies are found in close proximity to newly delivered mothers.

Direct maternal deaths or direct obstetric deaths are deaths resulting from complications of the pregnant state (pregnancy, labor, and after delivery) or from interventions, omissions, incorrect treatment, or a chain of events resulting from any of the above. An example would be a woman who dies from a ruptured uterus during prolonged obstructed labor.

An indirect obstetric or maternal death is a death resulting from previous existing disease or disease that developed during pregnancy and was not due to direct obstetric causes, but was aggravated by the physiologic effects of pregnancy. Examples would be a woman with diabetes, high blood pressure, tuberculosis, or HIV infection who dies during pregnancy or after delivery from complications of these conditions that were worsened by pregnancy.

morbidity. The condition or state of being diseased, or being caused by disease; physical or mental illness. A comorbidity is another condition or disease which is also present at the same time. Examples of comorbidities could include hypertension, anemia, and infection all present in the same patient at the same time.

multipara. See *parity.*

necrosis. Tissue death from disease, injury, or loss of blood supply.

negative predictive value. The probability that someone with a negative screening test actually does not have the disease or condition being tested for. Patients with a "false negative" test have a test result that says they do not have the condition when, in fact, they actually do have the condition.

neonatal death. Birth of a live baby who dies within 28 days of birth. See *perinatal mortality.*

nidus. A source or focus, often used for infection or concretion, as in the formation of a stone.

non-maleficence. The ethical obligation to avoid causing harm. In medicine this is the flip side of the obligation to do good, always to act in the patient's best interests. See also *beneficence.*

nullipara. See *parity.*

obstetric fistula. An abnormal opening between two body cavities that are not normally connected, such as between the bladder or rectum and the vagina, due to obstetric trauma. See also *fistula.*

oviduct. The tube through which eggs pass from an ovary. In humans, this is the Fallopian tube.

parietal bone. One of two large quadrangular bones that unite to form the midportion of the skull, separated in the midline by the sagittal suture.

parity. The condition of having given birth to a living or dead child, either vaginally or by Cesarean section. A nulliparous woman has never given birth, whereas a parous woman has. A primiparous women has given birth only once. A multiparous woman has given birth at least twice. A grand multipara is a woman who has given birth at least five times, sometimes many more.

parturient. A woman engaged in *parturition*; that is, a woman in *labor*.

parturition. The act of bringing forth young. See *labor*.

perinatal mortality. Perinatal death is a fetal death (stillbirth) or an early *neonatal death*. An early neonatal death is the death of a live-born infant within the first week of life. The perinatal mortality rate is calculated as the number of perinatal deaths (stillbirths + early neonatal deaths) per 1,000 total births. See also *neonatal death*.

perineal body. Defined/measured as the tissue between the posterior margin of the *genital hiatus* (hymen) to the midanal opening, in centimeters.

perineum. The tissues between the posterior border of the vaginal orifice and the anus.

peritoneal cavity. The space within the abdomen containing the intestines, stomach, pancreas, liver, and so on, surrounded by a thin membrane called the peritoneum.

pleural membrane. The outer covering of the lungs. When infected, the condition is known as pleurisy.

positive predictive value. The probability that someone with a positive screening test actually does have the disease or condition being tested for. A false positive test is a screening test that is positive in somebody who does not actually have the disease or condition being tested for. See also *negative predictive value*.

posterior. Situated at the back; situated behind or farther back than something else; denoting the hindmost of a pair or group of similar or related structures; opposite of anterior.

preeclampsia. A serious medical condition, unique to pregnancy, characterized by high blood pressure, swelling of peripheral tissues due to leakage of fluid from the capillary space (edema), and loss of protein in the urine (proteinuria). In the older obstetric literature, it is sometimes called "toxemia of pregnancy." The cause of the disease is unknown. In its most dramatic form, these signs are accompanied by grand mal seizures. When accompanied by seizures the condition is known as eclampsia, and the seizures are called eclamptic seizures or eclamptic fits. Women with eclamptic seizures may suffer brain hemorrhage and stroke, and they often die. Preeclampsia can progress to very severe manifestations, including failure of the blood to clot, respiratory failure from fluid collecting in the lungs (pulmonary edema), kidney failure, rupture of the liver, and fatal strokes. Severe preeclampsia and eclampsia require expert, meticulous medical management, which is often unavailable in poor countries. It is a common cause of maternal death among the bottom billion. The disease is more common in younger pregnant patients, especially during their first pregnancies. Preeclampsia/eclampsia is an extremely important obstetric disease.

presentation. Refers to the part of the fetus that lies lowest in the birth canal; that is, "what comes first." Usually this is the fetal head, but it could be the legs or buttocks (breech), or the shoulder (a transverse *lie*). An abnormal presentation is also called a *malpresentation*.

prevalence. The total number of cases (such as obstetric fistula) that are present in a given population at a particular time. See also *incidence*.

primipara. See *parity*.

prospectively. In medicine generally (and in medical research particularly) to do something prospectively means to collect data as you go forward, rather than attempting to look at things after they have occurred, such as by gathering information from a clinical chart review. Prospective studies imply that they are well thought out, that the categories of data to be collected have been determined in advance (for thoroughness) so that good decisions can be made and protocols altered on the basis of experience.

puerpera. A woman who has just had a baby. The six-week period after delivery is referred to as the "puerperium" and the adjective used to describe something related to this period is "puerperal." Puerperal fever is an infection of the uterus occurring during this time, a frequent cause of maternal death if antibiotics are not available.

recto-vaginal fistula. An abnormal opening between the rectum and the vagina, usually the result of obstetric trauma. See *fistula*.

sensitivity. If a person actually has a disease or condition, how often the screening test will be positive. This is a measure of the test's ability to pick up persons affected by a condition, the "true positive rate." You want screening tests with very high sensitivity and very high *specificity*, to avoid false positive and false negative rates. See also *negative predictive value* and *positive predictive value*.

sepsis. The response of the body to infection. In this book, sepsis is generally used to refer to advanced infections or systemic sepsis. Infections may progress from simple sepsis (characterized by elevated temperature, heart rate, respiration, and white blood cell count) to severe sepsis (with the beginning of organ failure) to septic shock, multisystem organ failure, and death from overwhelming infection. Because of its rich blood supply and the presence of amniotic fluid (a wonderful culture medium for bacteria) the pregnant uterus is particularly susceptible to infection if labor is prolonged.

series. In clinical medicine, a series refers to a collection of consecutive cases of some condition, usually collected for analysis; for example, a series of vesico-vaginal fistula cases.

specificity. If a person does not have the disease or condition, how often is the screening test negative; the true negative rate of a test. You want screening tests with very high specificity and very high *sensitivity* to avoid false positive and false negative rates. See *negative predictive value* and *positive predictive value*.

sphygmomanometer. A cuff wrapping around the arm used to measure blood pressure.

splenomegaly. Pathological enlargement of the spleen.

stages of labor. See *labor*.

stillbirth. A fetal death before the baby is born. See *perinatal mortality*.

stricture. A pathological narrowing of a canal, duct, or passage, such as of the urethra, vagina, or intestine. Strictures reduce the size of the passageway, often obstructing flow through it.

structural violence. As defined by James Gilligan, structural violence is "the increased rates of death and disability suffered by those who occupy the bottom rungs of society." Social scientists use the term to refer to how socioeconomic and political factors influence the unequal rates of death and disability found in any given society.

subpubic. Underneath the pubic bone.

suppuration. The process of pus formation in cases of infection.

suprapubic. Above the pubic bone.

symphysiotomy. A surgical operation in which the two pubic bones are transected at their cartilaginous point of union (pubic symphysis) in order to increase the diameter of the pelvic ring in difficult labor. Some surgeons tried to cut the pubic bone itself for similar purposes, an operation called pubiotomy. The operation is almost never done today in resource-rich countries. If done improperly, there can be serious complications.

tenesmus. A constant feeling of the need to empty the bowels or bladder, accompanied by straining, but with little or no discharge. A feeling of "blockage" of the bowels or bladder.

triage. A French world literally meaning "separating into three," which has entered medical use to refer to prioritizing patients for care based on the acuity of their conditions. It originated in military medicine as a process to separate battlefield casualties into groups composed of those who do not need immediate attention and can be dealt with later, those who needed immediate lifesaving interventions because they are likely to survive if such care is provided, and those who are so badly injured that care is likely to be futile in any case and should thus be diverted to cases with probable better outcomes.

uretero-vaginal fistula. A condition in which an abnormal communication develops between the tube carrying urine from the kidneys to the bladder (ureters) and the vagina due to obstetric trauma or surgical misadventure.

version. Refers to an obstetrical maneuver in which the fetus has a *malpresentation* (a breech or a transverse *lie*) and an attempt is made to turn the fetus into a more normal *presentation*. In the past, versions were done internally. The midwife or obstetrician would reach a hand up into the uterus to reposition the fetus. In difficult cases, attempts were made to turn the fetus completely around and to extract it as a breech, pulling on the legs for traction as the fetus was delivered. Before the discovery of anesthesia, this was an agonizing procedure for the pregnant woman, and the risk of injury or rupture of the uterus was great. It was only undertaken in serious cases. Today external version (by manipulation of the abdomen) is sometimes done, with ultrasound guidance, to turn a breech into a cephalic presentation. Internal versions are rarely done any more in modern obstetrics.

vesico-vaginal fistula. An abnormal opening between the bladder and the vagina, generally caused by trauma from prolonged obstructed labor. See also *fistula*.

ESSAY ON SOURCES

Prologue. Confronting Childbirth Injury among the World's Poorest Women

The maternal health statistics in this section are from *Trends in Maternal Mortality 1990–2015: Estimates by WHO, UNICEF, UNFPA, World Bank Group and the United Nations Population Division* (Geneva: World Health Organization, 2015). On the obstetric malpractice problem, see Jeffrey Klaghotz and Albert L. Strunk, "Overview of the 2009 ACOG Survey on Professional Liability," *ACOG Clinical Review* 14, no. 6 (2009); and Gary V. Hankins, Alastair MacLennan, Michael E. Speer, Albert Strunk, and Karin Nelson, "Obstetric Litigation Is Asphyxiating Our Maternity Services," *Obstetrics and Gynecology* 107 (2006): 1382–1385.

The quote from Josephine Baker is from S. J. Baker, "Maternal Mortality in the United States," *Journal of the American Medical Association* 89 (1927): 2016–2017.

The best historical treatment of maternal mortality is Irvine Loudon's magisterial book, *Death in Childbirth: An International Study of Maternal Care and Maternal Mortality, 1800–1950* (Oxford: Clarendon Press, 1992).

The 15 percent complication rate requiring transfer to a higher level of care for low-risk pregnancies is extrapolated from J. P. Rooks, N. L. Weatherby, and E. K. Ernst, "The National Birth Center Study: Part III—Intrapartum and Immediate Postpartum and Neonatal Complications and Transfers, Postpartum and Neonatal Care, Outcomes, and Client Satisfaction," *Journal of Nurse Midwifery* 37, no. 6 (1992): 361–397; and J. P. Rooks, N. L. Weatherby, E. K. Ernst, S. Stapleton, D. Rosen, and A. Rosenfield, "Outcomes of Care in Birth Centers: The National Birth Center Study," *New England Journal of Medicine* 321, no. 26 (1989): 1804–1811.

Various aspects of the obstetric fistula are covered at length in succeeding chapters of this book. For general surveys, see L. Lewis Wall, "Obstetric Vesicovaginal Fistula as an International Public-Health Problem," *Lancet* 368 (2006): 1201–1209; L. Lewis Wall, "Preventing Obstetric Fistulas in Low-Resource Countries: Insights from a Haddon Matrix," *Obstetrical and Gynecological Survey* 67 (2012): 111–121; and L. Lewis Wall, Steven D. Arrowsmith, Nimi D. Briggs, Andrew Browning, and Anyetei Lassey, "The Obstetric Vesicovaginal Fistula in the Developing World," *Obstetrical and Gynecological Survey* 60, no. S1 (2005): S1–S55.

The quote from Sherwood Washburn is in S. L. Washburn, "Tools and Human Evolution," *Scientific American* 203 (1960): 3–15.

On the subject of neglected tropical diseases, see Peter J. Hotez, Alan Fenwick, Lorenzo Savioli, and David H. Molyneux, "Rescuing the Bottom Billion through Control of Neglected Tropical Diseases," *Lancet* 373 (2009): 1570–1575; Doruk Ozgediz and Robert Riviello, "The 'Other' Neglected Diseases in Global Public Health: Surgical Conditions in Sub-Saharan Africa," *PLoS Medicine* 5, no. 6 (2008): e121; and L. Lewis Wall, "Obstetric Fistula Is a 'Neglected Tropical Disease,'" *PLoS Neglected Tropical Diseases* 6, no 8 (2012): e1769, doi:10.1371/journal.pntd.0001769 (online, open access).

Chapter 1. The Tragedy of Queen Henhenit

The story of Henhenit as I have told it is an imaginative historical reconstruction. We obviously do not have original medical records from Henhenit's labor and delivery, but everything I have described is grounded in solid historical research combined with what I consider reasonable interpolations from our knowledge of the pathophysiology of obstructed labor (which is further elaborated in chapter 2).

I have been fascinated by ancient Egypt for more than 50 years. For those readers who share this fascination and wish to pursue the background to Henhenit's story, there are many good introductions to ancient Egyptian civilization. Those unfamiliar with Egyptian history should understand that the Egyptian language was written without vowels. This means that Egyptian words and names must be reconstructed by scholarly guesswork, and there is often no consensus as to how a name should be written in English. Montuhotep, for example, can also be written as Mentuhotep, Mentuhetpe, and several other ways. The reader will find all of these variations in the sources below.

For a general survey of the ancient Egyptian worldview, there is no better place to start than Joyce Tyldesley's *The Penguin Book of Ancient Egyptian Myths and Legends* (London: Penguin Books, 2011). Good historical and cultural surveys can be found in Nicholas Grimal, *A History of Ancient Egypt* (Oxford: Blackwell, 1992); *The British Museum Book of Ancient Egypt* (London: British Museum Press, 2007); Barry J. Kemp, *Ancient Egypt: Anatomy of a Civilization* (New York: Routledge, 1989); B. G. Trigger, B. J. Kemp, D. O'Connor, and A. B. Lloyd, *Ancient Egypt: A Social History* (London: Cambridge University Press, 1983); Toby Wilkinson, *The Rise and Fall of Ancient Egypt* (New York: Random House, 2011); and Ian Shaw, ed., *The Oxford History of Ancient Egypt* (New York: Oxford University Press, 2000). An excellent general reference in three volumes is Donald B. Redford, ed., *The Oxford Encyclopedia of Ancient Egypt* (New York: Oxford University Press, 2001). On mummies and mummification, the reader is referred to a comprehensive and handsomely illustrated volume by Salima Ikram and Aidan Dodson, *The Mummy in Ancient Egypt: Equipping the Dead for Eternity* (New York: Thames and Hudson, 1998).

On the position of women in ancient Egypt, see Gay Robbins, *Women in Ancient Egypt* (Cambridge, MA: Harvard University Press, 1993); Joyce Tyldesley, *Daughters of Isis: Women of Ancient Egypt* (London: Penguin Books, 1994); and Carolyn Graves-Brown, *Dancing for Hathor: Women in Ancient Egypt* (New York: Continuum, 2010).

Much of the information about Montuhotep's temple in Deir el-Bahri comes from the original excavation report by Edouard Naville, *The XIth Dynasty Temple at Deir el-Bahari, Part I* (London: Egypt Exploration Fund, 1907), which also included chapters on the excavations by H. R. Hall and on the tombs by H. R. Hall and E. R. Ayrton. The quotations from the excavation report in this chapter are from pages 30 and 50.

For the Middle Kingdom at Thebes, the works of archaeologist Herbert Winlock are indispensable. In particular I have consulted his article "The Eleventh Egyptian Dynasty," *Journal of Near Eastern Studies* 3 (1943): 249–283; his book *The Rise and Fall of the Middle Kingdom in Thebes* (New York: Macmillan, 1947); and his report of *Excavations at Deir el Bahri, 1911–1931* (New York: Macmillan, 1942). In the latter book Winlock discussed his discovery, excavation, and interpretation of the mass tomb of the slain soldiers of Montuhotep II, mentioned briefly in this chapter. He elaborated more fully in a subsequent publication entitled *The Slain Soldiers of Neb-hepet-Re'-Mentu-Hotpe* (New York: Metropolitan Museum, 1945). The most detailed analysis of the reign of Montuhotep II is by Labib Habachi, "King Nebhepetre Mentuhotpe: His Monuments,

Place in History, Deification, and Unusual Representations in the Form of Gods," *Mitteilungen des Deutschen Archaologischen Instituts* 19 (1963): 16–52. More recent work on the history of the Middle Kingdom can be found in Wolfram Grajetzki's two books, *The Middle Kingdom of Ancient Egypt* (London: Duckworth, 2006); and *Court Officials of the Egyptian Middle Kingdom* (London: Duckworth, 2009).

On the goddess Hathor, see C. J. Bleeker, *Hathor and Thoth: Two Key Figures in the Ancient Egyptian Religion* (Leiden: E. J. Brill, 1973), from which I have also quoted. The lines to the hymn that Henhenit recited at the beginning of her labor are from an ancient papyrus preserved in Leiden, quoted by Bleeker on page 40 of his book. The hymn of the pharaoh dancing for Hathor is found on page 55 of the same work. On the priestesses of Hathor, see Robyn A. Gillam, "Priestesses of Hathor: Their Function, Decline, and Disappearance," *Journal of the American Research Center in Egypt* 32 (1995): 211–237.

For technical obstetric issues in ancient Egypt (insofar as we know anything about them), see Ann Macy Roth and Catherine H. Roehrig, "Magical Bricks and the Bricks of Birth," *Journal of Egyptian Archaeology* 88 (2002): 121–139; W. Benson Harer Jr., "Peseshkef: The First Special-Purpose Surgical Instrument," *Obstetrics and Gynecology* 83 (1994): 1053–1055; and Ann Macy Roth, "The PSS.KF and the Opening of the Mouth Ceremony: A Ritual of Birth and Rebirth," *Journal of Egyptian Archaeology* 78 (1992): 113–147. On amulets in childbirth, see Henri Frankfort, "A Note on the Lady of Birth," *Journal of Near Eastern Studies* 13, no. 3 (1943): 198–200.

The description of Henhenit's injuries is found in D. E. Derry, "Note on Five Pelves of Women of the Eleventh Dynasty in Egypt," *Journal of Obstetrics and Gynaecology of the British Empire* 42 (1935): 490–495. The photograph of Henhenit's mummy is taken from this article. It was Derry's opinion that Henhenit had died in childbirth. I disagree. Although, like him, I am confident that birth trauma was a precipitating cause for her death, it is improbable that she would have developed a fistula if she had died during the birth process itself. It usually takes some time for the fistula to form after the tissues have been injured. My reconstruction of Henhenit's last days is based on the assumption that she survived the birth of her child, developed a fistula, but succumbed to complications some time later. An appreciation of Derry's many contributions both to Egyptology and to Egyptian medical education can be found in his obituary in the *British Medical Journal* 1 (1961): 832–833.

Chapter 2. The Human Obstetrical Dilemma and Its Consequences

On reproductive problems in birds such as egg binding, dystocia, prolapsed oviducts, chronic egg laying, ectopic eggs, oviduct impaction, and other fascinating pathologies, see April Romagnano, "Avian Obstetrics," *Seminars in Avian and Exotic Pet Medicine* 5, no. 4 (1996): 180–188.

On doggy C-sections, see Katy M. Evans and Vicki J. Adams, "Proportion of Litters of Purebred Dogs Born by Caesarean Section," *Journal of Small Animal Practice* 51, no. 2 (2010): 113–118.

On the use of anesthesia in childbirth and the ensuing nineteenth-century religious tussle about its propriety, see Jack Cohen's article "Doctor James Young Simpson, Rabbi Abraham De Sola, and Genesis Chapter 3, Verse 16," *Obstetrics and Gynecology* 88 (1996): 895–898, which proves that in this, as in all of life's endeavors, the advice of a good rabbi is indispensable.

The scientific literature on bipedal locomotion is enormous. To delve into it, I suggest beginning with Anna Blackburn Wittman and L. Lewis Wall, "The Evolutionary Origins of Obstructed Labor: Bipedalism, Encephalization and the Human Obstetric Dilemma," *Obstetrical and Gynecological Survey* 62, no. 11 (2007): 739–748. Accessible general accounts can be found in Craig

Stanford's *Upright: The Evolutionary Key to Becoming Human* (Boston: Houghton Mifflin, 2003); and Jonathan Kingdon's *Lowly Origin: Where, When, and Why Our Ancestors First Stood Up* (Princeton, NJ: Princeton University Press, 2003). If you want to sample more technical fare, try David A. Raichlen, Adam D. Gordon, William E. H. Harcourt-Smith, Adam D. Foster, and William Randall Haas Jr., "Laetoli Footprints Preserve Earliest Direct Evidence of Human-Like Bipedal Biomechanics," *PLoS One* 3 (2010): e9769; Herman Pontzer, David A. Raichlen, and Michal D. Sokol, "The Metabolic Cost of Walking in Humans, Chimpanzees, and Early Hominins," *Journal of Human Evolution* 56 (2009): 43–54; and Mark Grabowski, John D. Polk, and Charles Roseman, "Divergent Patterns of Integration and Reduced Constraint in the Human Hip and the Origins of Bipedalism," *Evolution* 65, no. 5 (2011): 1336–1356.

The best current overview of human evolution has been produced by two of my colleagues from the Department of Anthropology at Washington University in St. Louis. I highly recommend Glenn C. Conroy and Herman Pontzer, *Reconstructing Human Origins*, 3rd ed. (New York: Norton, 2012).

The definitive book on obstetrical mechanics is Maurice Abitbol's *Birth and Human Evolution: Anatomical and Obstetrical Mechanics in Primates* (Westport, CT: Bergin and Garvey, 1996). Sherwood Washburn's famous statement of the human obstetrical dilemma is found in S. L. Washburn, "Tools and Human Evolution," *Scientific American* 203 (1960): 3–15.

On the fetal skull, see Eckhart J. Buchmann and Elena Libhaber, "Sagittal Suture Overlap in Cephalopelvic Disproportion: Blinded and Non-participant Assessment," *Acta Obstetricia et Gynecologica* 87 (2008): 731–737.

On brain development, see R. D. Martin, *Human Brain Evolution in an Ecological Context* (New York: American Museum of Natural History, 1983). See also Robert Martin, "Primate Reproduction," in *The Cambridge Encyclopedia of Human Evolution*, ed. Steve Jones, Robert Martin, and David Pilbeam (New York: Cambridge University Press, 1992), 86–90 (the quote is from page 87); and H. Coqueugniot, J. J. Hublin, F. Veillon, F. Houet, and T. Jacob, "Early Brain Growth in *Homo Erectus* and Implications for Cognitive Ability," *Nature* 431 (2004): 299–302.

An illuminating article on early Cesarean section (complete with illustrations of the kind of terribly distorted pelves that clinicians encountered in bygone eras) is M. H. Kaufman, "Caesarean Operations Performed in Edinburgh during the 18th Century," *British Journal of Obstetrics and Gynaecology* 102 (1995): 186–191.

On Cesarean delivery in resource-poor countries, see Carine Ronsmans, Vincent De Brouwere, Dominique Dubourg, and Greet Dieltiens, "Measuring the Need for Life-Saving Obstetric Surgery in Developing Countries," *BJOG: An International Journal of Obstetrics and Gynaecology* 111 (2004): 1027–1030; Alexandre Dumon, Luc de Bernis, Marie-Helen Bourvier-Colle, and Gerard Breart, "Caesarean Section Rate for Maternal Indication in Sub-Saharan Africa: A Systematic Review," *Lancet* 358 (2001): 1328–1334; and Carine Ronsmans, Sara Holtz, and Cynthia Stanton, "Socioeconomic Differentials in Caesarean Rates in Developing Countries: A Retrospective Analysis," *Lancet* 368 (2006): 1516–1523. My friend Professor E. Y. Kwawukume of the University of Ghana Medical School has produced an excellent synthesis of the problems of Cesarean delivery in his part of the world in "Caesarean Section in Developing Countries," *Best Practice & Research Clinical Obstetrics & Gynaecology* 15, no. 1 (2001): 165–178. For Cesarean rates and trends worldwide, see Yoshiko Niino, "The Increasing Cesarean Rate Globally and What We Can Do about It," *BioScience Trends* 5, no. 4 (2011): 139–150.

On bladder function during normal pregnancy, see John M. Thorp Jr., Peggy A. Norton, L. Lewis Wall, Jeffery A. Kuller, Barbara Eucker, and Ellen Wells, "Urinary Incontinence in Pregnancy and the Puerperium: A Prospective Study," *American Journal of Obstetrics and Gynecology* 181 (1999): 266–273.

Good general surveys of the obstetric fistula problem can be found in L. Lewis Wall, "Obstetric Vesicovaginal Fistula as an International Public Health Problem," *Lancet* 368 (2006): 1201–1209; and also in L. Lewis Wall, Steven D. Arrowsmith, Nimi D. Briggs, Andrew Browning, and Anyetei T. Lassey, "The Obstetric Vesicovaginal Fistula in the Developing World," supplement, *Obstetrical and Gynecological Survey* 60, no. S1 (2005): S1–S55.

Several large series detailing the clinical characteristics of women with obstetric fistulas and the results of surgical treatment have been published in the past few years. Among the more notable series are the following: L. Lewis Wall, Jonathan Karshima, Carolyn Kirschner, and Steven D. Arrowsmith, "The Obstetric Vesicovaginal Fistula: Characteristics of 899 Patients from Jos, Nigeria," *American Journal of Obstetrics and Gynecology* 190 (2004): 1011–1019; Mulu Muleta, Svein Rasmussen, and Torvid Kiserud, "Obstetric Fistula in 14,928 Ethiopian Women," *Acta Obstetricia et Gynecologica* 89 (2010): 945–951; Alyona Lewis, Melissa Kaufman, Christoper Wolder, Sharon Phillip, Darius Maggi, Leesa Condry, Roger Dmochowski, and Joseph A. Smith Jr., "Genitourinary Fistula Experience in Sierra Leone: Review of 505 Cases," *Journal of Urology* 181 (2009): 1725–1731; Paul Hilton and Ann Ward, "Epidemiological and Surgical Aspects of Urogenital Fistulae: A Review of 25 Years' Experience in Southeast Nigeria," *International Urogynecology Journal* 9 (1998): 189–194; Solbjorg Sjoveian, Siri Vangen, Denis Mukwege, and Mathias Onsrud, "Surgical Outcome of Obstetric Fistula: A Retrospective Analysis of 595 Patients," *Acta Obstetricia et Gynecologica Scandinavica* 90 (2011): 753–760.

On the psychosocial aspects of obstetric fistula, see Amina P. Alio, Laura Merrell, Kimberlee Roxburgh, Heather B. Clayton, Phillip J. Marty, Linda Bomboka, Salmatou Traore, and Hamis M. Salihu, "The Psychosocial Impact of Vesico-Vaginal Fistula in Niger," *Archives of Gynecology and Obstetrics* 284, no. 2 (2011): 371–378; Lilian T. Mselle, Karen Marie Moland, Bjorg Evjen Olsen, Abu Mvungi, and Thecia W. Kohi, " 'I Am Nothing': Experiences of Loss among Women Suffering from Severe Birth Injuries in Tanzania," *BMC Women's Health* 11, no. 49 (2011); E. P. Gharoro and K. N. Agholor, "Aspects of Psychosocial Problems of Patients with Vesico-Vaginal Fistula," *Journal of Obstetrics and Gynaecology* 29 no. 7 (1996): 644–647; S. Ahmed and S. A. Holtz, "Social and Economic Consequences of Obstetric Fistula: Life Changed Forever?," supplement, *International Journal of Gynecology and Obstetrics* 99, no. 1 (2007): S10–S15; M. Kabir, I. S. Abubaker, and U. I. Umar, "Medico-Social Problems of Patients with Vesico-Vaginal Fistula in Murtala Mohammed Specialist Hospital, Kano," *Annals of African Medicine* 2, no. 2 (2004): 54–57; Margaret Murphy, "Social Consequences of Vesico-Vaginal Fistula in Northern Nigeria," *Journal of Biosocial Science* 13, no. 2 (1981): 139–150; A. L. Islam and A. Begum, "A Psycho-Social Study on Genito-Urinary Fistula," *Bangladesh Medical Research Council Bulletin* 18, no. 2 (1992): 82–94; Judith T. W. Goh, K. M. Sloane, Hilda G. Krause, Andrew Browning, and S. Akhter, "Mental Health Screening in Women with Genital Tract Fistulae," *British Journal of Obstetrics and Gynaecology* 112 (2005): 1328–1330; K. A. Johnson, J. M. Turan, L. Hailermariam, E. Mengsteab, D. Jena, and M. L. Polan, "The Role of Counseling for Obstetric Fistula Patients: Lessons Learned from Eritrea," *Patient Education and Counselling* 80, no. 2 (2010): 262–265.

Subsequent obstetric performance among fistula patients in discussed in Andrew Browning, "Pregnancy Following Obstetric Fistula Repair, the Management of Delivery," *BJOG* 116 (2009): 1265–1267. The quotation is from page 1265.

The obstructed labor injury complex is described in Steven D. Arrowsmith, E. Catherine Hamlin, and L. Lewis Wall, "'Obstructed Labor Injury Complex': Obstetric Fistula Formation and the Multifaceted Morbidity of Maternal Birth Trauma in the Developing World," *Obstetrical and Gynecological Survey* 51 (1996): 568–574.

On Bandl's contraction rings, see Michele R. Lauria, Joan C. Barthold, Robert A. Zimmerman, and Mark A. Turrentine, "Pathological Uterine Ring Associated with Fetal Head Trauma and Subsequent Cerebral Palsy," *Obstetrics and Gynecology* 109, no. 2, part 2 (2007): 495–497; and also Mark A. Turrentine and R. L. Andres, "Recurrent Bandl's Ring as an Etiology for Failed Vaginal Birth after Cesarean Section," *American Journal of Perinataology* 11, no. 1 (1994): 65–66.

On urinary stones and fistulas, see K. Gingh, "An Unusual Complication of Vesical Stones," *International Urogynecology Journal* 13 (2002): 50–51; Apul Goel, S. N. Snakhwar, and Amita Pandey, "Genitourinary Stone in a Case of Vesicovaginal Fistula," *Urology* 68 (2006): 1342–1342; and also D. Dalela, Apul Goel, S. N. Shakhwar, and K. M. Singh, "Vesical Calculi with Unrepaired Vesicovaginal Fistula: A Clinical Appraisal of an Uncommon Association," *Journal of Urology* 170 (2003): 2206–2208.

On stress incontinence and urethral functioning after fistula repair, see L. Lewis Wall and Steven D. Arrowsmith, "The 'Continence Gap': A Critical Concept in Obstetric Fistula Repair," *International Urogynecology Journal* 18, no. 8 (2007): 843–844. See also Andrew Browning, "The Circumferential Obstetric Fistula: Characteristics, Management, and Outcomes," *BJOG: An International Journal of Obstetrics and Gynaecology* 114, no. 9 (2007): 1172–1176; and also his "A New Technique for the Surgical Management of Urinary Incontinence after Obstetric Fistula Repair," *BJOG: An International Journal of Obstetrics and Gynaecology* 113, no. 4 (2006): 475–478.

On postpartum pituitary necrosis (Sheehan's syndrome), see Alex H. Tessnow and Jean D. Wilson, "The Changing Face of Sheehan's Syndrome," *American Journal of the Medical Sciences* 340, no. 5 (2010): 402–406; E. U. Bieler and T. Schnable, "Pituitary and Ovarian Function in Women with Vesicovaginal Fistulae after Obstructed and Prolonged Labour," *South African Medical Journal* 50 (1976): 257–266; and O. O. Famuyiwa, A. F. Bella, and A. O. Akanji, "Sheehan's Syndrome in a Developing Country, Nigeria: A Rare Disease or Problem of Diagnosis?," *East African Medical Journal* 69, no. 1 (1992): 40–43.

My colleague Professor John DeLancey of the University of Michigan is the world authority on the obstetric injury to the levator ani muscle complex. Of particular interest are the following articles: Rohna Kearney, Myra Fitzpatrick, Sandra Brennan, Michael Behan, Janis Miller, Declan Keane, Colm O'Herlihy, and John O. L. DeLancey, "Levator Ani Injury in Primiparous Women with Forceps Delivery for Fetal Distress, Forceps for Second Stage Arrest, and Spontaneous Delivery," *International Journal of Gynecology and Obstetrics* 111, no. 1 (2010): 19–22; Janis Miller, Catherine Brandon, Jon Low, Lisa Kane, Ruth Zielinsky, James Ashton-Miller, and John O. L. DeLancey, "MRI Findings in Patients Considered High Risk for Pelvic Floor Injury Studied Serially after Vaginal Childbirth," *AJR, American Journal of Roentgenology* 195, no. 3 (2010): 786–791; James Ashton-Miller and John O. L. DeLancey, "Functional Anatomy of the Female Pelvic Floor," *Annals of the New York Academy of Sciences* 1101 (2007): 266–296; Rohna Kearney, Janis Miller, James Ashton-Miller, and John O. L. DeLancey, "Obstetric Factors Associated with Levator Ani Muscle Injury after Vaginal Birth," *Obstetrics and Gynecology* 107 (2006): 144–149; and

John O. L. DeLancey, Rohna Kearney, Queena Chou, Steven Speights, and Shereen Binno, "The Appearance of Levator Ani Muscle Abnormalities in Magnetic Resonance Images after Vaginal Delivery," *Obstetrics and Gynecology* 101 (2003): 46–53.

There is little contemporary scientific literature on foot drop and obstetric palsy, but see John Totterdale Cole, "Maternal Obstetric Paralysis," *American Journal of Obstetrics and Gynecology* 52 (1946): 372–386; M. E. Reif, "Bilateral Common Peroneal Nerve Palsy Secondary to Prolonged Squatting in Natural Childbirth," *Birth* 15 (1988):100–102; S. C. Colachis II, W. S. Pease, and E. W. Johnson, "A Preventable Cause of Foot Drop during Childbirth," *American Journal of Obstetrics and Gynecology* 171, no. 1 (1994): 270–272; O. Bademosi, B. O. Osuntokum, H. J. Van de Werd, A. K. Bademosi, and O. A. Ojo, "Obstetric Neuropraxia in the Nigerian African," *International Journal of Gynaecology and Obstetrics* 17 (1980): 611–614; and Kees Waaldijk and Thomas E. Elkins, "The Obstetric Fistula and Peroneal Nerve Injury: An Analysis of 947 Consecutive Patients," *International Urogynecology Journal* 5 (1994): 12–14.

The moving story of how Naguib Mahfouz decided to become an obstetrician-gynecologist is given in his book, *The Life of an Egyptian Doctor* (Edinburgh: E. & S. Livingstone, 1966), 52–53.

Chapter 3. The Conquest of Obstructed Labor

A wide variety of books on the history of childbirth may be found, with differing perspectives and of varying quality. Among the most notable are Palmer Findley, *The Story of Childbirth* (Garden City, NY: Doubleday, 1933); Edwin M. Jameson, *Obstetrics and Gynecology*, Clio Medica Series (New York: Paul B. Hoeber, 1936): Harvey Graham, *Eternal Eve: The History of Gynaecology and Obstetrics* (Garden City, NY: Doubleday, 1951); Richard W. Wertz and Dorothy C. Wertz, *Lying-In: A History of Childbirth in America* (New York: Free Press, 1977); Edward Shorter, *Women's Bodies: A Social History of Women's Encounter with Health, Ill-Health, and Medicine* (New Brunswick, NJ: Transaction, 1991); Judith Walzer Leavitt, *Brought to Bed: Childbearing in America, 1750–1950* (New York: Oxford University Press, 1986); and Jacques Gelis, *History of Childbirth: Pregnancy and Birth in Early Modern Europe* (New York: Polity Press, 1996).

On the contentious story of the rise of man-midwives and their rivalries with female contemporaries, see Jean Donnison, *Midwives and Medical Men: A History of Inter-Professional Rivalries and Women's Rights* (London: Heinemann, 1977); and Adrian Wilson, *The Making of Man-Midwifery: Childbirth in England, 1660–1770* (Cambridge, MA: Harvard University Press, 1995).

François Mauriceau's treatise was published in English as Francis Mauriceau, *The Diseases of Women with Child and in Child-bed*, translated from the French by Hugh Chamberlen and "reviewed, corrected, and enlarged, with the addition of the author's anatomy" (London: John Derby, 1683). Chamberlen's boast about his family's secret method of delivery is in his (unpaginated) translator's preface to Mauriceau's book. Mauriceau's diatribe against Cesareans section is on pages 275–285.

The history of the obstetrical forceps is detailed in Walter Radcliffe, *The Secret Instrument: The Birth of the Midwifery Forceps* (London: William Heinemann Medical Books, 1947); and also in J. H. Aveling, *The Chamberlens and the Midwifery Forceps: Memorials of the Family and an Essay on the Invention of the Instrument* (London: J. A. Churchill, 1882). The most comprehensive book on the instruments themselves is still Kedarnath Das, *Obstetric Forceps: Its History and Evolution* (Calcutta: Art Press, 1929; repr. Leeds: Medical Museum Publishing, 1993).

The cases of William Giffard are taken from his book *Cases in Midwifry* (London: Motte and Wotton, 1734). Case 59 is on pages 135–137; case 71 is on pages 161–166.

The career of the marvelous Scots physician William Smellie is covered in L. Lewis Wall, "William Smellie (1697–1763): The Father of Scientific Obstetrics," *Medical Heritage* 1 (1985): 158–167; John Glaister, *Dr. William Smellie and His Contemporaries: A Contribution to the History of Midwifery in the Eighteenth Century* (Glasgow: James Maclehouse and Sons, 1894); and R. W. Johnstone, *William Smellie: The Master of British Midwifery* (Edinburgh: E. and S. Livingstone, 1952).

Smellie's statistics on obstructed labor are found in William Smellie, *A Treatise on the Theory and Practice of Midwifery* (London: D. Wilson, 1752), 195.

Robert Bland's letter to Samuel Foart Simmons was published with the breathtaking title of "Some calculations of the number of accidents or deaths which happen in consequence of parturition; and of the proportion of male to female children, as well as of twins, monstrous productions, and children that are dead-born; taken from the midwifery reports of the Westminster General Dispensary: with an attempt to ascertain the chance of life at different periods, from infancy to twenty-six years of age; and likewise the proportion of natives to the rest of the inhabitants of London," *Philosophical Transactions of the Royal Society of London* 71 (1781): 355–371, doi:10.1098/rstl.1781.0046 (available online). The quotation about mortality is on page 360.

According the WHO statistics published in 2015, the maternal mortality ratio for the entire developing world was 239 deaths per 100,000 live births, and in sub-Saharan Africa specifically it was 546 maternal deaths per 100,000 live births. Comparable maternal mortality statistics (MMR) were Benin 405, Burkina Faso 371, Congo 442, Democratic Republic of the Congo 693, Ivory Coast 645, Ethiopia 353, Gambia 706, Ghana 319, Haiti 359, Kenya 510, Rwanda 290 and Afghanistan 396. See *Trends in Maternal Mortality 1990 to 2015: Estimates by WHO, UNICEEF, UNFPA, World Bank Group and the United Nations Population Division* (Geneva: World Health Organization, 2015).

The MOMA publications referred to are C. Vangeenerhuysen, A. Prual, and D. Ould el Joud, "Obstetric Fistulae: Incidence Estimates for Sub-Saharan Africa," *International Journal of Gynecology and Obstetrics* 73 (2001): 65–66; and Dahada Ould el Joud, Charles Vangeenderhuysen, Marie-Helen Bourvier-Cole, and the MOMA Group, "Epidemiological Features of Uterine Rupture in West Africa (MOMA Study)," *Paediatric and Perinatal Epidemiology* 16 (2002): 108–114.

The works of Thomas Denman cited are *An Essay On Difficult Labours, Part First* (London: J. Johnson, 1787); *An Essay on Difficult Labours, Part Second* (London: J. Johnson, 1790); and *An Essay on Difficult Labours, Part Third and Last* (London: J. Johnson, 1790). The quotations are from 1:97, 1:65, 2:20, and 3:40.

Quotes from Ramsbotham are from Francis Henry Ramsbotham, *The Principles and Practice of Obstetric Medicine and Surgery* (Philadelphia: Blanchard and Lea, 1859), 174, 195, 321, 322, 356. His views on anesthesia appear on page 174; his comments on exhaustion, collapse, and death on pages 321–323.

The quotes from Fielding Ould are from his book *A Treatise of Midwifery* (Dublin: Oliver Nelson, 1742), 198–203.

Blundell's remarks on giving "a fair trial of the full efforts of the uterus" and on Cesarean section for transverse lie are in James Blundell, *The Principles and Practice of Obstetric Medicine*, rev. and corrected by Alexander Cooper Lee and Nathaniel Rogers (London: Joseph Butler, Medical Bookseller and Publisher, 1840), 32, 151, and 165–166.

The controversy between William Simmons and John Hull is summarized nicely in J. H. Young, *The History of Caesarean Section* (London: H. K. Lewis, 1944), 58–64. The major sources are William Simmons, *Reflections on the Propriety of Performing the Caesarean Operation* (Manchester: Messrs Clarkes, 1978). The quote is from page 58. John Hull, *A Defence of the Cesarean Operation with Observations on Embryulcia* (Manchester: R. and W. Dean, 1798). The quote is from page 12. Simmons's reply is W. Simmons, *A Detection of the Fallacy of Dr. Hull's Defence of the Cesarean Operation* (Manchester: Sowler and Pussih, 1799). Hull's 480+page counterattack is John Hull, *Observations on Mr. Simmons's Detection &c, &c with a Defence of the Cesarean Operation* (Manchester: R. and W. Dean, 1799). The controversy was also waged in the correspondence pages, published in London, of the *Medical and Physical Journal* 2 (1799): 231–233 (William Simmons); 433–437 (John Sims); 437–441 (William Simmons); 472–476 (Charles White, Richard Hall, George Tomlinson, and John Thorp). Also see the article by William Wood, "A Case of Caesarean Section," *Memoirs of the Medical Society of London* 5 (1799): 463–476.

The best description of the early history of symphysiotomy is Philip D. Turner's paper "Symphysiotomy: Its Introduction, Decline and Revival" in the *Quarterly Medical Journal for Yorkshire and Adjoining Counties* 3 (1894): 358–372. Similar material is covered, in French, in Martial Dumont, "La longue et laborieuse naissance de la symphysiotomie ou de Severin Pineau à Jean-René Sigault," *Journal de gynecologie, obstetrique et biologie de la reproduction* 18 (1989): 11–21. American obstetrician Robert P. Harris treated the early clinical material comprehensively in "The Revival of Symphysiotomy in Italy, with Comparative Tables of the Early and Later Cases, Showing That the Operation Has Been More Frequently Performed in That Country in the Last Seventeen Years Than in All Europe in the Previous Eighty, and with Far Better Results," *American Journal of the Medical Sciences* 85 (1883): 17–32.

Jean Louis Baudelocque's work on symphysiotomy is found in his work, *A System of Midwifery*, trans. John Heath, 3 vols. (London: J. Parkinson and J. Murray; 1790), 3:236–350.

For more modern treatments of symphysiotomy from both the developing and industrialized world, see the following: Donald A. M. Gerbie; "Vacuum Extraction and Symphysiotomy in Difficult Vaginal Delivery in a Developing Country," *British Medical Journal* 2 (1966): 1490–1493; Y. B. Gordon, "An Analysis of Symphyseotomy in Baragwanath Hospital, 1964–1967," *South African Medical Journal* 43 (1969): 659–662; Glen D. L. Mola, "Symphysiotomy or Caesarean Section after Failed Trial of Assisted Delivery," *Papua New Guinea Medical Journal* 38 (1995): 172–177; Glen D. L. Mola, "Symphysiotomy: Technique, Problems and Pitfalls, and How to Avoid Them," *Papua New Guinea Medical Journal* 38 (1995): 231–238; G. L. Pape, "27 Symphysiotomies," *Tropical Doctor* 29 (1999): 248–249; C. B. Wykes, T. A. Johnston, S. Paterson-Brown, and R. B. Johanson, "Symphysiotomy: A Lifesaving Procedure," *BJOG: An International Journal of Obstetrics and Gynaecology* 110 (2003): 219–221; D. Maharaj and J. Moodley, "Symphysiotomy and Fetal Destructive Operations," *Best Practice and Research Clinical Obstetrics and Gynaecology* 16 (2002): 117–131; Kenneth Bjorkland, "Minimally Invasive Surgery for Obstructed Labour: A Review of Symphysiotomy during the Twentieth Century (Including 5,000 Cases)," *BJOG: An International Journal of Obstetrics and Gynaecology* 109 (2002): 236–248; I. M. Sunday-Adeoye, P. Okonta, and D. Twomey, "Symphysiotomy at the Mater Misericordiae Hospital Afikpo, Ebonyi State of Nigeria (1982–1999): A Review of 1013 Cases," *Journal of Obstetrics and Gynaecology* 24 (2004): 525–529; Douwe Arie Anne Verkuyl, "Think Globally Act Locally: The Case for Symphysiotomy," *PLoS Medicine* 4, no. 3 (2007): e71, doi:10.1371/journal.pmed.0040071; Subhadeep Basak, Shyama Kanugo, and Chaityanya Majhi, "Symphysiotomy: Is It Obsolete?" *Journal of Obstetrics and Gynaecology Research* 37 (2011): 770–774.

A terrific overview of infectious problems in Cesarean section is J. Robert Wilson, "The Conquest of Cesarean Section-Related Infections: A Progress Report," *Obstetrics and Gynecology* 72

(1988): 519–532. The quotation regarding mythology is on page 519. General overviews of the history of Cesarean section can be found in Harvey A. Gabert and Mohammed Bey, "History and Development of Cesarean Operation," *Obstetrics and Gynecology Clinics of North America* 15 (1988): 591–605; J. H. Young, *The History of Caesaren Section* (London: H. K. Lewis, 1944); Dyre Trolle, *The History of Caesarean Section* (Copenhagen: C. A. Reitzel Booksellers, 1982); and Samuel Lurie, *The History of Cesarean Section* (New York: Nova Science, 2013).

The "miraculous" nature of Cesarean delivery in the Middle Ages and Renaissance is covered nicely in Renate Blumenfeld Kosinski, *Not of Woman Born: Representations of Caesarean Birth in Medieval and Renaissance Culture* (Ithaca, NY: Cornell University Press, 1990). For the early contributions of Scipione Mercurio, see Herbert Thoms, *Classical Contributions to Obstetrics and Gynecology* (Springfield, IL: Charles C. Thomas, 1935): 105–112. The quotes are from Thoms's selection from Mercurio's treatise on how to perform a Cesarean section. Rousset's book has recently been translated into English as *Caesarean Birth: The Work of Francois Rousset in Renaissance France; A New Treatise on Hysterotomotokie or Caesarian Childbirth*, trans. Ronald M. Cyr and ed. with a commentary by Thomas F. Baskett (London: RCOG Press, 2010). The quotation that the suffering of a woman in obstructed labor "could scarcely fail to horrify even the most barbaric people in the world" is on page 26.

James Barlow's first case of Cesarean section is described in his book, *Essays on Surgery and Midwifery; with Practical Observations and Select Cases* (London: Baldwin, Carddock and Joy, 1822), 355–361. See also N. H. Naqvi, "James Barlow (1767–1839): Operator of the First Successful Cesarean Section in England," *British Journal of Obstetrics and Gynaecology* 92 (1985): 468–472.

On John Lambert Richmond's Cesarean section, see Arthur G. King, "America's First Cesarean Section," *Obstetrics and Gynecology* 37 (1971): 797–802; and John Lambert Richmond, "History of a Successful Case of Caesarian Operation," *Western Journal of Medicine and Physical Science* 3 (1830): 485–489.

The major publications of the indefatigable Robert Harris on Cesarean section are Robert P. Harris, "The Operation of Gastro-Hysterotomy (True Caesarean Section), Viewed in the Light of American Experience and Success; With the History and Results of Sewing Up the Uterine Wound; and a Full Tabular Record of the Caesarean Operations Performed in the United States, Many of Them Not Hitherto Reported," *American Journal of the Medical Sciences* 75 (1878): 313–343; Robert P. Harris, "Lessons from a Study of the Cesarean Operation in the City and State of New York, and Their Bearing upon the True Position of Gastro-Elytrotomy," *American Journal of Obstetrics and Diseases of Women and Children* 12 (1879): 82–91; Robert P. Harris, "A Study and Analysis of One Hundred Caesarean Operations Performed in the United States, during the Present Century, and Prior to the Year 1878," *American Journal of the Medical Sciences* 77 (1879): 43–63; Robert P. Harris, "Special Statistics of the Cesarean Operation in the United States, Showing the Successes and Failures in Each State," *American Journal of Obstetrics and Diseases of Women and Children* 14 (1881): 341–361; Robert P. Harris, "Progress of Obstetrical Surgery. Abdominal Deliveries in the United States during the Year 1880," *American Journal of the Medical Sciences* 83 (1882): 372–378; Robert P. Harris, "A Defence of the Caesarean Statistics of America," *American Journal of the Medical Sciences* 84 (1882): 155–156; and his most famous paper, Robert P. Harris, "Cattle-Horn Lacerations of the Abdomen and Uterus in Pregnant Women," *American Journal of Obstetrics and Disease of Women and Children* 20 (1887): 673–685.

On the short-lived operation of gastro-elytrotomy, see T. Gaillard Thomas, "Gastro-Elytrotomy: A Substitute for the Caesarean Section," *American Journal of Obstetrics and Diseases of Women and*

Children 3 (1871): 125–139; T. Gaillard Thomas, "Laparo-Elytrotomy: A Substitute for the Caesarean Section," *American Journal of Obstetrics and Diseases of Women and Children* 11 (1878): 225–247; and Henry J. Garrigues, "Remarks on Gastro-Elytrotomy," *Transactions of the American Gynecological Society* 3 (1879): 212–234. The quotation from Young is from J. H. Young, *The History of Caesarean Section* (London: H. K. Lewis, 1944), 207. The quote pertaining to the extreme conservatism of British obstetrics regarding Cesarean section is on page 79.

The work of Edoardo Porro is discussed at length in chapter 4 of J. H. Young's *The History of Caesarean Section* (London: H. K. Lewis, 1944), "The Porro Operation," 93–107; and by Harold Speert, "Edoardo Porro and Cesarean Hysterectomy," *Surgery, Gynecology and Obstetrics* 106 (1958): 245–250. As far as I know, Max Sanger's book has never been translated into English. The description of his operation is based on J. H. Young's *The History of Caesarean Section*, pages 136–146; and Sanger's paper "My Work in Reference to the Cesarean Operation: A Word of Protest in Reply to Henry J. Garrigues," *American Journal of Obstetrics and Diseases of Women and Children* 20 (1887): 593–617. A nice summary of Sanger's life is given in Erlend Hem and Per Bordahl, "Max Sanger—Father of the Modern Caesarean Section," *Gynecological and Obstetric Investigation* 55 (2003): 127–129. The quotation from Howard Kelly comes from his paper, "The Steps of the Cesarean Section—the Dos and Don'ts," *American Journal of Obstetrics and Diseases of Women and Children* 24 (1891): 532–544. The exhortatory quote to his colleagues at the end is from pages 543–544.

The quote from Grandin and Jarman is from Egbert H. Grandin and George W. Jarman, *Obstetric Surgery* (Philadelphia: F. A. Davis, 1895), 4–5.

The British data are from Amand Routh, "On Caesarean Section in the United Kingdom with Tables of 1,282 Cases of Caesarean Section by Over 100 Obstetricians and Gynaecologists of the United Kingdom, Who Were Living on June 1, 1910," *Journal of Obstetrics and Gynaecology of the British Empire* 19 (1911): 1–55; and Amand Routh, "The Indications for, and Technique of, Caesarean Section and Its Alternatives, in Women with Contracted Pelves, Who Have Been Long in Labour and Exposed to Septic Infection," *Journal of Obstetrics and Gynaecology of the British Empire* 19 (1911): 236–252.

The quotation from Joseph B. DeLee is from "An Illustrated History of the Low or Cervical Cesarean Section," *American Journal of Obstetrics and Gynecology* 10 (1925): 503–520.

Cesarean section statistics from Detroit are from W. E. Welz, "Abdominal Cesarean Section in Detroit in 1926," *American Journal of Obstetrics and Gynecology* 13 (1927): 361–374; and Ward F. Seely, "Abdominal Cesarean Sections in Detroit in 1930," *American Journal of Obstetrics and Gynecology* 24 (1932): 68–74. Welz's stunning statement that "one usually thinks of a maternal mortality of 2 per cent" is on page 373. The statistics from the Chicago Lying-In Hospital are from J. P. Greenhill, "An Analysis of 874 Cervical Cesarean Sections Performed at the Chicago Lying-In Hospital," *American Journal of Obstetrics and Gynecology* 19 (1930): 613–632. A later series from the same institution is W. J. Dieckmann and A. G. Seski, "Cesarean Section at the Chicago Lying-In Hospital 1931–1949," *Surgery, Gynecology and Obstetrics* 90 (1950): 443–450. The Boston Hospital for Women statistics are from Frederick D. Friggoletto Jr., Kenneth J. Ryan, and Mark Phillipe, "Maternal Mortality Rate Associated with Cesarean Section: An Appraisal," *Obstetrics and Gynecology* 136 (1980): 969–970.

My late friend Irvine Loudon was the world's foremost authority on the history of maternal mortality. The quotations come from his short paper "The Transformation of Maternal Mortality," *BMJ* 305 (1992): 1557–1560, page 1558. A much fuller discussion of the points he makes in this article can be found in his magisterial volume, *Death in Childbirth: An International Study of Maternal Care and Maternal Mortality 1800–1950* (Oxford: Clarendon Press, 1994). Specific parallels to developing countries are made in his paper "Maternal Mortality in the Past and Its Relevance to Developing Countries Today," supplement, *American Journal of Clinical Nutrition* 72 (2000): 241S–246S.

John Chassar Moir's career is briefly summarized in "Obituary: J. Chassar Moir," *BMJ* 2 (1977): 1551. The quotations are taken from Moir's publications "Vesico-Vaginal Fistulae as Seen in Britain," *Journal of Obstetrics and Gynaecology of the British Commonwealth* 80 (1973): 598–602; "Vesico-Vaginal Fistulae: Review of 100 Consecutive Cases," *Lancet* 1 (1954): 57–61; and "Injuries of the Bladder," *American Journal of Obstetrics and Gynecology* 82 (1961): 124–131. Though somewhat outdated today from a technical standpoint, Moir's book, *The Vesico-Vaginal Fistula*, 2nd ed. (London: Bailliere Tindall and Cassell, 1967), is an easy to read and an easy to understand introduction to obstetrical fistula surgery.

The entire meeting devoted to one Cesarean section is described in Frances H. Champneys, "A Case of Caesarean Section for Contracted Pelvis," *Transactions of the Obstetrical Society of London* 31 (1890): 136–160. For examples of the very rare case reports of obstructed labor and vesico-vaginal fistula in the United States today, see Allison Korell, Peter Argenta, and Janette Strathy, "Prolonged Obstructed Labor Causing a Severe Obstetric Fistula: A Case Report," *Journal of Reproductive Medicine* 52 (2007): 555–556; and Arielle Allen, Tracy Lakin, S. Abbas Shobeiri, and Mikio Nihira, "Transmural Vaginal-to-Bladder Injury from an Obstructed Labor Pattern," *Obstetrics and Gynecology* 117 (2011): 468–470.

On the current status of Cesarean delivery in the United States, see A. Pfuntner, L. M. Wier, and C. Stocks, "Most Frequent Procedures Performed in U.S. Hospitals, 2010," *HCUP Statistical Brief #149* (February 2013); and "Safe Prevention of the Primary Cesarean Delivery: Obstetric Care Consensus No. 1; American College of Obstetricians and Gynecologists," *Obstetrics and Gynecology* 123 (2014): 693–711.

Chapter 4. Dr. Sims Finds a Cure

The quotation from James Young Simpson is from *Clinical Lectures on Diseases of Women* (Philadelphia: Blanchard and Lea, 1863), 27. The quote from Velpeau is from Alfred Velpeau, *New Elements of Operative Surgery* (Philadelphia: Carey and Hart, 1844), 858. The quotation from Pancoast is from Joseph Pancoast, *Treatise on Operative Surgery* (Philadelphia: Carey and Hart, 1844), 339. Peter Kollock's work *History and Treatment of Vesico-Vaginal Fistula: A Report Read before the Medical Society of the State of Georgia, at Their Annual Meeting at Augusta, April 8th, 1857* (Augusta: McCafferty's Office, n.d.) is full of fascinating clinical details. The quotation about the fistula victim's "sad and disgusting picture" is on page 4. The quote from Robert Liston is from *Elements of Surgery*, 4th American ed. (Philadelphia: Barrington and Haswell, 1846), 556. Mortiz Schuppert, *A Treatise on Vesico-Vaginal Fistula* (New Orleans: Daily Commercial Bulletin Printers, 1866) contains a large number of interesting surgical cases. The quotation on "the amount of suffering and pain that human flesh is heir to" is on page 20. The case of Betsy is on pages 21–22. The quotation from Maurice Collis is from his paper "Cases of Vesico-Vaginal Fistula," *Dublin Quarterly Journal of Medical Science* 23 (1857): 119–132. The quote is from page 119.

The survey of methods of treatment of vesico-vaginal fistula is taken from J. M. Chelius, *A System of Surgery*, vol. 2 (Philadelphia: Lea and Blanchard, 1847), 188–197. The quotations are from pages 189 and 190. Keith's cases, including the remarkable use of a cork plug in the bladder by Mrs. Shirress, are described in William Keith, "Cases of Vesico-Vaginal Fistula, Complicated in One of the Cases by the Presence of Stone in the Bladder, Successfully Treated," *London and Edinburgh Monthly Journal of Medical Science* 23, no. 1 (1844): 12–16.

Good overviews of the early history of fistula surgery can be found in Howard A. Kelly, "The History of Vesicovaginal Fistula," *Transactions of the American Gynecological Society* 37 (1912): 3–29; Norman F. Miller, "Treatment of Vesicovaginal Fistulas," *American Journal of Obstetrics and Gynecology* 30 (1935): 675–695; and Robert Zacharin, *Obstetric Fistula* (New York: Springer-Verlag, 1988). Van Roonhuysen's report is in *Medico-Chirurgical Observations by Henry van Roon-huyse Practitioner of Physick and Chirurgery in Amsterdam. Englished out of the Dutch by a careful hand* (London: Printed by H. C. and to be sold by Moses Pitt at the Angel in St. Pauls Church-yard, 1676). A solid summary of the modern clinical literature is given in L. Lewis Wall, Steven D. Arrowsmith, Nimi D. Briggs, Andrew Browning, and Anyetei T. Lassey, "The Obstetric Vesicovaginal Fistula in the Developing World," supplement, *Obstetrical and Gynecology Survey* 60, no. 1 (2005): S1–S55.

Henry Earle's lecture was published as H. Earle, "Clinical Lecture on Vesico-Vaginal Fistula," *London Medical Gazette* 5 (1830): 198–202.

Gosset's operation was reported in a brief letter to the *Lancet* dated November 21, 1834, and entitled "Calculus in the Bladder: Incontinence of Urine; Vesico-Vaginal Fistula; Advantages of the Gilt-Wire Suture," *Lancet* 2 (1834): 345–346.

Hayward's case is reported in George Hayward, "Case of Vesico-Vaginal Fistula, Successfully Treated by an Operation," *American Journal of the Medical Sciences* 24 (1839): 283–288. Hayward's career and contributions are described in L. Lewis Wall, "Dr. George Hayward (1791–1863): A Forgotten Pioneer of Reconstructive Pelvic Surgery," *International Urogynecology Journal* 16 (2005): 330–333. It turned out that Dr. John Peter Mettauer of Virginia had previously cured a patient of vesico-vaginal fistula but did not report it until after Hayward's case appeared. See John P. Mettauer, "Vesico-Vaginal Fistula," *Boston Medical and Surgical Journal* 22 (1840): 154–155.

The quotation from Samuel D. Gross on the fistula sufferer being "an object of deepest commiseration" is from his *A System of Surgery; Pathological, Diagnostic, Therapeutic and Operative*, vol. 2 (Philadelphia: Blanchard and Lea, 1859), 1041.

There are two main resources for understanding the life and work of J. Marion Sims. The first of these is his own autobiography, published after his death: J. Marion Sims, *The Story of My Life* (New York: D. Appleton, 1884). Sims was working on this book when he died, and as a result it was incomplete, telling his story only up until 1863. The book was edited by his son, Dr. Harry Marion-Sims, and published posthumously, but its easy style and guileless narration of his life made it wildly popular, and it was a best seller in its day. The second source for Sims's life is the biography by Dr. Seale Harris, published in 1950: Seale Harris, *Woman's Doctor: The Life Story of J. Marion Sims* (New York: Macmillan, 1950). Harris's father, Dr. Charles Hooks Harris, was one of Sims's students and knew him personally. Harris also had access to personal reminiscences of Sims by a number of people who were still living when he was working on his book. *Woman's Surgeon* is carefully researched and well written but has been overly analyzed by modern critics who look upon it as an infallible narration of Sims's life rather than an interpretation influenced by the time and place in which it was written. Direct quotes in this chapter are taken from Sims's autobiography.

Another useful volume is Deborah Kuhn McGregor's book, *From Midwives to Medicine: The Birth of American Gynecology* (New Brunswick, NJ: Rutgers University Press, 1998). The reader should use this book with caution, as it contains numerous clinical inaccuracies, including a few major gaffes.

The Harris poll data on the prestige of occupations can be found at "Doctors, Military Officers, Firefighters, and Scientists Seen as among America's Most Prestigious Occupations," New York, September 10, 2104, http://www.theharrispoll.com/politics/Doctors__Military_Officers_ _Firefighters__and_Scientists_Seen_as_Among_America_s_Most_Prestigious_Occupations .html.

The best concise history of the transformation of medicine into a scientific endeavor is W. F. Bynum's *Science and the Practice of Medicine in the Nineteenth Century* (Cambridge: Cambridge University Press, 1994). Also useful is Guy Williams, *The Age of Miracles: Medicine and Surgery in the Nineteenth Century* (Chicago: Chicago Review Press, 2005). Typical medical practice in the South is well described in Steven M. Stowe, *Doctoring the South: Southern Physicians and Everyday Medicine in the Mid-nineteenth Century* (Chapel Hill: University of North Carolina Press, 2004).

The famous quote by Oliver Wendell Holmes is from his essay "Currents and Counter-currents in Medical Science," published in his book *Medical Essays 1842–1882* (Boston: Houghton, Mifflin, 1883), 203.

The quotation from Robert Liston is from his *Practical Surgery*, 4th ed. (London: John Churchill, 1846), 5.

Hunter's quote on the "necessary inhumanity" of surgery is from William Hunter, *Two Introductory Lectures, Delivered by William Hunter, to his Last Course of Anatomical Lectures at his Theatre in Windmill-Street* (London: J. Johnson, 1784), 67.

Sims wrote case reports of a number of his surgical operations from this period, including "Extraction of Foreign Bodies from the Meatus Auditorius Externus," *American Journal of the Medical Sciences* 9 (1845): 336–342; "Osteo-Sarcoma of the Lower Jaw: Resection of the Body of the Bone," *American Journal of the Medical Sciences* 11 (1846): 128–132; "Removal of the Superior Maxilla for a Tumor of the Antrum," *American Journal of the Medical Sciences* 13 (1847): 310–314; and "Osteo-Sarcoma of the Lower Jaw: Removal of the Body of the Bone," *American Journal of the Medical Sciences* 14 (1847): 310–314.

My discussion of Sims's operation for congenital double harelip is based on his autobiographical recollections and on his case report, "Double Congenital Hare-Lip—Absence of the Superior Incisors and Their Portion of Alveolar Process," *American Journal of Dental Science* 5 (1844): 51–56.

The history of urethral catheterization is covered succinctly in D. A. Bloom, E. J. McGuire, and J. Lapides, "A Brief History of Urethral Catheterization," *Journal of Urology* 151 (1994): 317–325. The development of the modern Foley balloon catheter is described in A. W. Zorgniotti, "Frederic E. B. Foley: Early Development of the Balloon Catheter," *Urology* 1 (1973): 75–80.

The basic description of his early operations in given in Sims's paper, "On the Treatment of Vesico-Vaginal Fistula," *American Journal of the Medical Sciences* 23 (1852): 59–82. Quotations are from this source unless otherwise specified. Sims described further fistula cases and his experiences with them in several other articles: "Two Cases of Vesicovaginal Fistula," *New York Medical Gazette* 5 (1854): 1–7; "A Case of Vesicovaginal Fistula with the Os Uteri Closed Up in the Bladder," *American Medical Monthly* 1 (1854): 109–112; "A Case of Vesicovaginal Fistula Resisting the Cautery for More Than Seven Years," *New York Medical Times* 3 (1854): 265–267; and *Silver Sutures in Surgery: The Anniversary Discourse before the New York Academy of Medicine* (New York: William Wood, 1858).

The quotation from Johannes Dieffenbach (1792–1847) is given by Moritz Schuppert in *A Treatise on Vesico-Vaginal Fistula* (New Orleans: Daily Commercial Bulletin Print, 1866), 36.

The most accessible account of the life and work of Thomas Addis Emmet is L. Lewis Wall, "Thomas Addis Emmet, the Vesicovaginal Fistula, and the Origins of Reconstructive Gynecologic Surgery," *International Urogynecology Journal* 13 (2002): 145–155. The description of Emmet's first meeting with Sims is from Thomas Addis Emmet, *Incidents of My Life, Professional—Literary—Social, with Services in the Cause of Ireland* (New York: G. P. Putnam's Sons, 1911). The quotation about fistula becoming his life's work is on page 166. The quotations concerning Emmet's fistula work are taken from Thomas Addis Emmet, *Vesico-Vaginal Fistula from Parturition and Other Causes: With Cases of Recto-Vaginal Fistula* (New York: William Wood, 1868), 13–22. The case of Mrs. R (no. 37) is found on pages 110–113. Howard Kelly's comments about the Sims-Emmet partnership are from "Thomas Addis Emmet," in *Dictionary of American Medical Biography: Lives of Eminent Physicians of the United States and Canada from the Earliest Times*, ed. H. A. Kelly and W. L. Burrage (New York: D. Appleton, 1928), 381–384.

The full reference for Sims's book is *Clinical Notes on Uterine Surgery, with Special Reference to the Management of the Sterile Condition* (London: Robert Hardwicke, 1866).

The subsequent history of fistula surgery is treated nicely in Robert Zacharin's book, *Obstetric Fistula* (New York: Springer-Verlag, 1988). Recent texts dealing with contemporary fistula surgery that the interested reader may peruse with profit include Brian Hancock, *First Steps in Vesico-Vaginal Fistula Repair* (London: Royal Society of Medicine, 2005); Brian Hancock and Andrew Browning, *Practical Obstetric Fistula Surgery* (London: Royal Society of Medicine, 2009); and Kees Waaldijk, *Step-by-Step Surgery of Vesicovaginal Fistulas* (Edinburgh: Campion Press, 1994). The latter book contains detailed clinical photographs of many varieties of obstetric fistula and the surgical operations to repair them, but it is not smooth reading. Hancock or Zacharin are better places to start.

Chapter 5. Structural Violence and Obstetric Fistula among the Hausa

Portions of this chapter appeared originally in L. Lewis Wall, "Dead Mothers and Injured Wives: The Social Context of Maternal Morbidity and Mortality among the Hausa of Northern Nigeria," *Studies in Family Planning* 29, no. 4 (1998): 341–359. The fistula song "Fitsari 'Dan Duniya" was originally published in L. Lewis Wall, "Fitsari 'Dan Duniya: An African (Hausa) Praise-Song about Vesico-Vaginal Fistulas," *Obstetrics and Gynecology* 100 (2002): 1328–1332.

For a general overview of Hausa village life and medical thinking, see L. Lewis Wall, *Hausa Medicine: Illness and Well-Being in a West African Culture* (Durham, NC: Duke University Press, 1988).

On the concept of structural violence, see James Gilligan, *Violence: Reflections on a National Epidemic*, Vintage Books ed. (New York: Vintage Books, 1997). The quote comes from page 192. See also Paul E. Farmer, Bruce Nizeye, Sara Stulac, and Salmaan Keshavjee, "Structural Violence and Clinical Medicine," *PLoS Medicine* 3, no. 10 (2006): 1686–1691.

Three important Hausa language references are Charles Henry Robinson, *Dictionary of the Hausa Language* (Cambridge: Cambridge University Press, 1925); G. P. Bargery, *A Hausa-English Dictionary and English-Hausa Vocabulary* (London: Oxford University Press, 1934); and R. C. Abraham, *Dictionary of the Hausa Language* (London: University of London Press, 1962).

There are now many works dealing with the Hausa diaspora throughout Africa. In particular, see Mahdi Adamu, *The Hausa Factor in West African History* (Zaria, Nigeria: Ahmadu Bello

University Press / Oxford University Press, 1978); Abner Cohen, *Custom and Politics in Urban Africa* (London: Routledge and Kegan Paul, 1969); John A. Works Jr., *Pilgrims in a Strange Land* (New York: Columbia University Press, 1976); C. Bawa Yamba, *Permanent Pilgrims: The Role of Pilgrimage in the Lives of West African Muslims in Sudan* (Washington, DC: Smithsonian Institution Press, 1995); and Deborah Pellow, *Strangers and Lodgers: Socio-Spatial Organization in an Accra Community* (New York: Prager, 2002).

On the histories of the Hausa city-states, see Finn Fuglestad, "A Reconsideration of Hausa History before the Jihad," *Journal of African History* 19 (1978): 319–339. Abdullahi Smith, "Some Considerations Relating to the Formation of States in Hausaland," *Journal of the Historical Society of Nigeria* 5 (1970): 329–346; and Michael G. Smith, *Government in Zazzau, 1800–1950* (London: International African Institute, 1960).

The Fulani jihad of Usman 'Dan Fodio and subsequent developments are treated in Mervyn Hiskett, *The Sword of Truth: The Life and Times of Shehu Usuman Dan Fodio* (London: Oxford University Press, 1973); Murray Last, *The Sokoto Caliphate* (London: Longman, 1967); R. H. Dusgate, *The Conquest of Northern Nigeria* (London: Frank Cass, 1985); D. J. M. Muffett, *Concerning Brave Captains: Being a History of the British Occupation of Kano and Sokoto and the Last Stand of the Fulani Forces* (London: Andre Deutsch, 1964).

Basic information on Hausa social organization is given in M. G. Smith, "The Hausa System of Social Status," *Africa* 29 (1959): 239–251; E. R. Yeld, "Islam and Social Stratification in Northern Nigeria," *British Journal of Sociology* 11 (1960): 112–128; Polly Hill, *Rural Hausa: A Village and a Setting* (New York: Cambridge University Press, 1972); J. C. Moughtin, "The Traditional Settlements of the Hausa People," *Town Planning Review* 35 (1964): 21–34; J. C. Moughtin, *Hausa Architecture* (London: Ethnographica, 1985); A. D. Goddard, "Changing Family Structures among the Rural Hausa," *Africa* 43 (1973): 207–218; J. Trevor, "Family Change in Sokoto, a Traditional Moslem Fulani/Hausa City," in *Population Growth and Socioeconomic Change in West Africa*, ed. J. C. Caldwell (New York: Columbia University Press, 1975), 236–253.

The lives of Hausa women are discussed in the following: Renee Pittin, "Migration of Women in Nigeria: The Hausa Case," *International Migration Review* 18 (1984): 1293–1314. The quotation about "this God-given system of unrelenting spatial constraint" is on page 1297. Barbara J. Callaway, *Muslim Hausa Women in Nigeria: Tradition and Change* (Syracuse, NY: Syracuse University Press, 1987). The extended quotation about life in the Hausa compound is on page 35. Jean Trevor, "Family Change in Sokoto, a Traditional Moslem Fulani/Hausa City," in *Population Growth and Socioeconomic Change in West Africa*, ed. J. C. Caldwell (New York: Columbia University Press, 1975), 236–253 (the quotation about maternal death is on page 259); H. Papanek, "Purdah: Separate Worlds and Symbolic Shelter," *Comparative Studies in Society and History* 15 (1973): 289–325; Richard Longhurst, "Resource Allocation and the Sexual Division of Labor: A Case Study of a Moslem Hausa Village in Northern Nigeria," in *Women and Development: The Sexual Division of Labor in Rural Societies*, ed. L. Beneria (New York: Praeger, 1982), 95–117; Polly Hill, "Hidden Trade in Hausaland," *Man*, n.s., 4 (1969): 392–409; Jerome H. Barkow, "Hausa Women and Islam," *Canadian Journal of African Studies* 6 (1972): 317–328; Yakubu Zakaria, "Entrepreneurs at Home: Secluded Muslim Women and Hidden Economic Activities in Northern Nigeria," *Nordic Journal of African Studies* 10, no. 1 (2001): 107–123; Catherine VerEecke, " 'It Is Better to Die Than to Be Shamed': Cultural and Moral Dimensions of Women's Trading in an Islamic Nigerian Society," *Anthropos* 88 (1993): 403–417; Frank A. Salamone, "The Arrow and the Bird: Proverbs in the Solution of Hausa Conjugal Conflicts," *Journal of Anthropological Research* 32, no. 4 (1976): 358–371; Mary Smith, *Baba of Karo: A Woman of the Muslim Hausa* (New York: Philosophical Society, 1955); Barbara J. Callaway, "Ambiguous Consequences of the Socialisation and Seclusion of Hausa Women," *Journal of Modern African Studies* 22 (1984): 429–450; Elizabeth Dry, "The Social Development of the Hausa Child," in *Proceedings of the Third International West African Conference, Ibadan, December 12–21* (Ibadan: Nigerian Museum, 1949), 164–170; C. Coles, "The Older Woman in Hausa Society: Power and Authority in Urban Nigeria," in *The Cultural Context of Aging*, ed. J. Sokolovsky (Westport, CT: Bergin and Garvey, 1990), 58–81; N. Rehan, "Knowledge, Attitude and Practice of Family Planning in Hausa Women," *Social Science and Medicine* 18 (1984): 839–844; Enid Schildkrout, "Widows in Hausa Society: Ritual Phase or Social Status?," in *Widows in African Societies: Choices and Constraints*, ed. B. Potash (Stanford, CA: Stanford University Press, 1986), 131–152; A. J. N. Tremearne, "Marital Relations of the Hausas as Shown in Their Folk-Lore," *Man* 14 (1914): 23–26, 137–139, 148–156; Jean Trevor, "Western Education and Muslim Fulani/Hausa Women in Sokoto, Northern Nigeria," in *Conflict and Harmony in Education in Tropical Africa*, ed. G. N. Brown and M. Hiskett (Rutherford, NJ: Fairleigh Dickinson University Press, 1976), 247–270 (the quote is from page 259); C. Coles, "The Older Woman in Hausa Society: Power and Authority in Urban Nigeria," in *The Cultural Context of Aging*, ed. J. Sokolovsky (Westport, CT: Bergin and Garvey, 1990), 289–325; Renee Pittin, "Houses of Women: A Focus on Alternative Life-Styles in Katsina City," in *Female and Male in West Africa*, ed. C. Oppong (London: George Allen and Unwin, 1983), 291–302; Annabel Erulkar and Mairo Bello, *The Experience of Married Adolescent Girls in Northern Nigeria* (New York: Population Council, 2007); Marg Csapo, "Religious, Social and Economic Factors Hindering the Education of Girls in Northern Nigeria," *Comparative Education* 17, no. 3 (1981): 311–319; Elsbeth Robson, "The 'Kitchen' as Women's Space in Rural Hausaland, Northern Nigeria," *Gender, Place and Culture* 13, no. 6 (2006): 669–676; Elsbeth Robson, "Wife Seclusion and the Spatial Praxis of Gender Ideology in Nigerian Hausaland," *Gender, Place, and Culture* 7, no. 2 (2000): 179–199; Kelsey A. Harrison, "The Importance of the Educated Healthy Woman in Africa," *Lancet* 349 (1997): 644–647; Nimi D. Briggs, "Illiteracy and Maternal Health: Educate or Die," *Lancet* 341 (1993): 1063–1064.

There are an increasing number of books and articles dealing with the status of women in Islamic law. Two useful references are Joseph Schacht, *An Introduction to Islamic Law* (Oxford: Clarendon Press, 1964); and D. Hinchcliffe, "The Status of Women in Islamic Law," in *Conflict and Harmony in Education in Tropical Africa*, ed. G. N. Brown and M. Hiskett (Rutherford, NJ: Fairleigh Dickinson University Press, 1976), 455–466.

Introductory materials on maternal mortality can be found in World Health Organization, *Trends in Maternal Mortality 1990–2015: Estimates by WHO, UNICEF, UNFPA, World Bank Group and the United Nations Population Division* (Geneva: World Health Organization, 2015); Andrea A. Creanga, Cynthia J. Berg, Carla Syverson, Kristi Seed, F. Carol Bruce, and William M. Callaghan, "Pregnancy-Related Mortality in the United States, 2006–2010," *Obstetrics and Gynecology* 125 (2015): 5–12; M. Waterstone, S. Bewley, and C. Wolf, "Incidence and Predictors of Severe Obstetric Morbidity: Case-Control Study," *BMJ* 322 (2001): 1080–1094; and Erica Royston and Sue Armstrong, *Preventing Maternal Deaths* (Geneva: World Health Organization, 1989).

On childbirth and maternal health in Hausaland, the place to start is Kelsey Harrison's groundbreaking study from 1985: K. A. Harrison, "Child-Bearing, Health and Social Priorities: A Survey of 22,774 Consecutive Hospital Births in Zaria, Northern Nigeria," supplement,

British Journal of Obstetrics and Gynaecology 92, no. 5 (1985): 1–119. His comment about the low status of women is from page 5, and his moving conclusion about "large numbers of women are born into a cycle of deprivation" is on page 116. A succinct overview of the maternal health problems in Nigeria can be found in Kelsey Harrison, "The Struggle to Reduce High Maternal Mortality in Nigeria," *African Journal of Reproductive Health* 13, no. 9 (2009): 9–20. Harrison's autobiography is also full of illuminating information: Kelsey Harrison, *An Arduous Climb: From the Creeks of the Niger Delta to Leading Obstetrician and University Vice-Chancellor* (London: Adonis and Abbey, 2006).

Of special interest are the following sections of Harrison's larger report: K. A. Harrison, A. F. Fleming, N. D. Briggs, and C. E. Rossiter, "Growth during Pregnancy in Nigerian Teenage Primigravidae," supplement, *British Journal of Obstetrics and Gynaecology* 92, no. 5 (1985): 32–39; K. A. Harrison, U. G. Lister, C. E. Rossiter, and H. Chong, "Perinatal Mortality," supplement, *British Journal of Obstetrics and Gynaecology* 92, no. 5 (1985): 86–99; K. A. Harrison, "Mode of Delivery with Notes on Rupture of the Gravid Uterus and Vesicovaginal Fistula," supplement, *British Journal of Obstetrics and Gynaecology* 92, no. 5 (1985): 61–71.

Unfortunately, there is no shortage of publications documenting the terrible maternal health conditions in northern Nigeria and southern Niger. Harrison's findings from 30 years ago have been supplemented by numerous other works, which have been used in the compilation of table 5.1: B. A. Ekele, L. R. Audu, and S. Muyibi, "Uterine Rupture in Sokoto, Northern Nigeria: Are We Winning?," *African Journal of Medical Sciences* 29 (2000): 191–193; Y. Ahmend, C. E. Shehu, E. I. Nwobodo, and B. A. Ekele, "Reducing Maternal Mortality from Ruptured Uterus: The Sokoto Initiative," *African Journal of Medical Sciences* 33 (2004): 135–138; M. K. Kisekkea, C. C. Ekwempu, E. S. Essien, and B. M. Olorukoba, "Determinants of Maternal Mortality in Zaria Area," in *Women's Health Issues in Nigeria*, ed. Mere Nakateregga Kisekka (Zaria, Nigeria: Tamaza, 1992), 51–65; I. A. O. Ujab, O. A. Aisien, J. T. Mutihir, D. J. Wanderjagt, R. H. Glew, and V. E. Uguru, "Factors Contributing to Maternal Mortality in North-Central Nigeria: A Seventeen Year Review," *African Journal of Reproductive Health* 9, no. 3 (2005): 27–40; P. I. Onwuhafua, A. On-wuhafua, and J. Adze, "The Challenge of Reducing Maternal Mortality in Nigeria," *International Journal of Gynecology and Obstetrics* 71 (2000): 211–213; I. R. Audu and B. A. Ekele, "A Ten Year Review of Maternal Mortality in Sokoto, Northern Nigeria," *West African Journal of Medicine* 21, no. 1 (2002): 74–76; D. J. Shehu, "Socio-Cultural Factors in the Causation of Maternal Mortality and Morbidity in Sokoto," in *Women's Health Issues in Nigeria*, ed. Mere Nakateregga Kisekka (Zaria, Nigeria: Tamaza, 1992), 203–214; Y. M. Audu, M. H. Salihu, N. Sathikumar, and G. R. Alexander, "Maternal Mortality in Northern Nigeria: A Population-Based Study," *European Journal of Obstetrics & Gynecology and Reproductive Medicine* 109 (2003): 153–159; O. O. Adetoro and A. Agah, "The Implications of Childbearing in Postpubertal Girls in Sokoto, Nigeria," *International Journal of Gynecology and Obstetrics* 27 (1988): 73–77; L. R. Airede and B. A. Ekele, "Adolescent Maternal Mortality in Sokoto, Nigeria," *Journal of Obstetrics and Gynaecology* 23, no. 2 (2003): 163–165 (their bleak conclusions about adolescent deaths being the result of poverty, powerlessness, and neglect is on page 164); A. A. Kullima, M. B. Kawuwa, A. D. Geidam, and A. G. Mairiga, "Trends in Maternal Mortality in a Tertiary Institution in Northern Nigeria," *Annals of African Medicine* 8, no. 4 (2009): 221–224; J. Tukur and T. A. Jido, "Maternal Mortality in Rural Northern Nigeria," *Tropical Doctor* 38 (2008): 35–36; H. V. Doctor, A. Olatunji, S. E. Findley, G. Y. Afenyadu, A. Abdulwahab, and A. Jumare, "Maternal Mortality in Northern Nigeria: Findings of the Health and Demographic Surveillance System in Zamfara State, Nigeria," *Tropical*

Doctor 42 (2012): 140–143; E. I. Nwobo and A. Pantin,"Adolescent Maternal Mortality in North-west Nigeria," *West African Journal of Medicine* 32, no. 4 (2012): 224–226; M. K. Kisekka, C. C. Ekwempu, E. S. Essien, and B. M. Olorukoba, "Determinants of Maternal Mortality in Zaria Area," in *Women's Health Issues in Nigeria,* ed. Mere Nakateregga Kisekka (Zaria, Nigeria: Tamaza, 1992), 224–226.

Additional social and cultural aspects of childbirth among the Hausa are covered in the following: N. Rehan, "Knowledge, Attitude and Practice of Family Planning in Hausa Women," *Social Science and Medicine* 18 (1984): 839–844; N. E. Rahan and S. Sani, "Obstetric Behaviour of Hausa Women," *Journal of Obstetrics and Gynaecology of East and Central Africa* 5 (1986): 21–25; Lorna A. Trevitt, "Attitudes and Customs in Childbirth amongst Hausa Women in Zaria City," *Savannah* 2 (1973): 223–226; Kelsey A. Harrison, "Traditional Birth Attendants," *Lancet* 2 (1980): 43–44; D. A. Ityavyar, "A Traditional Midwife Practice, Sokoto State, Nigeria," *Social Science and Medicine* 18 (1984): 497–501; B. U. Ezem and J. A. Otubu, "A Complication of a Traditional Puerperal Practice in Nigeria," *International Journal of Gynecology and Obstetrics* 18 (1980): 383–384; O. A. Mabogunje, "Burn Injuries during the Puerperium in Zaria, Nigeria," *International Journal of Gynecology and Obstetrics* 30 (1989): 133–137; Z. Iliyasu, M. Kabir, H. S. Galadanci, I. S. Abubakar, H. M. Salihu, and M. H. Aliyu, "Postpartum Beliefs and Practices in Danbare Village, Northern Nigeria," *Journal of Obstetrics and Gynaecology* 26, no. 3 (2006): 211–215; H. M. Salihu, Y. M. Adamu, Z. Y. Aliya, and M. H. Aliyu, "Pregnancy-Associated Morbidity in Northern Nigeria," *Journal of Obstetrics and Gynaecology* 24, no. 4 (2004): 367–371; A. Prual, D. Huguet, O. Garvin, and G. Rabe, "Severe Obstetric Morbidity of the Third Trimester, Delivery, and Early Puerperium in Niamey (Niger)," *African Journal of Reproductive Health* 2, no. 1 (1998): 10–19; H. V. Doctor and T. Dahiru, "Utilization of Non-skilled Birth Attendants in Northern Nigeria: A Rough Terrain to the Health-Related MDGs," *African Journal of Reproductive Health* 14, no. 2 (2010): 37–45; H. V. Doctor, S. E. Findley, G. Cometto, and G. Y. Afenyadu, "Awareness of Critical Danger Signs of Pregnancy and Delivery, Preparations for Delivery, and Utilization of Skilled Birth Attendance in Nigeria," *Journal of Health Care for the Poor and Underserved* 24 (2013): 152–170; E. Okereke, S. Aradeon, A. Akerele, M. Tanko, I. Yisa, and B. Obonyo, "Knowledge of Safe Motherhood among Women in Rural Communities in Northern Nigeria: Implications for Maternal Mortality Reduction," *Reproductive Health* 10 (2013): 57, doi:10.1186/1742-4755-10 57: H. V. Doctor, S. E. Findley, A. Ager, G. Cometto, G. Y. Afenyadu, and C. Green, "Using Community-Based Research to Shape the Design and Delivery of Maternal Health Services in Northern Nigeria," *Reproductive Health Matters* 20, no. 9 (2012): 104–112; C. C. Ekwempu, D. Maine, M. B. Olorukoba, E. S. Essien, and M. N. Kisseka, "Structural Adjustment and Health in Africa," *Lancet* 336 (1990): 56–57; Prevention of Maternal Mortality Network, "Situation Analyses of Emergency Obstetric Care: Examples from Eleven Operations Research Projects in West Africa," *Social Science and Medicine* 40, no. 5 (1995): 657–667; H. Galadanci, W. Kunzel, O. Shittu, R. Zinser, M. Gruhl, and S. Adams, "Obstetric Quality Assurance to Reduce Maternal and Fetal Mortality in Kano and Kaduna State Hospitals in Nigeria," *International Journal of Gynecology and Obstetrics* 114 (2011): 23–28.

On birthweights and sex distribution of newborns, see N. E. Rehan, "Sex Ratio of Live-Born Hausa Infants," *British Journal of Obstetrics and Gynaecology* 89, no. 2 (1982): 136–141; M. G. Arenne, "Sex Ratios at Birth in African Populations: A Review of Survey Data," *Human Biology* 74, no. 6 (2002): 889–900; N. E. Rehan and D. S. Tafida, "Birth Weight of Hausa Infants in Northern Nigeria," *British Journal of Obstetrics and Gynaecology* 86 (1979): 443–449; and M. T.

Abena-Obama, V. W. Shasha, J. Fodjo, F. Bonongkaho, J. Mbede, and J. Kamdom Moyo, "Foetal Macrosomia in Cameroon: Prevalence, Risk Factors and Complications," *West African Journal of Medicine* 14 (1995): 249–254.

Peripartum cardiomyopathy is relatively rare in the United States but almost epidemic in northern Nigeria. See J. Abboud, Y. Murad, C. Chen-Scarabelli, L. Saravolatz, and T. M. Scarabelli, "Peripartum Cardiomyopathy: A Comprehensive Review," *International Journal of Cardiology* 118 (2007): 295–303; F. G. Cunningham, J. A. Pritchard, G. D. V. Hankins, P. L. Anderson, M. J. Lucas, and K. F. Armstrong, "Peripartum Heart Failure: Idiopathic Cardiomyopathy or Compounding Cardiovascular Events?," *Obstetrics and Gynecology* 67 (1986): 157–168; E. H. O. Parry, N. M. Davidson, G. O. A. Ladipo, and H. Watkins, "Seasonal Variation of Cardiac Failure in Northern Nigeria," *Lancet* 1 (1977): 1023–1025; S. A. Iseuzo and S. A. Abubakar, "Epidemiologic Profile of Peripartum Cardiomyopathy in a Tertiary Care Hospital," *Ethnicity & Disease* 17 (2007): 228–233; N. M. Davidson and E. H. O. Parry, "Peri-partum Cardiac Failure," *Quarterly Journal of Medicine*, n.s., 47 (1978): 431–461; N. M. Davidson, L. Trevitt, and E. H. O. Parry, "Peripartum Cardiac Failure: An Explanation for the Observed Geographic Distribution in Nigeria," *Bulletin of the World Health Organization* 51 (1974): 203–208.

Because these injuries are so numerous in northern Nigeria, there is now a fairly robust literature on obstetric fistula in this part of the world: K. Ampofo, B. A. Omotara, T. Otu, and G. Uchebo, "Risk Factors of Vesico-Vaginal Fistulae in Maiduguri, Nigeria: A Case-Control Study," *Tropical Doctor* 20 (1990): 138–139; F. Tahzib, "Epidemiological Determinants of Vesico-vaginal Fistulas," *British Journal of Obstetrics and Gynaecology* 90 (1983): 387–391; F. Tahzib, "Vesicovaginal Fistula in Nigerian Children," *Lancet* 2 (1985): 1291–1293; L. Lewis Wall, Jonathan Karshima, Carolyn Kirschner, and Steven D. Arrowsmith, "The Obstetric Vesicovaginal Fistula: Characteristics of 899 Patients from Jos, Nigeria," *American Journal of Obstetrics and Gynecology* 190 (2004): 1011–1119; Kelsey A. Harrison, "Obstetric Fistula: One Social Calamity Too Many," *British Journal of Obstetrics and Gynaecology* 90 (1983): 385–386; Margaret Murphy, "Social Consequences of Vesico-Vaginal Fistula in Northern Nigeria," *Journal of Biosocial Science* 13 (1981): 139–150; M. Murphy and T. M. Baba, "Rural Dwellers and Health Care in Northern Nigeria," *Social Science and Medicine* 15A (1981): 265–271; K. Ampofo, T. Otu, and G. Uchebo, "Epidemiology of Vesico-Vaginal Fistulae in Northern Nigeria," *West African Journal of Medicine* 9 (1990): 98–102; S. D. Arrowsmith, "Genitourinary Reconstruction in Obstetric Fistulas," *Journal of Urology* 152 (1994): 403–406; D. P. Ghatak, "A Study of Urinary Fistulae in Sokoto, Nigeria," *Journal of the Indian Medical Association* 90, no. 1 (1992): 285–287; M. Kabir, I. S. Iliyasu, and U. I. Umar, "Medico-Social Problems of Patients with Vesico-Vaginal Fistula in Murtala Mohammed Specialist Hospital, Kano," *Annals of African Medicine* 3, no. 2 (2003): 54–57; D. N. Onolemhemhen, *A Social Worker's Investigation of Childbirth Injured Women in Northern Nigeria* (Lanham, MD: University Press of America, 2005); G. S. Melah, A. A. Massa, U. R. Yahaya, M. Bukar, D. D. Kizaya, and A. U. El-Nafaty, "Risk Factors for Obstetric Fistulae in North-Eastern Nigeria," *Journal of Obstetrics and Gynaecology* 27, no. 8 (2007): 819–823; Kees Waaldijk, "The (Surgical) Management of Bladder Fistula in 775 Women in Northern Nigeria" (PhD Thesis, Nijmegen, Holland, 1989); O. Ojanuga and M. Johnson, "Hausa Families and Health Care Choices: Birth Injuries in African Communities," *Family Systems Medicine* 10 (1992): 413–421.

On the Hausa cultural practice of *gishiri* cutting and its consequences, see F. Tahzib, "Vesicovaginal Fistula in Nigerian Children," *Lancet* 2 (1985): 1291–1293; and J. Tukur, T. A. Jido, and

C. C. Uzoho, "The Contribution of *Gishiri* Cut to Vesicovaginal Fistula in Birnin Kudu, Northern Nigeria," *African Journal of Urology* 12 (2006): 121–125.

As the problem with radical Islamic groups such as Boko Haram grows, so does the literature on this topic. For starters, see Virginia Comelli, *Boko Haram: Nigeria's Islamist Insurgency* (London: C. Hurst, 2015); and Mike Smith, *Boko Haram: Inside Nigeria's Holy War* (London: I. B. Tauris, 2015). On Boko Haram's war on women, see Jacob Zenn and Elizabeth Pearson, "Women, Gender and the Evolving Tactics of Boko Haram," *Journal of Terrorism Research* 5, no. 1 (2014): 46–57. Also timely and useful is Charlotte Alfred, "10 Must-Reads for Understanding Boko Haram's War on Women," *Huffington Post*, April 14, 2016, http://www.huffingtonpost.com /entry/boko-haram-women_us_57096e82e4b0836057a17194.

The quotation by Nimi Briggs is from "Illiteracy and Maternal Health: Educate or Die," *Lancet* 341 (1993): 1063–1064.

Chapter 6. Deadly Delays in Deciding to Seek Care

Portions of this chapter originally appeared as L. Lewis Wall, "Overcoming Phase 1 Delays: The Critical Component of Obstetric Fistula Prevention Programs in Resource-Poor Countries," *BMC Pregnancy and Childbirth* 12 (2012): 68, http://www.biomedcentral.com/1471-2393/12/68, an open access publication. I am grateful for permission to reuse this material.

The quote from Thomas Addis Emmet is from *Vesico-Vaginal Fistula from Parturition and Other Causes: With Cases of Recto-Vaginal Fistula* (New York: William Wood; 1868), 20.

The three mechanisms for reducing maternal death are described in J. McCarthy and D. Maine, "A Framework for Analyzing the Determinants of Maternal Mortality," *Studies in Family Planning* 23 (1992): 23–33. This framework has been adapted to obstetric fistula in L. Lewis Wall, "A Framework for Analyzing the Determinants of Obstetric Fistula Formation," *Studies in Family Planning* 43, no. 4 (2012): 255–272.

The value of family planning in attacking problems of obstetric morbidity and mortality is discussed in J. A. Fortney, "The Importance of Family Planning in Reducing Maternal Mortality," *Studies in Family Planning* 18 (1987): 109–114.

The importance of nutrition and the role of pelvic growth in obstructed labor is discussed in A. O. Tsui, A. A. Creanga, and S. Ahmed, "The Role of Delayed Childbearing in the Prevention of Obstetric Fistulas," supplement, *International Journal of Gynecology and Obstetrics* 99, no. 1 (2007): S98–S107; and in M. L. Moerman, "Growth of the Birth Canal in Adolescent Girls," *American Journal of Obstetrics and Gynecology* 143, no. 5 (1982): 528–532.

The problems with the risk assessment approach to maternal mortality and the difficulties of using screening tests to assess the risk of obstructed labor are covered in the following references: J. A. Fortney, "Antenatal Risk Screening and Scoring: A New Look," supplement, *International Journal of Gynecology and Obstetrics* 50, no. 2 (1995): S53–S58; E. A. Yuster, "Rethinking the Role of the Risk Approach and Antenatal Care in Maternal Mortality Reduction," supplement, *International Journal of Gynecology and Obstetrics* 50, no. 2 (1995): S59–S61; A. Prual, A. Toure, D. Huguet, and Y. Aurent, "The Quality of Risk Factor Screening during Antenatal Consultations in Niger," *Health Policy and Planning* 15 (2000): 11–16; B. Dujardin, G. Clarysse, M. Mentens, I. De Schampheleire, and R. Kulker, "How Accurate Is Maternal Height Measurement in Africa?," *International Journal of Gynecology and Obstetrics* 41 (1993): 139–145; B. Dujardin, R. Van Cutsem, and T. Lamrechts, "The Value of Maternal Height as a Risk Factor of Dystocia: A Meta-analysis," *Tropical Medicine and International Health* 1 (1996): 510–521; B. Moller and G. Lindmark, "Short

Stature: An Obstetric Risk Factor? A Comparison of Two Villages in Tanzania," *Acta Obstetricia et Gynecologica Scandinavica* 76 (1997): 394–397; M. V. Zaretsky, J. M. Alexander, D. D. McIntire, M. R. Hatab, D. M. Twickler, and K. J. Leveno, "Magnetic Resonance Imaging Pelvimetery and the Prediction of Labor Dystocia," *Obstetrics and Gynecology* 106 (2005): 919–926; A. O. Awonuga, Z. Merhi, M. T. Awonuga, T. A. Samuels, and J. Waller, D. Pring, "Anthropometric Measurements in the Diagnosis of Pelvic Size: An Analysis of Maternal Height and Shoe Size and Computed Tomography Pelvimetric Data," *Archives of Gynecology and Obstetrics* 276 (2007): 523–528; Kasongo Project Team, "Antenatal Screening for Fetopelvic Dystocias: A Cost-Effectiveness Approach to the Choice of Simple Indicators for Use by Auxiliary Personnel," *Journal of Tropical Medicine and Hygiene* 87 (1984): 173–183.

Access to emergency obstetric care is the lynchpin of attempts to reduce maternal mortality and severe obstetric morbidity. These two references make this point clearly: C. Ronsmans, J. F. Etard, G. Walraven, L. Hoj, A. Dumont, L. de Bernis, and B. Kodio, "Maternal Mortality and Access to Obstetric Services in West Africa," *Tropical Medicine and International Health* 8 (2003): 940–948; and A. Paxton, D. Maine, L. Freedman, D. Fry, and L. Lobis, "The Evidence for Emergency Obstetric Care," *International Journal of Gynecology and Obstetrics* 88 (2005): 181–191.

There are many controversies regarding Cesarean section in the world obstetrical literature. What is not in dispute is the cost-effectiveness of Cesarean section in preventing obstetric fistulas: B. C. Alkire, T. R. Vincent, C. Turlington-Burns, I. S. Metzler, P. E. Farmer, and J. G. Meaara, "Obstructed Labor and Caesarean Delivery: The Cost and Benefit of Surgical Intervention," *PloS One* 7, no. 4 (2012): e34595, doi:10.1371/journal.pone.0034595.

The concept of phases of delay was first articulated by Sereen Thaddeus and Deborah Maine in their classic article, "Too Far to Walk: Maternal Mortality in Context," *Social Science and Medicine* 38, no. 8 (1994): 1091–1110. Related articles include the following: Deborah Maine and the Prevention of Maternal Mortality Network, "Barriers to Treatment of Obstetric Emergencies in Rural Communities of West Africa," *Studies in Family Planning* 23, no. 5 (1992): 279–291; Deborah Maine and the Prevention of Maternal Mortality Network, "Situation Analyses of Emergency Obstetric Care: Examples from Eleven Operations Research Projects in West Africa," *Social Science and Medicine* 40, no. 5 (1995): 657–667; Sabine Gabrysch and Oona M. R. Campbell, "Still Too Far to Walk: Literature Review of the Determinants of Delivery Service Use," *BMC Pregnancy and Childbirth* 9 (2009): 34; J. Stekelenburg, S. Kyanamina, M. Mukelabai, I. Wolffers, and J. van Roosmalen, "Waiting Too Long: Low Use of Maternal Health Services in Kalabo, Zambia," *Tropical Medicine and International Health* 9, no. 3 (2004): 390–398; Godfrey Mbaruku, Jos van Roosmalen, Iluminata Kimondo, Filigona Bilango, and Staffan Bergstrom, "Perinatal Audit Using the 3-Delays Model in Western Tanzania," *International Journal of Gynecology and Obstetrics* 106 (2009): 85–88; and Deborah Barnes-Josiah, Cynthia Myntti, and Antoine Augustin, "The 'Three Delays' as a Framework for Examining Maternal Mortality in Haiti," *Social Science and Medicine* 46, no. 8 (1998): 981–993.

Two excellent references on the transformation of maternal mortality in Honduras are I. Danel, *Maternal Mortality Reduction, Honduras, 1990–1997: A Case Study* (Washington, DC: World Bank, 1998); and J. Shiffman, C. Stanton, and A. P. Salazar, "The Emergence of Political Priority for Safe Motherhood in Honduras," *Health Policy and Planning* 19, no. 6 (2004): 380–390.

The story of how Sri Lanka and Malaysia dramatically dropped their maternal mortality ratios is told in I. Pathmanathan, J. Liljestrand, J. M. Martins, L. C. Rajapaksa, C. Lissner, A. de

Silva, S. Selvaraju, and P. J. Singh, *Investing in Maternal Health: Learning from Malaysia and Sri Lanka* (Washington, DC: World Bank, 2003).

The quote from Edward de Bono is from his book *Serious Creativity: Using the Power of Lateral Thinking to Create New Ideas* (New York: HarperBusiness, 1992), 58.

Risk factors are characteristics of patients or population groups that make them more susceptible to certain diseases, conditions, or maladies. The factors that put women at risk for developing an obstetric fistula are discussed in the following: P. M. Tebeu, L. de Bernis, A. Doh, A. Sama, C. H. Rochat, and T. Delvaux, "Risk Factors for Obstetric Fistula in the Far North Province of Cameroon," *International Journal of Gynecology and Obstetrics* 107 (2009): 12–15; L. Lewis Wall, Jonathan A. Karshima, Carolyn Kirschner, and Steven D. Arrowsmith, "The Obstetric Vesicovaginal Fistula: Characteristics of 899 Patients from Jos, Nigeria," *American Journal of Obstetrics and Gynecology* 190 (2004): 1011–1019; M. Muleta, S. Rasmussen, and T. Kiserud, "Obstetric Fistula in 14,928 Ethiopian Women," *Acta Obstetricia et Gynecologica* 89 (2010): 945–951; A. Lewis, M. R. Kaufman, C. E. Wolder, S. E. Phillips, D. Maggi, L. Condry, R. R. Dmochowski, and J. A. Smith Jr., "Genitourinary Fistula Experience in Sierra Leone: Review of 505 Cases," *Journal of Urology* 181 (2009): 1725–1731; P. Hilton and A. Ward, "Epidemiological and Surgical Aspects of Urogenital Fistulae: A Review of 25 Years' Experience in Southeast Nigeria," *International Urogynecology Journal* 9 (1998): 189–194; S. Sjoveian, S. Vangen, D. Mukwege, and M. Onsrud, "Surgical Outcome of Obstetric Fistula: A Retrospective Analysis of 595 Patients," *Acta Obstetricia et Gynecologica Scandinavica* 90 (2011): 753–760.

In every society there are competing pathways to access care that are open to all patients. In African settings in particular, culturally traditional forms of therapy compete with more recently introduced biomedical therapies. Examples of how such systems interact can be found in John Janzen, *The Quest for Therapy: Medical Pluralism in Lower Zaire* (Berkeley: University of California Press, 1982); and Carolyn F. Sargent, *The Cultural Context of Therapeutic Choice: Obstetrical Care Decision among the Bariba of Benin* (Boston: D. Reidel, 1982).

There is a huge literature on the duration of labor. The basics are covered in World Health Organization, *Educational Material for Teachers of Midwifery: Midwifery Education Modules; Managing Prolonged and Obstructed Labour*, 2nd ed. (Geneva: World Health Organization, 2008). The anecdotes about prolonged labor in West Africa are from the Prevention of Maternal Mortality Network, "Barriers to Treatment of Obstetric Emergencies in Rural Communities of West Africa," *Studies in Family Planning* 23 (1992): 279–291.

The quotation about risk is from M. Douglas and A. Wildavsky, *Risk and Culture: An Essay on the Selection of Technical and Environmental Dangers* (Los Angeles: University of California Press, 1982), 1. Further thoughts on risk, blame, time, and false labor can be found in the following: Mary Douglas, *Risk and Blame: Essays in Cultural Theory* (New York: Routledge, 1992); C. M. Obermeyer, "Risk, Uncertainty, and Agency: Culture and Safe Motherhood in Morocco," *Medical Anthropology* 19 (2000): 173–201; C. McCourt, ed., *Childbirth, Midwifery and Concepts of Time* (New York: Berghahn Books, 2009); C. W. Schauberger, "False Labor," *Obstetrics and Gynecology* 68 (1986): 770–772; M. Mathai, "The Partograph for the Prevention of Obstructed Labor," *Clinical Obstetrics and Gynecology* 52 (2009): 256–269; and A. B. Caughey, "Is There an Upper Time Limit for the Management of the Second Stage of Labor?," *American Journal of Obstetrics and Gynecology* 201 (2009): 337–338.

The term "authoritative knowledge" has been used to refer to the repository within a particular culture where expert information about a particular issue or problem is thought to reside.

To say that so-and-so is the local "expert" on obstructed labor (for example) means only that she or he is so regarded as having authoritative knowledge within that culture or community; it says nothing about whether such knowledge or treatment is actually efficacious in alleviating the obstructed mechanics within a particular labor. This is part of the problem of perception and deciding where to go when obstetrical problems arise. There may be many "false starts" before a woman actually gets the care she needs. See R. E. Davis-Floyd and C. F. Sargent, eds., *Childbirth and Authoritative Knowledge: Cross-Cultural Perspectives* (Los Angeles: University of California Press, 1997); J. A. Adetunji, "Church-Based Obstetric Care in a Yoruba Community, Nigeria," *Social Science and Medicine* 35 (1992): 1171–1178; E. J. Udoma, E. E. J. Asuqu, and M. I. Ekott, "Maternal Mortality from Obstructed Labor in South-Eastern Nigeria: The Role of Spiritual Churches," *International Journal of Gynecology and Obstetrics* 67 (1999): 103–105.

The quotation regarding West Africa is from the Prevention of Maternal Mortality Network, "Barriers to Treatment of Obstetric Emergencies in Rural Communities of West Africa," *Studies in Family Planning* 23 (1992): 279–291.

The quotation concerning the Essan is from F. I. Omorodion, "The Socio-Cultural Context of Health Behavior among Esan Communities, Edo State, Nigeria," *Health Transition Review* 3 (1993): 125–136. The quotation regarding prolonged labor among the Nyakyusa is from M. Wilson, *Rituals of Kinship among the Nyakyusa* (London: Oxford University Press for the International African Institute, 1957), 144.

The quotation from Denise Allen is from her book *Managing Motherhood, Managing Risk: Fertility and Danger in West Central Tanzania* (Ann Arbor: University of Michigan Press, 2002), 205.

The quotations from Chapman's work in Mozambique are from Rachel R. Chapman, *Family Secrets: Risking Reproduction in Central Mozambique* (Nashville, TN: Vanderbilt University Press, 2010), 125 and 215.

The quotation about social strife and prolonged labor in Guatemala is from Nicole S. Berry, *Unsafe Motherhood: Mayan Maternal Mortality and Subjectivity in Post-war Guatemala* (New York: Berghahn Books, 2010), 171.

There is an internal logic to traditional midwifery practice in other cultures, but it is often built on different assumptions and presuppositions from those of modern scientific biology. This can have unfortunate consequences for patients. See B. A. Anderson, E. N. Anderson, T. Franklin, and A. Dzib-Xhium de Cen, "Pathways of Decision Making among Yucatan Mayan Traditional Birth Attendants," *Journal of Midwifery and Women's Health* 49 (2004): 312–319; and also D. A. Ityavyar, "A Traditional Midwife Practice, Sokoto State, Nigeria," *Social Science and Medicine* 18, no. 6 (1984): 497–501.

The use and abuse of medications to enhance uterine contractions is described in the following papers: M. Kamatenesi-Mugisha and H. Oryem-Origa, "Medicinal Plants Used to Induce Labour during Childbirth in Western Uganda," *Journal of Ethnopharmacology* 109 (2007): 1–9; B. Dujardin, M. Boutsen, I. De Schampheleire, R. Kulker, J. P. Manshande, J. Bailey, E. Wollast, and P. Buekens, "Oxytocics in Developing Countries," *International Journal of Gynecology and Obstetrics* 50 (1995): 243–251; and M. Sharan, D. Strobino, and S. Ahmed, "Intrapartum Oxytocin Use for Labor Acceleration in Rural India," *International Journal of Gynecology and Obstetrics* 90 (2005): 251–257.

Gender equity and contraceptive use is variously discussed in the following references: C. E. E. Okojie, "Gender Inequalities of Health in the Third World," *Social Science and Medicine* 39, no. 9 (1994): 1237–1247; L. Doyal, "Gender Equity in Health: Debates and Dilemmas," *Social*

Science and Medicine 51 (2000): 931–939; E. M. Murphy, "Being Born Female Is Dangerous for Your Health," American Psychologist 58 (2003): 205–210; A. Riyami, M. Afifi, and R. M. Mabry, "Women's Autonomy, Education and Employment in Oman and Their Influence on Contraceptive Use," Reproductive Health Matters 12, no. 3 (2004): 144–154; U. D. Upadhyay and M. J. Hindin, "Do Higher Status and More Autonomous Women Have Longer Birth Intervals? Results from Cebu, Philippines," Social Science and Medicine 60 (2005): 2641–2655; M. C. Duze and I. Z. Mohammed, "Male Knowledge, Attitudes and Family Planning Practices in Northern Nigeria," African Journal of Reproductive Health 10 (2006): 53–65; B. Audu, S. Yahya, A. Geidam, H. Abdussalam, I. Takai, and O. Kyari, "Polygamy and the Use of Contraceptives," International Journal of Gynecology and Obstetrics 101 (2008): 88–92.

The famous anecdote about the woman in labor who lived next door to the hospital and who nevertheless developed a fistula is from the Prevention of Maternal Mortality Network, "Barriers to Treatment of Obstetric Emergencies in Rural Communities of West Africa," Studies in Family Planning 23 (1992): 279–291.

Issues of women's agency and its impact on health, especially in northern Nigeria, are discussed in L. Lewis Wall, "Dead Mothers and Injured Wives: The Social Context of Maternal Morbidity and Mortality among the Hausa of Northern Nigeria," Studies in Family Planning 29 (1998): 341–359; C. Delaney, The Seeds and the Soil: Gender and Cosmology in Turkish Village Society (Berkeley: University of California Press, 1991); H. Papanek, "Purdah: Separate Worlds and Symbolic Shelter," Comparative Studies in Society and History 15 (1973): 289–325; C. VerEecke, "'It Is Better to Die Than to Be Shamed': Cultural and Moral Dimensions of Women's Trading in an Islamic Nigerian Society," Anthropos 88 (1993): 403–417; B. J. Callaway, "Ambiguous Consequences of the Socialization and Seclusion of Hausa Women," Journal of Modern African Studies 22 (1984): 429–450; L. M. Solivetti, "Marriage and Divorce in a Hausa Community: A Sociological Model," Africa 64 (1994): 252–271; Polly Hill, "Hidden Trade in Hausaland," Man, n.s., 4 (1969): 392–409; and Renee Pittin, "Women, Work and Ideology in Nigeria," Review of African Political Economy 52 (1991): 38–52.

Educating girls and women is important. This is demonstrated in the following papers: C. McAlister and T. F. Baskett, "Female Education and Maternal Mortality: A Worldwide Survey," Journal of Obstetrics and Gynecology of Canada 28 (2006): 983–990; and especially eloquently by Kelsey Harrison in "The Importance of the Educated Healthy Woman in Africa," Lancet 349 (1997): 644–647.

The important paper quoted here is A. Weeks, T. Lavender, E. Nazziwa, and F. Mirembe, "Personal Account of 'Near-Miss' Maternal Mortalities in Kampala, Uganda," BJOG: An International Journal of Obstetrics and Gynaecology 112 (2005): 1302–1307.

The paper dealing with garukayo in Uganda is G. B. Kyomuhendo, "Low Use of Rural Maternity Services in Uganda: Impact of Women's Status, Traditional Beliefs and Limited Resources," Reproductive Health Matters 11, no. 21 (2003): 16–26.

Difficulties with acceptance and performance of Cesarean section (including the widespread African belief that a woman who has one is "not really a woman") are discussed in the following: X. De Muylder, "Caesarean Section Morbidity at District Level in Zimbabwe," Journal of Tropical Medicine and Hygiene 92 (1989): 89–92; E. Y. Kwawukume, "Caesarean Section in Developing Countries," Best Practice and Research in Clinical Obstetrics and Gynaecology 15 (2001): 165–178; O. T. Oladapo, M. A. Lamina, and A. O. Sule-Odu, "Maternal Morbidity and Mortality Associated with Elective Caesarean Delivery at a University Hospital in Nigeria," Australia New Zealand

Journal of Obstetrics and Gynaecology 47 (2007): 110–114; X. De Muylder and P. de Waals, "Poor Acceptance of Caesarean Section in Zimbabwe," *Tropical and Geographic Medicine* 41 (1989): 230–233; C. O. Chigbu and G. C. Ilobachie, "The Burden of Caesarean Section Refusal in a Developing Country Setting," *BJOG: An International Journal of Obstetrics and Gynaecology* 114 (2007): 1261–1263; H. E. Onah, "Formal Education Does Not Improve the Acceptance of Cesarean Section among Pregnant Nigerian Women," *International Journal of Gynecology and Obstetrics* 76 (2002): 321–323; H. E. Onah and P. O. Nkwo, "Caesarean Section or Symphysiotomy for Obstructed Labour for Developing Countries? Need to Ascertain Women's Preferences," *Journal of Obstetrics and Gynaecology* 23 (2003): 594–595; J. O. Parkhurst and S. A. Rahman, "Life Saving or Money Wasting? Perceptions of Caesarean Sections among Users of Services in Rural Bangladesh," *Health Policy* 80 (2007): 392–401.

The quotations from Nicole Berry are from *Unsafe Motherhood: Mayan Maternal Mortality and Subjectivity in Post-war Guatemala* (New York: Berghahn Books, 2010), 174 and 182.

The studies from Gabon and China referred to in the chapter are S. Mayi-Tsonga, L. Oksana, I. Ndombi, T. Diallo, M. H. de Sousa, and A. Faoundes, "Delay in the Provision of Adequate Care to Women Who Died from Abortion-Related Complications in the Principal Maternity Hospital of Gabon," *Reproductive Health Matters* 17, no. 34 (2009): 65–70; and S. E. Short and F. Zhang, "Use of Maternal Health Services in Rural China," *Population Studies* 58 (2004): 3–19.

Americans are very conscious of the costs of healthcare, and for good reasons. It comes as a shock to many to realize that these concerns are just as pressing even for the rural poor in Africa and Asia. There is a growing literature on health costs and their impact in low-income countries. The quotation about the struggles of patients to gather financial resources during emergencies in Bangladesh is from Kaosar Afsana, "The Tremendous Cost of Seeking Hospital Obstetric Care in Bangladesh," *Reproductive Health Matters* 12, no. 214 (2004): 171–180. These other articles round out the economic dimensions of emergency care in poor countries: B. Abel-Smith and P. Rawal, "Can the Poor Afford 'Free' Health Services? A Case Study of Tanzania," *Health Policy and Planning* 7 (1992): 329–342; M. Kowalewski, P. Mujinja, and A. John, "Can Mothers Afford Maternal Health Care Costs? User Costs of Maternity Services in Rural Tanzania," *African Journal of Reproductive Health* 6 (2002): 65–73; T. T. Su, B. Kouyate, and S. Flessa, "Catastrophic Household Expenditure for Health Care in a Low-Income Society: A Study from Nouna District, Burkina Faso," *Bulletin of the World Health Organization* 84 (2006): 21–27; J. Borghi, K. Hanson, C. A. Acquah, G. Ekanmian, V. Filippi, C. Ronsmans, R. Brugha, E. Browne, and E. Alihonou, "Cost of Near-Miss Obstetric Complications for Women and Their Families in Benin and Ghana," *Health Policy and Planning* 18 (2003): 383–390; J. Borghi, T. Ensor, B. D. Neupane, and S. Tiwari, "Financial Implications of Skilled Attendance at Delivery in Nepal," *Tropical Medicine and International Health* 11 (2006): 228–237; S. Nahar and A. Costello, "The Hidden Cost of 'Free' Maternity Care in Dhaka, Bangladesh," *Health Policy and Planning* 13 (1998): 417–422; T. A. J. Houweling, C. Ronsmans, O. M. R. Campbell, and A. Kunst, "Huge Poor-Rich Inequalities in Maternity Care: An International Comparative Study of Maternity and Child Care in Developing Countries," *Bulletin of the World Health Organization* 85 (2007): 745–754; J. Borghi, N. Sabina, L. S. Blum, H. E. Hoque, and C. Ronsmans, "Household Costs of Healthcare during Pregnancy, Delivery, and the Postpartum Period: A Case Study from Matlab, Bangladesh," *Journal of Health, Population and Nutrition* 24 (2006): 446–455; L. Say and R. Rainse, "A Systematic Review of Inequalities in the Use of Maternal Health Care in Developing Countries: Examining the Scale of the Problem and the Importance of Context," *Bulletin of the World Health Organization* 85

(2007): 812–819; K. Afsana, "The Tremendous Cost of Seeking Hospital Obstetric Care in Bangladesh," *Reproductive Health Matters* 12, no. 24 (2004): 171–180; J. K. Mbugua, G. H. Bloom, and M. M. Segall, "Impact of User Charges on Vulnerable Groups: The Case of the Kibwezi in Rural Kenya," *Social Science and Medicine* 41 (1995): 829–835; P. Nanda, "Gender Dimensions of User Fees: Implications for Women's Utilization of Health Care," *Reproductive Health Matters* 10, no. 20 (2002): 127–134; K. Xu, D. B. Evans, P. Kadama, J. Nabyonga, P. O. Ogwal, P. Nabukhonzo, and A. M. Aguilar, "Understanding the Impact of Eliminating User Fees: Utilization and Catastrophic Health Expenditures in Uganda," *Social Science and Medicine* 62 (2006): 866–876; M. E. Kruk, G. Mbaruku, P. C. Rockers, and S. Galea, "User Fee Exemptions Are Not Enough: Out-of-Pocket Payments for 'Free' Delivery Services in Rural Tanzania," *Tropical Medicine and International Health* 13 (2008): 1442–1451; M. Lewis, "Informal Payments and the Financing of Health Care in Developing and Transition Countries," *Health Affairs* 26 (2007): 984–997; A. Khan and S. Zaman, "Costs of Vaginal Delivery and Caesarean Section at a Tertiary Level Public Hospital in Islamabad, Pakistan," *BMC Pregnancy Childbirth* 10, no. 2 (2010): doi:10.1186/1471-2393-10-2; D. McIntyre, M. Thiede, G. Dahlgren, and M. Whitehead, "What Are the Economic Consequences for Households of Illness and Paying for Health Care in Low- and Middle-Income Country Contexts?," *Social Science and Medicine* 62 (2006): 858–865; C. Ronsmans, S. Holtz, and C. Stanton, "Socioeconomic Differentials in Caesarean Rates in Developing Countries: A Retrospective Analysis," *Lancet* 368 (2006): 1516–1523; S. Russell, "Ability to Pay for Health Care: Concepts and Evidence," *Health Policy and Planning* 11 (1996): 219–237; P. Fofana, O. Samai, A. Kebbie, and P. Sengeh, "Promoting the Use of Obstetric Services through Community Loan Funds, Bo, Sierra Leone," supplement, *International Journal of Gynecology and Obstetrics* 59, no. 2 (1997): S225–S230; R. Sauerborn, A. Nougtara, M. Hien, and H. J. Diesfeld, "Seasonal Variations of Household Costs of Illness in Burkina Faso," *Social Science and Medicine* 43, no. 3 (1996): 281–290; E. Pitchforth, E. van Teijlingen, W. Graham, M. Dixon-Woods, and M. Chowdhury, "Getting Women to Hospital Is Not Enough: A Qualitative Study of Access to Emergency Obstetric Care in Bangladesh," *Quality and Safety in Health Care* 15 (2006): 214–219; P. Renaudin, A. Prual, C. Vangeenderhuysen, M. Ould Abdelkader, M. Ould Mohammed Vall, and D. Ould el Joud, "Ensuring Financial Access to Emergency Obstetric Care: Three Years of Experience with Obstetric Risk Insurance in Nouakchott, Mauritania," *International Journal of Gynecology and Obstetrics* 99 (2007): 183–190; Odi' U. J. Umeora, Joseph O. Mbazor, and Boniface N. Ejikeme, "The Hidden Cost of 'Free Maternity Care' in a Low-Resource Setting in South-Eastern Nigeria," *Tropical Journal of Obstetrics and Gynaecology* 24, no. 1 (2007): 21–24; Sophie Witter, Daniel Kojo Arhinful, Anthony Kusi, and Sawudatu Zakariah-Akoto, "The Experience of Ghana in Implementing a User Fee Exemption Policy to Provide Free Delivery Care," *Reproductive Health Matters* 15, no. 30 (2007): 61–71; Attiak Khan and Shakila Zaman, "Costs of Vaginal Delivery and Caesarean Section at a Tertiary Level Public Hospital in Islamabad, Pakistan," *BMC Pregnancy and Childbirth* 10 (2010): 10:2, http://www.biomedcentral.com/1471-2393/10/2; Mohammed Enamul Hoque, Sushil Kanta Dasgupta, Evan Naznin, and Abdullah Al Mamun, "Household Coping Strategies for Delivery and Related Healthcare Cost: Findings from Rural Bangladesh," *Tropical Medicine and International Health* 20, no. 10 (2015): 1368–1375; Aslihan Kes, Sheila Ogwang, Rohini Prabha Pande, Zayid Doughals, Robinson Karuga, Frank O. Odhiambo, Kayla Laserson, and Kathleen Schaffer, "The Economic Burden of Maternal Mortality on Households: Evidence from Three Sub-counties in Rural Western Kenya," supplement, *Reproductive Health* 12, no. 1 (2015): S3; K. T. Storeng, R. F. Baggaley, R. Ganaba, F. Ouattara, M. S.

Akoum, and V. Filippi, "Paying the Price: The Cost and Consequences of Emergency Obstetric Care in Burkina Faso," *Social Science and Medicine* 66 (2008): 545–557. The quote about inequities in maternal mortality being shaped by social, economic, and political vulnerabilities of the world's poor is from page 546.

Chapter 7. Deadly Delays in Getting to a Place of Care

The Farafenni study from Gambia is A. M. Greenwood, B. M. Greenwood, A. K. Bradley, K. Williams, F. C. Shelton, S. Tulloch, P. Byass, and F. S. J. Oldfield, "A Prospective Survey of the Outcome of Pregnancy in a Rural Area of the Gambia," *Bulletin of the World Health Organization* 65, no. 5 (1987): 635–643.

The challenges of distance and geography in access to emergency obstetric care are discussed in Claudia Hanson, Jonathan Cox, Godfrey Mabruku, Fatuma Manzi, Sabine Gabrysch, David Schellenberg, Marcel Tanner, Carine Ronsmans, and Joanna Schellenberg, "Maternal Mortality and Distance to Facility-Base Obstetric Care in Rural Southern Tanzania: A Secondary Analysis of Cross-Sectional Census Data in 226,000 Households," *Lancet Global Health* 385 (2015): e387–e395; Linda Barlett, Shairose Mawji, Sara Whitehead, Chadd Crouse, Suray Dalil, Denish Ionete, Peter Salama, and the Afghan Maternal Mortality Study Team, "Where Giving Birth Is a Forecast of Death: Maternal Mortality in Four Districts of Afghanistan, 1999–2002," *Lancet* 365 (2005): 864–870; Sabein Gabrysch, Simon Cousen, Jonathan Cox, and Oona M. R. Campbell, "The Influence of Distance and Level of Care on Delivery Place in Rural Zambia: A Study of Linked National Data in a Geographic Information System," *PloS Medicine* 8, no. 1 (2011): e1000394; Sabine Gabrysch, Virginia Simush, and Oona M. R. Campbell, "Availability and Distribution of, and Geographic Access to Emergency Obstetric Care in Zambia," *International Journal of Gynecology and Obstetrics* 114 (2011): 174–179.

The recommended distribution of emergency obstetrical services is discussed in UNICEF, WHO, and UNFPA, *Guidelines for Monitoring the Availability and Use of Obstetric Services* (New York: United Nations Children's Fund, 1997).

Rural/urban maternal mortality discrepancies are discussed in C. Ronsmans, J. F. Etard, G. Walraven, L. Joh, A. Dumont, and L. de Bernis, "Maternal Mortality and Access to Obstetric Services in West Africa," *Tropical Medicine and International Health* 8 (2003): 940–948.

Deborah Maine's scenario-building exercise for cost-effectiveness in averting maternal mortality is found in Deborah Maine, *Safe Motherhood Programs: Options and Issues* (New York: Center for Population and Family Health, Columbia University, 1991).

The study of the distribution of comprehensive emergency obstetric care in Bangladesh is M. Mahmud Khan, Disha Ali, Zohra Ferdousy, and Abdullah Al-Mamum, "A Cost-Minimization Approach to Planning the Geographical Distribution of Health Facilities," *Health Policy and Planning* 16, no. 3 (2001): 264–272.

The transformation of maternal mortality in Honduras is discussed in I. Danel, *Maternal Mortality Reduction, Honduras, 1990–1997: A Case Study* (Washington, DC: World Bank, 1998); and also in Jeremy Shiffman, Cynthia Stanton, and Patricia Salazar, "The Emergence of Political Priority for Safe Motherhood in Honduras," *Health Policy and Planning* 19, no. 6 (2004): 380–390. The importance of infrastructure development as a key component in reducing maternal mortality is discussed in I. I. Pathmanathan, J. Liljestrand, J. M. Martins, L. C. Rajapaksa, C. Lissner, A. de Silva, S. Selvaraju, and P. J. Singh, *Investing in Maternal Health: Learning from Malaysia and Sri Lanka* (Washington, DC: World Bank, 2003).

Everyone involved in maternal health issues in poor countries recognizes the importance of transportation systems and how they link to healthcare. Among the important articles are the following: Annie Wilson, Sarah Hillman, Mikey Rosato, John Skelton, Anthony Costello, Julia Hussein, Christine MacArthur, and Arri Coomarasamy, "A Systematic Review and Thematic Analysis of Qualitative Studies on Maternal Emergency Transport in Low- and Middle-Income Countries," *International Journal of Gynecology and Obstetrics* 122 (2013): 192–201; Susan F. Murphy and Stephen C. Pearson, "Maternity Referral Systems in Developing Countries: Current Knowledge and Future Research Needs," *Social Science and Medicine* 62 (2006): 2205–2215; K. Krasovec, "Auxiliary Technologies Related to Transport and Communication for Obstetric Emergencies," supplement, *International Journal of Gynecology and Obstetrics* 85, no. 1 (2004): S14–S23; Thomas Schmid, Omari Kanenda, Indu Ahluwalia, and Michelle Kouletio, "Transportation for Maternal Emergencies in Tanzania: Empowering Communities through Participatory Problem-Solving," *American Journal of Public Health* 91, no. 10 (2001): 1589–1590; E. Essien, D. Ifenne, K. Sabitu, A. Musa, M. Alti-Mu'azu, V. Adidiu, N. Golji, and M. Mikaddas, "Community Loan Funds and Transport Services for Obstetric Emergencies in Northern Nigeria," supplement, *International Journal of Gynecology and Obstetrics* 59, no. 2 (1997): S237–S244; D. Shehu, A. T. Ikeh, and M. J. Kuna, "Mobilizing Transport for Obstetric Emergencies in Northwestern Nigeria," supplement, *International Journal of Gynecology and Obstetrics* 59, no. 2 (1997): S173–S180; O. Sami and P. Senegh, "Facilitating Emergency Obstetric Care through Transportation and Communication, Bo, Sierra Leone," supplement, *International Journal of Gynecology and Obstetrics* 59, no. 2 (1997): S157–S164;

The Malawi motorcycle experiment is described in Jan J. Hofman, Chris Dzimadzi, Kingsley Lung, Esther Y. Ratsman, and Julia Hussein, "Motorcycle Ambulances for Referral of Obstetric Emergencies in Rural Malawi: Do They Reduce Delay and What Do They Cost?," *International Journal of Gynecology and Obstetrics* 102 (2008): 191–197.

The development of a protocol to handle obstructed labor in Guinea is described in M. D. Balde and G. Bastert, "Decrease in Uterine Rupture in Conakry, Guinea by Improvements in Transfer Management," *International Journal of Gynecology and Obstetrics* 31 (1990): 21–24.

Communications technology in maternal healthcare is discussed in Paul Bossyns, Ranaou Abache, Mahaman Sani Abdoulaye, and Wim Van Lerberghe, "Unaffordable or Cost-Effective: Introducing an Emergency Referral System in Rural Niger," *Tropical Medicine and International Health* 10, no. 9 (2005): 879–887; A. Camielle Nooerdam, Barbar M. Kuepper, Jelle Stekelenburg, and Anneli Milen, "Improvement of Maternal Health Services through the Use of Mobile Phones," *Tropical Medicine and International Health* 16, no. 5 (2011): 622–626; Stine Lund, Brigitte B. Nielsen, Maryam Hemed, Ida M. Boas, Azzah Said, Khadija Said, Mkoko M. Makungu, and Vibeke Rasch, "Mobile Phone Improve Antenatal Care Attendance in Zanzibar: A Cluster Randomized Controlled Trial," *BMC Pregnancy and Childbirth* 14 (2014): 29; S. Lund, M. Hemed, B. B. Nielsen, S. Said, K. Said, M. H. Makungu, and V. Rasch, "Mobile Phones as a Health Communication Tool to Improve Skilled Attendance at Delivery in Zanzibar: a Cluster-Randomized Controlled Study," *BJOG: An International Journal of Obstetrics and Gynaecology* 119 (2012): 1256–1264; and Alison N. Fiander and Tom Vanneste, "TransportMYpatient: An Initiative to Overcome the Barrier of Transport Costs for Patients Accessing Treatment of Obstetric Fistula and Cleft Lip in Tanzania," *Tropical Doctor* 42 (2012): 77–79.

Assessing the risk of poor obstetrical outcome was, for a long time, a foundation of safe motherhood initiatives. This approach failed because of the lack of sensitivity and specificity of the screening tests that were used. The problems of antenatal risk assessment are discussed in World Health Organization, *Risk Approach for Maternal and Child Health Care: A Managerial Strategy to Improve the Coverage and Quality of Maternal and Child Health/Family Planning Services Based on the Measurement of Individual and Community Risk*, WHO Offset Publication No. 39 (Geneva: WHO, 1978); Allan Rosenfield, Caroline J. Min, and Lynn P. Freedman, "Making Motherhood Safe in Developing Countries," *New England Journal of Medicine* 356, no. 14 (2007): 1395–1397; E. A. Yuster; "Rethinking the Role of the Risk Approach and Antenatal Care in Maternal Mortality Reduction," supplement, *International Journal of Gynecology and Obstetrics* 50, no. 2 (1995): S59–S61; Odile A. van den Heuvel, Wouter G. de Mey, Henk Buddingh, and Michiel L. Bots, "Use of Maternal Care in a Rural Area of Zimbabwe: A Population-Based Study," *Acta Obstetricia et Gynecologica Scandinavica* 78 (1999): 838–846; J. A. Fortney, "Antenatal Risk Screening and Scoring: A New Look," supplement, *International Journal of Gynecology and Obstetrics* 50, no. 2 (1995): S53–S58; Kasongo Project Team, "Antenatal Screening for Fetopelvic Dystocias: A Cost-Effectiveness Approach to the Choice of Simple Indicators for Use by Auxiliary Personnel; The Kasongo Project Team," *Journal of Tropical Medicine & Hygiene* 87, no. 4 (1984): 173–183; World Health Organization, "Maternal Anthropometry and Pregnancy Outcomes: A WHO Collaborative Study," supplement, *Bulletin of the World Health Organization* 73 (1995): 1–47; A. Kelly, J. Kevany, M. de Onis, and P. M. Shah, "A WHO Collaborative Study of Maternal Anthropometry and Pregnancy Outcomes," *International Journal of Gynecology and Obstetrics* 53 (1996): 219–233.

The maternity waiting home concept is an appealing concept on its surface, but there are substantial problems: how to screen, who to send there, and how to make the home work in practical terms. See J. K. Knowles, "A Shelter That Saves Mothers' Lives," *World Health Forum* 9 (1988): 387–388; L. van Lonkhuijzen, J. Stekelenburg, and J. van Roosmalen, "Maternity Waiting Facilities for Improving Maternal and Neonatal Outcome in Low-Resource Countries," *Cochrane Database of Systematic Reviews*, no. 10 (2012): Art. No. CD006759, doi:10.1002/14651858. CD006759.pub3; Irene Figa-Talamanca, "Maternal Mortality and the Problem of Accessibility to Obstetric Care: The Strategy of Maternity Waiting Homes," *Social Science and Medicine* 42, no. 10 (1996): 1381–1390; Kayli Wild, Lesley Barclay, Paul Kelly, and Nelson Martins, "The Tyranny of Distance: Maternity Waiting Homes and Access to Birthing Facilities in Rural Timor-Leste," *Bulletin of the World Health Organization* 90 (2012): 97–103; D. Chandramohan, F. Cutts, and R. Chandra, "Effects of a Maternity Waiting Home on Adverse Maternal Outcomes and the Validity of Antenatal Risk Screening," *International Journal of Gynecology and Obstetrics* 46 (1994): 279–284; Lazarus Mramba, Faiza Ahmed Nassir, Charles Ondieki, and Davies Kimanga, "Reasons for Low Utilization of a Maternity Waiting Home in Rural Kenya," *International Journal of Gynecology and Obstetrics* 108 (2010): 152–160.

The Ghana case study is described in J. B. Wilson, A. H. K. Collison, D. Richardson, G. Kwofie, K. A. Senah, and E. K. Tinkorang, "The Maternity Waiting Home Concept: The Nsawam, Ghana Experience," supplement, *International Journal of Gynecology and Obstetrics* 59, no. 2 (1997): S165–S172.

Chapter 8. Deadly Delays in Receiving Care

The comparative study of maternal mortality between Zambia and Chicago is Sarah J. Kilpatrick, Karen E. Crabtree, Andrea Kemp, and Stacie Geller, "Preventability of Maternal Deaths: Comparison between Zambian and American Referral Hospitals," *Obstetrics and Gynecology* 100

(2002): 321–326. Surveys of the problem of phase 3 delays can be found in the following: T. K. Sundari, "The Untold Story: How the Health Care Systems in Developing Countries Contribute to Maternal Mortality," *International Journal of Health Services* 22, no. 3 (1992): 513–528; F. L. Cavallardo and T. J. Marchant, "Responsiveness of Emergency Obstetric Care Systems in Low- and Middle-Income Countries: A Critical Review of the 'Third Delay,'" *Acta Obstetricia et Gynecological Scandinavica* 92 (2013): 496–507; H. E. Knight, A. Self, and S. H. Kennedy, "Why Are Women Dying When They Reach Hospital on Time? A Systematic Review of the 'Third Delay,'" *PLoS One* 8, no. 5 (2013): e63846; H. E. Onah, J. M. Okaro, U. Umeh, and C. O. Chigbu, "Maternal Mortality in Health Institutions with Emergency Obstetric Care Facilities in Enugu State, Nigeria," *Journal of Obstetrics and Gynaecology* 25, no. 6 (2005): 569–574; B. L. Sorensen, P. Elsass, B. B. Nielsen, S. Massawe, J. Nyakina, and V. Rasch, "Substandard Emergency Obstetric Care: A Confidential Enquiry into Maternal Deaths at a Regional Hospital in Tanzania," *Tropical Medicine and International Health* 15, no. 8 (2010): 894–900; and M. H. Bouvier-Cole, C. Ouedraogo, A. Dumont, C. Vangeenderhuysen, B. Salanve, and C. Decam for the MOMA Group, "Maternal Mortality in West Africa: Rates, Causes, and Substandard Care from a Prospective Survey," *Acta Obstetricia et Gynecologica Scandinavica* 80 (2001): 113–119.

Specific examples of facility-related problems impacting obstetric care in poor countries—and some local solutions—are discussed in these articles: K. Sabitu, M. Alti-Mu'azu, A. A. Musa, D. I. Ifenne, E. S. Essien, N. G. Golji, V. Adidu, and M. Mukaddas, "The Effect of Improving Maternity Services in a Secondary Facility, Zaria, Nigeria: The Zaria PMM Team," supplement, *International Journal of Gynaecology and Obstetrics* 59, no. 2 (1997): S99–S106; J. O. Djan, S. Kyei-Faried, S. Twum, J. B. Danquah, M. Ofori, and E. N. Brown, "Upgrading Obstetric Care at the Health Center Level, Juaben, Ghana: The Kumasi PMM Team," supplement, *International Journal of Gynaecology and Obstetrics* 59, no. 2 (1997): S83–S90; and D. Ifenne, E. Essien, N. Golji, K. Sabitu, M. Alti-Mu'azu, A. Musa, V. Adidu, and M. Mukaddas, "Improving the Quality of Obstetric Care at the Teaching Hospital, Zaria, Nigeria," supplement, *International Journal of Gynaecology and Obstetrics* 159, no. 2 (1997): S37–S46.

Kelsey Harrison's description of the conditions at Emuoha Hospital are from his autobiography, *An Arduous Climb: From the Creeks of the Niger Delta to Leading Obstetrician and University Vice-Chancellor* (London: Adonis and Abbey, 2006), 272–275. His description of clinical conditions at Ahmadu Bello University Teaching Hospital is taken from "Background Information," supplement, *British Journal of Obstetrics and Gynaecology* 92, no. 5 (1985): 3–13. The supplement as a whole is entitled "Child-Bearing, Health and Social Priorities: A Survey of 22774 Consecutive Hospital Births in Zaria, Northern Nigeria," and it is 119 pages long. It is a landmark publication in the history of safe motherhood initiatives.

Fake and counterfeit drugs have emerged as a major problem in poor countries. See Bernard Pecoul, Pierre Chirac, Patrice Trouiller, and Jacques Pinel, "Access to Essential Drugs in Poor Countries: A Lost Battle?," *Journal of the American Medical Association* 281 (1999): 361–367; C. S. Gautam, A. Utreja, and G. L. Singal, "Spurious and Counterfeit Drugs: A Growing Industry in the Developing World," *Postgraduate Medical Journal* 85 (2009): 251–256; A. Seiter, "Health and Economic Consequences of Counterfeit Drugs," *Nature* 85, no. 6 (2009): 576–578; and Paul Newton, Abdinasir Amin, Chris Bird, Phillip Passmore, Graham Dukes, Goran Tomson, Bright Simons, Roger Bate, Philippe Guerin, and Nicholas White, "The Primacy of Public Health Considerations in Defining Poor Quality Medicines," *PLoS Medicine* 8, no. 12 (2011): e1001139.

The health statistics on personnel shortages, delivery coverage, and Cesarean sections come from World Health Organization, *World Health Statistics 2015* (Geneva: WHO, 2015). Overviews on the shortages of trained healthcare personnel in poor countries can be found in Marge Koblinsky, Zoe Matthews, Julia Hussein, Dileep Mavalankar, Malay Mrigha, Iqbal Anwar, Endan Achadi, Sam Adjei, P. Padmanabham, and Wim van Lerberghe on behalf of the Lancet Maternal Survival Series steering group, "Maternal Survival 3: Going to Scale with Professional Skilled Care," *Lancet* 368 (2006): 1377–1386; and Alexander K. Rowe, Don de Savigny, Claudio Lanata, and Cesar Victora, "How Can We Achieve and Maintain High-Quality Performance of Health Workers in Low-Resource Settings?," *Lancet* 366 (2005): 1026–1035.

The problems of blood banking and blood shortages in developing countries are described in I. Bates, G. K. Chapotera, S. McKew, and N. van den Broek, "Maternal Mortality in Sub-Saharan Africa: The Contribution of Ineffective Blood Transfusion Services," *BJOG: An International Journal of Obstetrics and Gynaecology* 115 (2008): 1331–1339.

The use of trained nonphysicians to perform Cesarean sections is covered in Sharon White, Roger Thorpe, and Deborah Maine, "Emergency Obstetric Surgery Performed by Nurses in Zaire," *Lancet* 2 (1987): 612–613; M. E. Kruk, C. Pereira, F. Vaz, S. Bergstrom, and S. Galea, "Economic Evaluation of Surgically Trained Assistant Medical Officers in Performing Major Obstetric Surgery in Mozambique," *BJOG: An International Journal of Obstetrics and Gynaecology* 114 (2007): 1253–1260; and Amie Wilson, David Lissauer, Shakila Thanagratinam, Khalid Khan, Christine MacArthur, and Arri Coomarasamy, "A Comparison of Clinical Officers with Medical Doctors on Outcomes of Caesarean Section in the Developing World: Meta-analysis of Controlled Studies," *BMJ* 342 (2011): d2600.

Tom Elkins made many contributions to obstetrics and gynecology in his short life. The most important was the development of the successful Ghanaian residency training program in obstetrics and gynecology. This program is admirably described in this series of papers: J. O. Martey, Thomas E. Elkins, J. B. Wilson, Sydney W. K. Adedevoh, John MacVicar, and John J. Sciarra, "Innovative Community-Based Postgraduate Training for Obstetrics and Gynecology in West Africa," *Obstetrics and Gynecology* 85 (1995): 1042–1046; J. O. Martey and C. N. Hudson, "Training Specialists in the Developing World: Ten Years on, a Success Story for West Africa," *British Journal of Obstetrics and Gynaecology* 106 (1999): 91–94; Cecil A. Klufio, E. Y. Kwaukume, K. A. Danso, John J. Sciarra, and Timothy Johnson, "Ghana Postgraduate Obstetrics/Gynecology Collaborative Residency Training Program: Success Story and Model for Africa," *American Journal of Obstetrics and Gynecology* 189 (2003): 692–696; Frank W. J. Anderson, Ian Mutchnick, E. Y. Kwawukume, K. A. Danso, C. A. Klufio, Y. Clinton, Luke Lu Yen, and Timothy R. B. Johnson, "Who Will Be There When Women Deliver? Assuring Retention of Obstetric Providers," *Obstetrics and Gynecology* 110 (2007): 1012–1016; and Yvette Clinton, Frank W. Anderson, and E. Y. Kwawukume, "Factors Related to Retention of Postgraduate Trainees in Obstetrics-Gynecology at the Korle-Bu Teaching Hospital in Ghana," *Academic Medicine* 85 (2010): 1564–1570.

The abuse and neglect of women during labor and delivery is tied up with many other issues relating to staffing, facilities, clinical workloads, and so on, but especially with the way women are valued in particular societies. The specific examples cited in the chapter are Innocent I. Okafor, Emmanuel O. Ugwu, and Samuel N. Obi, "Disrespect and Abuse during Facility-Based Childbirth in a Low-Income Country," *International Journal of Gynecology and Obstetrics* 128 (2015): 110–113 (from Enugu, Nigeria); Shannon A. McMahon, Asha S. George, Joy J. Chebet,

Idda H. Mosha, Rose N. M. Mpembeni, and Peter J. Winch, "Experiences of and Responses to Disrespectful Maternity Care and Abuse during Childbirth: A Qualitative Study with Women and Men in Morogoro Region, Tanzania," *BMC Pregnancy and Childbirth* 14 (2014): 268; Cheryl A. Moyer, Philip B. Adongo, Raymond A. Aborigo, Abraham Hodgson, and Cyril M. Engmann, "'They Treat You like You Are Not a Human Being': Maltreatment During Labour and Delivery in Rural Northern Ghana," *Midwifery* 30 (2014): 262–268; and Anteneh Asefa and Delayehu Bekele, "Status of Respectful and Non-abusive Care during Facility-Based Childbirth in a Hospital and Health Centers in Addis Ababa, Ethiopia," *Reproductive Health* 12 (2015): 12:33.

Here is a list of articles introducing this problem: M. A. Bohren, J. P. Vogel, E. C. Hunter, O. Lutsiv, S. K. Makh, J. P. Souza, C. Aguiar, F. S. Coneglian, A. L. A Diniz, Ö. Tunçalp, D. Javadi, O. T. Oladapo, R. Khosla, M. J. Hindin, and A. M. Gülmezoglu, "The Mistreatment of Women during Childbirth in Health Facilities Globally: A Mixed-Methods Systematic Review," *PLoS Medicine* 12, no. 6 (2015): e1001847, doi:10.1371/journal.pmed.1001847; Roxana Behruzi, Marie Hatem, Lise Goulet, William Fraser, and Chizuru Misago, "Understanding Childbirth Practices as an Organizational Cultural Phenomenon: A Conceptual Framework," *BMC Pregnancy and Childbirth* 13 (2013): 205; Rachel Jewkes and Loveday Penn-Kekana, "Mistreatment of Women in Childbirth: Time for Action on This Important Dimension of Violence against Women," *PLoS Medicine* 12, no. 6 (2015): e1001849, doi:10.1371/journal.pmed.1001849; Ana d'Oliveira, Simone Diniz, and Lilia Schraiber, "Violence against Women in Health-Care Institutions: An Emerging Problem," *Lancet* 359 (2002): 1681–1685; Diana Bowser and Kathleen Hill, *Exploring Evidence for Disrespect and Abuse in Facility-Based Childbirth: Report of a Landscape Analysis* (Chevy Chase, MD: USAID-TRAction Project, Harvard School of Public Health, 2010).

Specific institutional studies of the mistreatment of women in labor can be found in the following: Carolyn Sargent and Joan Rawlins, "Transformations in Maternity Services in Jamaica," *Social Science and Medicine* 35, no. 10 (1992): 1225–1232; Rachel Jewkes, Naeemah Abrahams, and Zodumo Mvo, "Why Do Nurses Abuse Patients? Reflections from South African Obstetric Services," *Social Science and Medicine* 47, no. 11 (1998): 1781–1795; J. Ruminjo, C. Cordero, K. J. Beattie, and M. N. Wegner, "Quality of Care in Labor and Delivery: A Paradox in the Dominican Republic; Commentary," *International Journal of Gynecology and Obstetrics* 82 (2003): 115–119; S. Miller, M. Cordero, A. L. Coleman, J. Figueroa, S. Brito-Anderson, R. Dabagh, V. Calderon, F. Caceres, A. J. Fernandez, and M. Nunez, "Quality of Care in Institutionalized Deliveries: The Paradox of the Dominican Republic," *International Journal of Gynecology and Obstetrics* 82 (2003): 89–103; L. P. Freeman, "Human Rights, Constructive Accountability and Maternal Mortality in the Dominican Republic: A Commentary," *International Journal of Gynecology and Obstetrics* 82 (2003): 111–114; Rita Khayat and Oona Campbell, "Hospital Practices in Maternity Wards in Lebanon," *Health Policy and Planning* 15, no. 3 (2000): 270–278; Lucia d'Ambruoso, Mercy Abbey, and Julia Hassein, "Please Understand When I Cry Out in Pain: Women's Account of Maternity Services during Labour and Delivery in Ghana," *BMC Public Health* 5 (2005): 140; Charlotte Warren, Rebecca Njuki, Timothy Abuya, Charity Ndwifa, Grace Maingi, Jane Serwanga, Faith Mbvehero, Louis Muteti, Anne Njeru, Joseph Karanja, Joyce Olenja, Lucy Gitonga, Chris Rakuom, and Ben Bellows, "Study Protocol for Promoting Respectful Maternity Care Initiative to Assess, Measure and Design Interventions to Reduce Disrespect and Abuse during Childbirth in Kenya," *BMC Pregnancy and Childbirth* 13 (2013): 21; C. Misago, C. Kendall, P. Freitas, K. Haneda, D. Silveira, D. Onuki, T. Mori, T. Sadamori, and T. Umenai, "From 'Culture of Dehumanization of Childbirth' to 'Childbirth as a Transformative

Experience': Changes in Five Municipalities in North-East Brazil," supplement, *International Journal of Gynecology and Obstetrics* 75, no. 1 (2001): S67–S72;

Properly implemented, the partograph is one of the most useful low-technology tools for the improvement of childbirth and the prevention of obstetric fistulas. Proper use of the partograph requires training, commitment, and supervision. There is a large literature on this subject. The basic documents are three World Health Organization publications (Geneva, Switzerland: WHO, 1994) entitled *Preventing Prolonged Labor: A Practical Guide. The Partograph Part I: Principles and Strategy*; *Part II: User's Manual*; and *Part III: Facilitator's Guide*. The large multicenter trial is described in the paper authored by Barbara E. Kwast, "World Health Organization Partograph in Management of Labour," *Lancet* 1 (1994): 1399–1404. Another good review is Matthews Mathai, "The Partograph for the Prevention of Obstructed Labor," *Clinical Obstetrics and Gynecology* 52 (2009): 256–269. The latter article has an extensive bibliography of relevant clinical studies.

The article on uterine rupture at Kenyatta National Hospital is V. M. Lema, S. B. Ojwang, and S. H. Wanjala, "Rupture of the Gravid Uterus: A Review," *East African Medical Journal* 68, no. 6 (1991): 430–441. The paper from rural Nigeria is Ugochukwu O. J. Umeora, Brown N. Ejikeme, and Vincent E. Egwuatu, "Contribution of Ruptured Uterus to Maternal Mortality in Rural South Eastern Nigeria," *Tropical Journal of Obstetrics and Gynaecology* 22, no. 2 (2005): 184–188. The best current overview of uterine rupture in poor countries is Yibrah Berhe and L. Lewis Wall, "Uterine Rupture in Resource-Poor Countries," *Obstetrical and Gynecological Survey* 69, no. 1 (2014): 695–707.

On treatment protocols for obstructed labor, see J. B. Lawson, "Obstructed Labor," in *Obstetrics and Gynaecology in the Tropics and Developing Countries*, ed. J. B. Lawson and D. B. Stewart (London: Edward Arnold, 1967), 172–202; E. J. Kongnyuy and N. van den Broek, "A Criterion Based Audit of the Management of Obstructed Labour in Malawi," *Archives of Gynecology and Obstetrics* 279 (2009): 649–654; and P. T. Wagaarachchi, W. J. Graham, G. C. Penney, A. McCaw-Burns, K. Y. Antwi, and M. H. Hall, "Holding Up a Mirror: Changing Obstetric Practice through Criterion-Based Clinical Audit in Developing Countries," *International Journal of Gynecology and Obstetrics* 74 (2001): 119–130; and O. M. R. Campbell, W. J. Graham, and the Lancet Maternal Survival Series steering group, "Maternal Survival 2: Strategies for Reducing Maternal Mortality; Getting On with What Works," *Lancet* 368 (2006): 1284–1299. The quotation is from page 1285.

The reference to Peter Singer's book is Peter Singer, *How Are We to Live? Ethics in an Age of Self Interest* (Amherst, NY: Prometheus Books, 1995).

A huge effort went into reducing maternal mortality in the Western world in the twentieth century, and, as a result, there is a robust literature on clinical audits and maternal mortality reviews. For an introduction, see Gwyneth Lewis, "Reviewing Maternal Deaths to Make Pregnancy Safer," *Best Practice and Research Clinical Obstetrics and Gynecology* 22, no. 3 (2008): 447–463. Gwyneth has led the Confidential Enquiry into Maternal Deaths (now called the Confidential Enquiry into Maternal and Child Health) in England and Wales for years. Her work is generally regarded as the gold standard for maternal death reviews around the world.

The quotation is from E. J. Kongnyuy and N. van den Broek, "Audit for Maternal and Newborn Health Services in Resource-Poor Countries," *BJOG: An International Journal of Obstetrics and Gynaecology* 116 (2009): 7–10. The maternity audit in Burkina Faso is described in F. Richard, C. Ouedraogo, V. Zongo, F. Ouattara, S. Zongo, M. E. Gruenais, and V. De Brouwere, "The Difficulty of Questioning Clinical Practice: Experience of Facility-Based Case Reviews in

Ouagadougou, Burkina Faso," *BJOG: An International Journal of Obstetrics and Gynaecology* 116 (2009): 38–44. Additional papers on maternal mortality of relevance include the following: Cynthia Berg, "From Identification and Review to Action—Maternal Mortality Review in the United States," *Seminars in Perinatology* 36 (2012): 7–13; Gillian Penney and Victoria Brace, "Near Miss Audit in Obstetrics," *Current Opinion in Obstetrics and Gynecology* 19 (2007): 145–150; Pius Okong, Josaphat Byamgisha, Florence Mirembe, Romano Byaruhanga, and Staffan Bergstrom, "Audit of Severe Maternal Morbidity in Uganda—Implications for Quality of Obstetric Care," *Acta Obstetricia et Gynecologica* 85 (2006): 797–804; Fathima Paruk and Jack Moodley, "Severe Obstetric Morbidity," *Current Opinion in Obstetrics and Gynecology* 13 (2001): 563–568; Veronique Filippi, Fabienne Richard, Isabelle Lange, and Fatoumata Ouattara, "Identifying Barriers from Home to the Appropriate Hospital through Near-Miss Audits in Developing Countries," *Best Practice and Research Clinical Obstetrics and Gynaecology* 23 (2009): 389–400; Veronique Filippi, Carine Ronsmans, Valeri Gohou, Sorou Goufodji, Mohamed Lardi, Amina Sahel, Jacques Saizonou, and Vincente de Brouwere, "Maternity Wards or Emergency Obstetric Rooms? Incidence of Near-Miss Events in African Hospitals," *Acta Obstetricia et Gynecologica Scandinavica* 84 (2005): 11–16; and Michael Reichenheim, Flavio Zylbersztajn, Claudia Moraes, and Gustavo Lobato, "Severe Acute Obstetric Morbidity (Near-Miss): A Review of the Relative Use of Its Diagnostic Indicators," *Archives of Gynecology and Obstetrics* 280 (2009): 337–343.

A useful practical review on a specific clinical topic is Eugene Justine Kongnyuy, Grace Mlava, and Nynke van den Broek, "A Criterion Based Audit of the Management of Obstructed Labour in Malawi," *Archives of Gynecology and Obstetrics* 279 (2009): 649–654.

The story of Godfrey Mbaruku and the Kigoma Hospital turnaround is detailed in Godfrey Mbaruku and Staffan Bergstrom, "Reducing Maternal Mortality in Kigoma, Tanzania," *Health Policy and Planning* 10, no. 1 (1995): 71–79. The quotation is from page 77 of this work. Dr. Mbaruku has gone on to a distinguished career investigating health systems factors in maternal mortality and morbidity.

The quotation for Tarek Meguid is from his article "Lack of Political Will Is a Clinical Issue," *BMJ* 338 (2009): 1013. See also Jeremy Shiffman's work, especially "How to Advocate for Political Change on Obstetrical and Gynaecological Issues Facing Low-Income Countries," supplement, *BJOG* 116 (2009): 84–85.

The Millennium Development Goals can be found at http://www.who.int/topics/millennium _development_goals/en/.

The book by Kwame Anthony Appiah is *The Honor Code: How Moral Revolutions Happen* (New York: Norton, 2010). The quotation is from page xvii.

On trust, see Margaret Kruk, Peter C. Rockers, Godfrey Mbaruku, Magdalena Paczkowski, and Sandro Galea, "Community Health System Factors Associated with Facility Delivery in Rural Tanzania: A Multilevel Analysis," *Health Policy* 97 (2010): 209–216. Also see the article by MacMahon from Tanzania referred to earlier in this chapter.

Chapter 9. Compassion, Respect, and Justice

On organizational culture, see Edgar H. Schein, *Organizational Culture and Leadership*, 4th ed. (San Francisco: John Wiley and Sons/Jossey-Bass, 2010). On the nature of compassion, see particularly Tenzin Gyatso (the fourteenth Dalai Lama), *The Compassionate Life* (Boston: Wisdom, 2003); Thubten Jinpa, *A Fearless Heart: How the Courage to Be Compassionate Can Transform Our Lives* (New York: Hudson Press-Random House, 2015); and Matthieu Ricard, *Altruism: The*

Power of Compassion to Change Yourself and the World, trans. Charlotte Mandell and Sam Gordon (New York: Little, Brown, 2015).

The quotations from Adam Smith come from "Of Sympathy," in *The Theory of Moral Sentiments* (Indianapolis, IN: Liberty Fund, 1984), 9–13 (repr. of vol. 1 of *The Glasgow Edition of the Works and Correspondence of Adam Smith* [Oxford: Oxford University Press, 1976]).

The quotation from David Hume is from the first chapter of his treatise *An Essay concerning the Principles of Morals*, ed. Tom L. Beauchamp (New York: Oxford University Press, 1998), 79.

The quotations from Frans de Waal come from his paper "The Antiquity of Empathy," *Science* 336 (2012): 874–876. These ideas are elaborated more fully in his books *The Age of Empathy: Nature's Lessons for a Kinder Society* (New York: Broadway Books / Random House, 2010); and *The Bonobo and the Atheist: In Search of Humanism among the Primates* (New York: Norton, 2013). His book *Chimpanzee Politics: Power and Sex among Apes* (Baltimore: Johns Hopkins University Press, 2007) is a primatological and ethological classic. On the neurophysiology of altruistic behavior, see Donald W. Pfaff, *The Altruistic Brain: How We Are Naturally Good* (New York: Oxford University Press, 2015).

The Golden Rule is discussed in detail in Jeffrey Wattles, *The Golden Rule* (New York: Oxford University Press, 1996).

The famous quotation from Dr. Francis W. Peabody is from "The Care of the Patient," *Journal of the American Medical Association* 88, no. 12 (1927): 877–882. There is a huge literature on the placebo effect, but useful summaries relevant to the main point of this chapter are the following: W. Grant Thompson, *The Placebo Effect and Health: Combining Science and Compassionate Care* (Amherst, NY: Prometheus Books, 2005). The definition of the placebo effect given in this chapter is from page 50 of his book. See also Ted J. Kaptchuk, "Placebo Studies and Ritual Theory: A Comparative Analysis of Navajo, Acupuncture and Biomedical Healing," *Philosophical Transactions of the Royal Society B* 366 (2011): 1849–1858; Elisa Carlino, Antonella Pollo, and Fabrizio Benedetti, "The Placebo in Practice: How to Use It in Clinical Routine," *Current Opinion in Supportive and Palliative Care* 6, no. 2 (2012): 220–225; Elisa Carlino, Antonella Pollo, and Fabrizio Benedetti, "Placebo Analgesia and Beyond: A Melting Pot of Concepts and Ideas for Neuroscience," *Current Opinion in Anesthesia* 24 (2011): 540–544; Karin Meissner, Ulrike Bingel, Luana Colloca, Tor D. Water, Alison Watson, and Magne Arve Flaten, "The Placebo Effect: Advances from Different Methodological Perspectives," *Journal of Neuroscience* 31, no. 45 (2011): 16117–16124; Karin Meissner, Niko Kohls, and Luana Colloca, "Introduction to Placebo Effects in Medicine: Mechanisms and Clinical Implications," *Transactions of the Royal Society B* 366 (2011): 1783–1789; and Luana Colloca and Franklin G. Miller, "The Nocebo Effect and Its Relevance for Clinical Practice," *Psychosomatic Medicine* 73 (2011): 598–603.

On snakebite, see David A. Warrell, "Snake Bite," *Lancet* 375 (2010): 77–88; Barry S. Gold, Richard C. Dart, and Robert A. Barish, "Bites of Venomous Snakes," *New England Journal of Medicine* 347 (2002): 347–356; and H. Alistair Reid, "Snakebite in the Tropics," *British Medical Journal* 3 (1968): 359–362.

The quotation from the Dalai Lama is from his lovely book, *The Compassionate Life* (Boston, Wisdom, 2003), 10.

Walter B. Canon's famous paper is "Voodoo Death," *American Anthropologist* 44 (1942): 169–181.

As one might imagine, there is an enormous literature on pain and pain management during labor. Recent review articles of merit pertaining to this chapter include the following: Nancy K.

Lowe, "The Nature of Labor Pain," *American Journal of Obstetrics and Gynecology* 186 (2002): S16–S24; Ellen Hodnett, "Pain and Women's Satisfaction with the Experience of Childbirth: A Systematic Review," *American Journal of Obstetrics and Gynecology* 186 (2002): S160–S172; Helen Schnol, Nicole Paul, and Inna Belfer, "Labor Pain Mechanisms," *International Anesthesiology Clinics* 52, no. 3 (2014): 1–17; Judith P. Rooks, "Labor Pain Management Other Than Neuraxial: What Do We Know and Where Do We Go Next?" *Birth* 39, no. 4 (2012): 318–322; Penny Simkin and April Bolding, "Update on Nonpharmacologic Approaches to Relieve Labor Pain and Prevent Suffering," *Journal of Midwifery and Women's Health* 49 (2004): 489–504;Terhi Saisto and Erja Halmesmaki, "Fear of Childbirth: A Neglected Dilemma," *Acta Obstetricia et Gynecologica Scandinavica* 82 (2003): 201–208; Debra Pascali-Bonaro and Mary Kroeger, "Continuous Female Companionship during Childbirth: A Crucial Resource in Times of Stress or Calm," supplement, *Journal of Midwifery and Women's Health* 49, no. 1 (2004): 19–27. See also the amusing cross-species rumination of Dana Raphael, in "Uncle Rhesus, Auntie Pachyderm, and Mom: All Sorts and Kinds of Mothering," *Perspectives in Biology and Medicine* 12, no. 2 (1969): 290–297.

The quotation about childbirth in Arab Palestine is from Hilda Granqvist, *Birth and Childhood among the Arabs: Studies in a Muhammadan Village in Palestine* (Helsingfors, Finland: Soderstom, 1947), 62.

The citations are from John Rawls, *A Theory of Justice* (Cambridge, MA: Harvard University Press, 1971), 14–15, and 140.

I have explored the concept of obstetric fistula as a neglected tropical disease in L. Lewis Wall, "Obstetric Fistula Is a 'Neglected Tropical Disease,'" *PLoS Neglected Tropical Diseases* 6, no. 8 (2012): e1769, doi:10.1371/journal.pntd.0001769. This is an open access publication, easily available on the Internet.

The quotation from James Gilligan, *Violence: Reflections on a National Epidemic,* Vintage Books ed. (New York: Vintage Books, 1997), 192.

On Cesarean section, see World Health Organization, "Appropriate Technology for Birth," *Lancet* 326 (1985): 436–437, for the citation on an optimal Cesarean section rate of 10–15 percent. The paper by Alexandre Dumont, Luc de Bernis, Marie-Helen Bouriver Colle, Gerard Breart, and the MOMA Study Group, "Caesarean Section Rate for Maternal Indication in Sub-Saharan Africa: A Systematic Review," *Lancet* 358 (2001): 1328–1333, provoked a lively correspondence subsequently published in *Lancet* 359 (2002): 974–976. See also Anton Kunst and Tanja Houweling, "A Global Picture of Poor-Rich Differences in the Utilization of Delivery Care," *Studies in Health Services Organization and Policy* 71 (2001): 293–311; Carine Ronsmans, Vincent De Brouwere, Dominique Dubourg, and Greet Dieltiens, "Measuring the Need for Life-Saving Obstetric Surgery in Developing Countries," *BJOG: An International Journal of Obstetrics and Gynaecology* 111 (2004): 1027–1030. The paper from which I have redrawn the graphs is Carine Ronsmans, Sara Holtz, and Cynthia Stanton, "Socioeconomic Differentials in Caesarean Rates in Developing Countries: A Retrospective Analysis," *Lancet* 368 (2006): 1516–1523. Luz Gibbons, Jose M. Belizan, Jeremy Lauer, Ana Betran, Mario Merialdi, and Fernando Althabe, *The Global Numbers and Costs of Additionally Needed and Unnecessary Caesarean Sections Performed per Year: Overuse as a Barrier to Universal Coverage,* World Health Report, Background Paper 30 (Geneva: World Health Organization, 2010), estimates that an annual expenditure of $432 million was required to cover the unmet but yet needed burden of Cesarean sections in poor countries in that year—a pittance in the world economy.

On vulnerabilities, the work I have found most useful is Kenneth Kipnis, "Vulnerability in Research Subjects: An Analytical Approach," in *The Variables of Moral Capacity*, ed. D. C. Thomasma and D. N. Weisstub (Boston: Kluwer, 2004), 217–231. I have explored these issues with respect to the obligation to provide fistula patients with a "just deal" in L. Lewis Wall, "Ethical Concerns Regarding Operations by Volunteer Surgeons on Vulnerable Patient Groups: The Case of Women with Obstetric Fistulas," *HEC Forum* 23 (2011): 115–127; and also in L. Lewis Wall, "A Bill of Rights for Patients with Obstetric Fistula," *International Journal of Gynecology and Obstetrics* 127 (2014): 301–304; and in L. Lewis Wall, Jeffrey Wilkinson, Steven D. Arrowsmith, Oladosu Ojengbede, and Hillary Mabeya, "A Code of Ethics for the Fistula Surgeon," *International Journal of Gynecology and Obstetrics* 101 (2008): 84–87. In this chapter I have reordered Kipnis's categories of vulnerability and modified them slightly, but the fundamental framework is the same. I am grateful to the publishers for permission to reuse this material from my three articles.

A robust bibliography on economic costs and the consequences of obstetric emergencies in poor countries can be found at the end of the reading list for chapter 6.

The best account of the travails of the traveling fistula victim is my graduate student Alison W. Heller's doctoral dissertation in anthropology, "Interrogating the Superlative Sufferer: Experiencing Obstetric Fistula and Treatment Seeking in Niger" (Department of Anthropology, Washington University in St. Louis, May 2015). Other pertinent references are the following: Margaret Murphy, "Social Consequences of Vesico-Vaginal Fistula in Northern Nigeria," *Journal of Biosocial Science* 13 (1981): 139–150; M. Kabir, Z. Iliyasu, I. S. Abubakar, and U. I. Umar, "Medico-Social Problems of Patients with Vesico-Vaginal Fistula in Murtala Mohammed Specialist Hospital, Kano," *Annals of African Medicine* 2, no. 2 (2003): 54–57; Marissa Pine Yeakey, Effie Chipeta, Frank Taulo, and Amy O. Tsui, "The Lived Experience of Malawian Women with Obstetric Fistula," *Culture, Health, and Sexuality* 11, no. 5 (2009): 499–513; Lisa M. Nathan, Charles H. Rochat, Bogdan Gigorescu, and Erika Banks, "Obstetric Fistulae in West Africa: Patient Perspectives," *American Journal of Obstetrics and Gynecology* 200, no. 5 (2009): e40–e42; Anne M. Khisa and Isaac K. Nyamongo, "Still Living with Fistula: An Exploratory Study of the Experience of Women with Obstetric Fistula Following Corrective Surgery in West Pokot, Kenya," *Reproductive Health Matters* 20, no. 40 (2012): 59–66, doi:10.1016/S0968-8080(12)40661-9; Nathalie Maulet, Mahamoudou Keita, and Jean Macq, "Medico-Social Pathways of Obstetric Fistula Patients in Mali and Niger: An 18-Month Cohort Follow-Up," *Tropical Medicine and International Health* 18, no. 5 (2013): 524–533; Lanne L. Gjerde, Guri Rortveit, Mulu Muleta, and Astrid Blystad, "Silently Waiting to Heal: Experiences among Women Living with Urinary Incontinence in Northwest Ethiopia," *International Urogynecology Journal* 24 (2013): 953–958; Lilian T. Mselle, Karen Marie Moland, Bjorg Evjen-Olsen, Abu Mvungi, and Thecla W. Kohi, "'I Am Nothing': Experiences of Loss among Women Suffering from Severe Birth Injuries in Tanzania," *BMC Women's Health* 11 (2011): 49; Lilian T. Mselle, Thecla W. Kohi, Abu Mvungi, Bjorg Evjen-Olsen, and Karen Marie Moland, "Waiting for Attention and Care: Birthing Accounts of Women in Rural Tanzania Who Developed Obstetric Fistula as an Outcome of Labour," *BMC Pregnancy and Childbirth* 11 (2011): 75.

On perceptions of Cesarean section and on seeing Cesarean delivery as being a "failure" as a woman, see O. C. Ezechi, O. B. Fasubaa, B. E. K. Kola, C. A. Nwokoro, and L. O. Obiese, "Caesarean Delivery: Why the Aversion?" *Tropical Journal of Obstetrics and Gynaecology* 21, no. 2 (2004): 164–167; M. Aziken, L. Omogo-Aghoja, and F. Okonofua, "Perceptions and Attitudes of Pregnant Women towards Caesarean Section in Urban Nigeria," *Acta Obstetricia et Gynecologica* 86

(2007): 42–47; C. O. Chibu and G. C. Ilobachie, "The Burden of Caesarean Section Refusal in a Developing Country Setting," *BJOG: An International Journal of Obstetrics and Gynaecology* 114 (2007): 1261–1265; and F. Richard, S. Zongo and F. Ouattara, "Fear, Guilt, and Debt: An Exploration of Women's Experience and Perception of Cesarean Birth in Burkina Faso, West Africa," *International Journal of Women's Health* 6 (2014): 469–478.

The social and infrastructural vulnerabilities of childbearing women in poor countries are nicely described in several good ethnographies, including Denise Roth Allen, *Managing Motherhood, Managing Risk: Fertility and Danger in West Central Tanzania* (Ann Arbor: University of Michigan Press, 2002); Cecilia van Hollen, *Birth on the Threshold: Childbirth and Modernity in South India* (Berkeley: University of California Press, 2003); Patricia Jeffrey, Roger Jeffrey, and Andrew Lyon, *Labour Pains and Labour Power: Women and Childbearing in India* (London: Zed Press, 1989); Nicole S. Berry, *Unsafe Motherhood: Mayan Maternal Mortality and Subjectivity in Post-war Guatemala* (New York: Berghahn Books, 2010); Marcia C. Inhorn, *Quest for Conception: Gender, Infertility, and Egyptian Medical Traditions* (Philadelphia: University of Pennsylvania Press, 1994); and Rachel R. Chapman, *Family Secrets: Risking Reproduction in Central Mozambique* (Nashville, TN: Vanderbilt University Press, 2010).

The view of women as fields to be tilled by men, who plant their seed and reap the harvest, is common. It is definitely the view held by Hausa villagers in northern Nigeria. Carol Delaney has written extensively about this in the context of Turkish village society: *The Seed and the Soil: Gender and Cosmology in Turkish Village Society* (Berkeley: University of California Press, 1991). The principle is explicitly stated in the Koran (2:223): "Your wives are a place of sowing of seed for you, so come to your place of cultivation however you wish and put forth [righteousness] for yourselves." See http://corpus.quran.com/translation.jsp?chapter=2&verse=223.

Information on the Worldwide Fistula Fund and the Danja Fistula Center can be found on the website www.worldwidefistulafund.org. The work of the Danja Fistula Center is recounted in Itengre Ouedraogo, Christopher Payne, Rahel Nardos, Avril J. Adelman, and L. Lewis Wall, "Obstetric Fistula in Niger: Six-Month Post-operative Follow-Up on 384 Patients from the Danja Fistula Center," *International Urogynecology Journal* (in press). Deepest thanks are due to Nick Kristof of the *New York Times*, whose story "New Life for the Pariahs," *New York Times*, November 1, 2009, described the struggle of the fistula patient and our hope to build the Danja Fistula Center. His article generated more than $500,000 in donations from readers, and, without him, the Danja Fistula Center would never have become a reality.

Chapter 10. The Vision of Hamlin Fistula

The work of Hamlin Fistula is internationally known and widely acclaimed. It is supported by charities in the United States, Australia, Britain, New Zealand, the Netherlands, Germany, Sweden, Switzerland, and Japan. I have drawn heavily on Catherine's published autobiographical memoir (*The Hospital by the River*) for much of this chapter and also on many personal visits to the Addis Ababa Fistula Hospital and its affiliated institutions over 20 years, including detailed conversations with Catherine Hamlin herself and with many other people associated with the hospital, both in Ethiopia and around the world. Many of the anecdotes in the book have been conveyed to me independently by other sources; some of the anecdotes in this chapter are not recounted in the book. The quotation from Margaret Fitzherber that "the fistula patients will break your heart" is on page 10. The quotation about the first fistula patient is on page 85. The catastrophic case studies are on pages 142–143.

The major published materials on the hospital are Robert Zacharin, *Obstetric Fistula* (New York: Springer-Verlag, 1988), especially chapter 5, "The Hamlins and the Second Fistula Hospital," 110–119; Catherine Hamlin, with John Little, *The Hospital by the River: A Story of Hope*, rev. ed. (Sydney: Pan McMillan, 2016 [2002]); and John Little's *Catherine's Gift: Stories of Hope from the Hospital by the River* (Oxford: Monarch Books, 2010). Unless otherwise attributed, quotations are from *The Hospital by the River*. The moving depiction of the plight of the fistula patient is from R. H. J. Hamlin and E. Catherine Nicolson, "Experiences in the Treatment of 600 Vaginal Fistulas and in the Management of 80 Labours Which Have Followed the Repair of These Injuries," *Ethiopian Medical Journal* 4, no 5 (1966): 189–192. The Ethiopian famine and its aftermath are discussed by Jonathan Dimbleby (who brought it to the world's attention) in "Feeding on Ethiopia's Famine," *Independent*, Monday, December 7, 1998.

The remarkable story of Mamitu Goshi is told in Judith T. W. Goh, *Mamitu: A Life in Ethiopia* (Pittsburgh, PA: Dorrance, 2003), as well as in Catherine's memoirs.

The complete story of the 17-year struggle of the Ethiopian people to free themselves from the tyranny of Mengistu and the Derg remains to be written. Of special interest are John Young's *Peasant Revolution in Ethiopia: The Tigray People's Liberation Front, 1975–1991* (New York: Cambridge University Press, 1997); and Jenny Hammond's *Fire from the Ashes: A Chronicle of the Revolution in Tigray, Ethiopia, 1975–1991* (Lawrenceville, NJ: Red Sea Press, 1999). Visitors to Ethiopia should not miss the opportunity to visit the Red Terror Martyr's Museum in Addis Ababa, established and run by victims of the Derg. The museum guides are former prisoners of the Mengistu regime. A fitting "bookend" to such a visit is a trip to Mekelle, in the Tigray Region of northern Ethiopia, to the magnificent monument and museum to the Tigray People's Liberation Front, which tells the story of the overthrow of the dictatorship from the point of view of the oppressed.

The research paper on characteristics and patient outcomes at the Addis Ababa Fistula Hospital is Mulu Muleta, Svein Rasmussen, and Torvid Kiserud, "Obstetric Fistula in 14,928 Ethiopian Women," *Acta Obstetricia et Gynecologica* 89 (2010): 945–951. The significance of the "continence gap" is discussed in L. Lewis Wall and Steven D. Arrowsmith, "The 'Continence Gap': A Critical Concept in Obstetric Fistula Repair," *International Urogynecology Journal* 18 (2007): 843–844. Ethical issues associated with urinary diversion in the fistula patient are discussed in L. Lewis Wall, Steven D. Arrowsmith, and Brian Hancock, "Ethical Aspects of Urinary Diversion for Women with Irreparable Obstetric Fistulas in Developing Countries," *International Urogynecology Journal* 19, no. 7 (2009): 1027–1030, doi:10.1007/s00192-008-0559-1.

Midwifery and maternal health statistics given in this chapter are taken from *The State of the World's Midwifery, 2014* (Geneva: World Health Organization, 2014), 96–97, on Ethiopia; and from *Trends in Maternal Mortality 1990–2015: Estimates by WHO, UNICEF, UNFPA, World Bank Group and the United Nations Population Division* (Geneva: World Health Organization, 2015). The maternal mortality ratio of 567 represents the upper limits of confidence for this 2015 estimate, the middle range of which was 353 maternal deaths per 100,000 live births. See also Tegbar Yigzaw, Firew Ayalew, Young-Mi Kim, Mintwab Gelagay, Daniel Dejene, Hannah Gibson, Aster Teshome, Jacqueline Broerse, and Jelle Stekelenburg, "How Well Does Pre-service Education Prepare Midwives for Practice: Competence Assessment of Midwifery Students at the Point of Graduation in Ethiopia," *BMC Medical Education* 15 (2015): 130, doi:10.1186/s12909-015-0410-6.

The maternal mortality ratio of 38 deaths per 100,000 deliveries for patients under the care of Hamlin-trained midwives is based on information provided to me by Zelalem Belete, the dean of the Hamlin College of Midwives. These statistics are a remarkable tribute to the work he has done in directing this educational institution.

Economic and population statistics in this chapter are from the World Bank (http://www .worldbank.org/en/country/ethiopia/overview) and the *CIA World Factbook* (https://www.cia.gov /library/publications/the-world-factbook/geos/et.html). The data on pelvic organ prolapse are from Karen Ballard, Fekade Ayenachew, Jeremy Wright, and Hatamu Atnafu, "The Prevalence of Obstetric Fistula and Symptomatic Pelvic Organ Prolapse in Rural Ethiopia," *International Urogynecology Journal* 27 (2016): 1063–1067.

Film and video treatments of the Hamlin story include the BBC's pioneering documentary, *Walking Back to Happiness* (London: British Broadcasting Corporation, 1993). This aired on the program *QED* and prompted more than £500,000 in spontaneous donations to the hospital. Also of note is the later documentary produced by Engel Entertainment, *A Walk to Beautiful* (2007), which subsequently aired in an edited version on the PBS program *Nova* (2008).

Further information on the work of Hamlin Fistula—including how to donate to the cause— can be found on the website, www.hamlinfistula.org. Please note that Hamlin Fistula USA is the only charity authorized to raise funds in the United States on behalf of the Addis Ababa Fistula Hospital and Hamlin Fistula Ethiopia.

Epilogue. Lessons Learned and the Way Forward

The last two paragraphs of the epilogue appeared previously in L. Lewis Wall, "Fitsari 'Dan Duniya: An African (Hausa) Praise-Song about Vesicovaginal Fistulas," *Obstetrics and Gynecology* 100 (2002):1328–1332. I am grateful for permission from the publisher to reuse this material.

Acknowledgments

The quote from Albert Schweitzer's *Out of My Life and Thought* (New York: New American Library, 1953), is on page 70.

Appendix. The Controversy concerning Sims's Experimental Surgeries on Slaves

The passages from J. Chassar Moir are from *The Vesico-Vaginal Fistula*, 2nd ed. (London: Bailliere Tindall and Cassell, 1968), 15–16.

Barker-Benfield's book is G. J. Barker-Benfield, *The Horrors of the Half-Known Life: Male Attitudes toward Women and Sexuality in Nineteenth-Century America* (New York: Harper and Row). The three reviews cited in the text are Michael Gordon, review of *The Horrors of the Half-Known Life: Male Attitudes toward Women and Sexuality in Nineteenth-Century America*, by G. J. Barker-Benfield, *Contemporary Sociology* 6, no. 1 (January 1977): 89–90; Anita Clair Fellman and Michael Fellman, "Man Amuck," review of *The Horrors of the Half-Known Life: Male Attitudes toward Women and Sexuality in Nineteenth-Century America*, by G. J. Barker-Benfield, *Reviews in American History* 4, no. 4 (December 1976): 558–564; and Regina Markell Morantz, review of *The Horrors of the Half-Known Life: Male Attitudes toward Women and Sexuality in Nineteenth-Century America*, by G. J. Barker-Benfield, *Bulletin of the History of Medicine* 51, no. 3 (1977): 307–310.

The term "zombie idea" and the quotation come from Paul Krugman, "The Ultimate Zombie Idea," *New York Times*, November 3, 2012.

On "truthiness," see the press release from the American Dialect Society, "Truthiness Voted 2005 Word of the Year by American Dialect Society," January 6, 2006, http://www.americandialect .org/truthiness_voted_2005_word_of_the_year. Butterfield's marvelous excursion into the philosophy of history is Herbert Butterfield, *The Whig Interpretation of History* (London: G. Bell and Sons, 1950). The quotations are from pages 52, 62, and 119.

In addition to Barker-Benfield's work, the current "anti-Sims" position is exemplified by Mary Daly, *Gyn/Ecology: The Metaethics of Radical Feminism* (Boston: Beacon Press, 1978); Harriet Washington, *Medical Apartheid: The Dark History of Medical Experimentation on Black Americans from Colonial Times to the Present* (New York: Doubleday, 2006); W. Michael Bird and Linda A. Clayton, *An American Health Dilemma*, vol. 1, *A Medical History of African Americans and the Problem of Race: Beginning to 1900* (New York: Routledge, 2000); Diana E. Axelson, "Women as Victims of Medical Experimentation: J. Marion Sims' Surgery on Slave Women, 1845–1850," *Sage* 2, no. 2 (1985): 10–13; David A. Richardson, "Ethics in Gynecological Surgical Innovation," *American Journal of Obstetrics and Gynecology* 170 (1994): 1–6; Jeffery S. Sartin, "J. Marion Sims, the Father of Gynecology: Hero or Villain?," *Southern Medical Journal* 97 (2004): 500–505; Durrenda Ojanuga, "The Medical Ethics of the 'Father of Gynecology,' Dr. J. Marion Sims," *Journal of Medical Ethics* 19 (1993): 28–31; and Sara Spettel and Mark D. White, "The Portrayal of J. Marion Sims' Controversial Surgical Legacy," *Journal of Urology* 195 (2011): 2424–2427.

Writers with a more sympathetic view of Sims include C. M. de Costa, "James Marion Sims: Some Speculations and a New Position," *Medical Journal of Australia* 178 (2003): 660–663; J. P. O'Leary, "J. Marion Sims: A Defense of the Father of Gynecology," *Southern Medical Journal* 97, no. 5 (2004): 427–429; L. Lewis Wall; "The Medical Ethics of Dr. J. Marion Sims: A Fresh Look at the Historical Record," *Journal of Medical Ethics* 32 (2006): 346–350; L. Lewis Wall, "Did J. Marion Sims Deliberately Addict His First Fistula Patients to Opium?," *Journal of the History of Medicine and Allied Sciences* 62 (2006): 336–356; J. M. Straughn Jr., R. E. Gandy, and Charles B. Rodning, "The Core Competencies of James Marion Sims, MD," *Annals of Surgery* 256, no. 1 (2012): 193–202; and Robert Baker, *Before Bioethics: A History of American Medical Ethics from Colonial Times to the Bioethics Revolution* (New York: Oxford University Press, 2013).

Kees Waaldijk's modern advocacy of fistula repair without the use anesthesia is found in his paper "The Immediate Surgical Management of Fresh Obstetric Fistulas with Catheter and/or Early Closure," *International Journal of Gynecology and Obstetrics* 45 (1994): 11–16. While this would have been a reasonable point of view in 1847 (and one that was, in fact, held by many surgeons at that time), doing this in the twenty-first century is completely unethical and cannot be condoned.

The introduction of anesthesia and the controversies surrounding its early use are admirably treated by Martin S. Pernick, *A Calculus of Suffering: Pain, Professionalism, and Anesthesia in Nineteenth Century America* (New York: Columbia University Press, 1985). The quotation is from page 35.

The account of Simpson's experiments with chloroform is taken from chapter 10, "Chloroform," in Morrice McCrae, *Simpson: The Turbulent Life of a Medical Pioneer* (Edinburgh: John Donald, 2010), 117–137. The quotation is from page 117.

The quotation from Thomas Addis Emmet on the use of anesthesia at the Woman's Hospital is from his "Reminiscences of Founders of the Woman's Hospital Association," *New York Journal of Gynecology and Obstetrics* 3 (1893): 353–369.

INDEX

Denman, Thomas, 58–59, 61
depression, 16, 36, 38, 44, 59
Derry, Douglas E., 5–6, 17
Desta Mender, 264–65, 267
de Waal, Frans, 216
diagnosis of obstructed labor, 30, 46, 158, 159, 161, 180, 181, 194, 196, 229
Dictionary of American Medical Biography (Kelly), 120
Dictionary of the Hausa Language (Robinson), 125
Dieckmann, J., 84
Dieffenbach, Johannes, 110–11
Dimbleby, Jonathan, 254
Diseases of Women with Child and in Child-bed, The (Mauriceau), 49
divorce or separation, 36, 38, 44, 165, 170, 235; in Ethiopia, 261, 262, 265–66; in Hausaland, 125, 132, 136, 149
dose-response curve, 48, 297
Douglas, M., 162
doula, 220. *See also* midwives
dwarves, 64, 68, 75, 77
dystocia, 19, 20, 47, 163, 168, 297

Earle, Henry, 92–93
eclampsia/preeclampsia, 73, 275, 301–2; in Hausaland, 142, 143–44, 146, 150
economic barriers to care, 168–70, 187, 188, 206, 231–35, 275, 276. *See also* poverty
economic resources, 182, 204, 208, 231, 242, 275, 276
egg-binding, 19–20
egg fertilization, 19, 41, 297
Egypt, 8, 44–46, 249; Queen Henhenit's story, 5–18
Ekwendeni Hospital, Malawi, 182
Elkins, Tom, 192
emergency obstetric care, 2, 18; basic or comprehensive, 173–75, 189; champions for, 200–203; with compassion, respect, and justice, 209–46; cultural barriers to, 151, 208; delays in getting to, 171–83, 209; delays in receiving, 184–208, 209, 210; delays in seeking, 157–70, 207, 209; drugs, supplies, and equipment for, 190–91; economic barriers to, 168–70, 187, 188, 206, 231–35, 275, 276; in Ethiopia, 251–52; facilities and infrastructure for, 173–74, 188–90; inadequacy of, 185–87; management, guidelines, and policies for, 194–99; in Nigeria, 185–87; patients' trust in, 206–8; phases of delay and, 159–60, 207; political will and, 203–6; referral systems for, 178; requirements for, 187; responsive institutional ethic of care and, 199–200;

shortages of staff/supplies, 153, 160, 185, 188, 191–92, 200–203, 208, 237; staffing for, 191–94; substandard, 199–200, 209, 210, 234
Emigrant Refuge Hospital, New York, 116, 117
Emmet, Thomas Addis, 116–22, 157
empathy, 210, 215–16, 217, 219, 220, 221, 225, 255
Emuoha Hospital, Nigeria, 185, 201
encephalization, 23–24, 297
endomyometritis, 39, 297
Enugu State University Teaching Hospital Parklane, Nigeria, 194
epidemiology of obstetric fistula, 122, 160; in Ethiopia, 261–62
episiotomy, 141, 167, 297
ergot, 48
Esan people, Nigeria, 163
ethical principles, 204, 211, 222, 239, 272, 276; for fistula surgeon, 239–43; institutional, 187, 199–200; for staff, 191
Ethiopia, 175, 194, 246, 247–73; analysis of fistula cases in, 261–63; beyond the eradication of fistula in, 270–73; Hamlin College of Midwifery in, 267–69, 272; Hamlins's establishment of fistula hospital in, 248–73; intractable fistulas and Desta Mender in, 263–65, 267; Mamitu's story, 247, 256–58, 260, 266; Mengistu and the Derg in, 254–56, 258–59; regionalized care in, 266–67, 270
Evangel Hospital, Nigeria, 41, 123, 127, 161
evolutionary pressures, 3, 19–25, 219, 274

Fallopian tubes, 41, 300; fimbriated ends of, 41, 297
fear, 218–19; delays in seeking care due to, 167–68
fecal incontinence, 2, 35, 38, 42, 89–90, 126, 147, 237, 257
fetal head/skull: in breech delivery, 87, cephalopelvic disproportion and, 296; during childbirth, 26–28, 42, 219; compression of lumbosacral nerve plexus by, 43, 223, 265; cranial sutures of, 25–26; craniotomy of, 56, 76, 79, 81–82, 296–97; encephalization of, 23–24, 297; forceps delivery and, 50, 53, 67; "lessening" of, 48, 52, 53–56, 58, 296; normal presentation of, 299, 302; obstructed labor and impaction of, 3, 14, 31, 32–33, 37, 52–53, 74, 87, 103, 159, 198, 298
fetal lie, 299; transverse, 28, 58, 62, 299, 302, 304
fetal maceration, 13, 31, 172, 214
fetal malpresentation, 28, 58, 158, 299; version maneuvers for, 304
fetal presentation, 302. *See also* breech presentation

Mangochi District Hospital, Malawi, 177
Martin, Robert, 26
Martius, Heinrich, 249
maternal height, 158, 181, 262
maternal morbidity, 299; and access to emergency
services, 158, 173, 181, 203; Cesarean section–
related, 61, 76, 81–84; in Ethiopia, 267, 269; in
Hausaland, 130, 143, 149, 150, 152, 153; historical, 57–58; severe, 142–43; social-structural
violence and, 128; in West Africa, 58
maternal mortality, 1, 4, 275, 276, 299; and access to emergency services, 158, 162, 163, 170,
172–75, 178, 184, 190, 191, 238; causes of, 86,
142, 143, 146, 150, 190, 227, 275; Cesarean
section–related, 71, 72, 75–78, 80–84; clinical
audit of, 199–200; direct and indirect, 300; in
Ethiopia, 267–69; in Ghana, 192; in Hausaland,
130, 139, 142–47, 149–51, 153, 156, 208; historical, 57–58; in industrialized countries, 2, 142;
from obstructed labor, 20, 31, 37; poverty and,
2; prevention of, 130, 142, 159, 162, 163, 173–74,
184; risk approach to, 180; social-structural
violence and, 128; in sub-Saharan Africa, 2, 57,
142, 144, 191; in Tanzania, 200–203; twentieth-
century decline in, 84–86, 275; UN goal for
reduction of, 204; in West Africa, 58; in Zambia
vs. Chicago, 184–85
maternity waiting homes, 179–83
Mauriceau, François, 49–50, 61–62
Mbaruku, Godfrey, 201–3, 205, 207, 210, 221
McClellan, George, 99, 100, 101
McMahon, S. A., 194, 207
medical vulnerability, 236–37
Meguid, Tarek, 203, 204
Mengistu Haile Mariam, 255, 258–59
menstrual problems, 38, 40, 94, 141, 148; in Hausa
women, 133, 134, 138, 141, 148
Mercurio, Scipione, 70–72
midwives, 47, 128, 171, 200, 208; in Afghanistan,
173; delays in receiving care by, 186–87, 188;
delays in seeking treatment and, 159, 163, 164,
165; in Ethiopia, 249, 262, 270, 272, 273; in
Gambia, 172; Hamlin College of Midwifery,
267–69, 272; Hausa, 138–39, 141; man-
midwives, 49–52, 57; "meddlesome," 59, 76, 81,
83; mobile phone contact in Africa and, 179; for
Queen Henhenit, 11, 12, 13; respectful and ethical care by, 220, 222, 276; role of, in building
political will, 204, 205, 206; for Safiya, 212–14,
222; shortage of, 191; in Tanzania, 202, 203
"mixing of men," 164
mobile phones in Africa, 179
Moir, J. Chassar, 86–88, 249

morality, 204, 205, 215–16, 225
morbidity. *See* maternal morbidity
mortality. *See* maternal mortality
Moyer, C. A., 194
Mozambique, 164
Mulago Hospital, Uganda, 166
mummification process, 6, 16
Murphy, Margaret, 149
muscle contractions, 219

Naville, Edouard, 6, 9
necrosis, 33, 40–41, 42, 87, 148, 240, 300
negative predictive value, 300
neglected tropical diseases (NTDs), 4, 228
neglect or abuse of patients, 193, 194
neonatal death, 41–42, 300, 301
New Elements of Operative Surgery (Velpeau), 89
Nicholson, Jock, 264
Niger, 175, 178, 243, 244, 246, 276
Nigeria, 41, 244; antenatal care in, 208; delays in
seeking care in, 163–64, 166; emergency obstetric services in, 185–86, 188–89, 194, 197, 198,
201; Hausaland, 122–56; Safiya's story, 210–14,
219, 221, 222–25, 228, 229–30, 231, 235, 238,
243–46; transportation in, 176–77
nocebo effect, 218–19
non-maleficence, 239, 300
Nyakyusa people, East Africa, 164

obstetrical mechanics, 3, 18, 20, 24, 26–28, 274;
in obstructed labor, 30–31, 36, 37, 48, 161, 207,
236, 256, 269
obstetric fistula, 298, 300; causes, 3, 122, 128–30,
157; cure of (*see* vesico-vaginal fistula surgery);
incidence of, 36; labor duration and, 33; persistence of, 4, 122, 229, 267; reducing risk factors
for, 157–58; twentieth-century decline in, 46,
84–88; unrepaired, 3, 36, 37, 160, 206. *See also*
specific types
obstetrics and gynecology, discipline of, 86
Obstetric Surgery (Grandin and Jardin), 81
O'Neill, Tip, 204
On the Origin of Species (Darwin), 20
orangutans, 26, 27, 298
Ould, Fielding, 62
oviduct, 19, 300
ovulation, 41
oxytocic drugs, 165, 189, 190

Pakistan, 169
Pancoast, Joseph, 89, 90
Papanek, Hannah, 134
parietal bones, 25, 26, 28, 29, 214, 301

sepsis, 38, 39; Cesarean section and, 61, 72, 81, 83; maternal death due to, 143–44, 158
Serving in Mission (SIM), 246
Seski, A. G., 84
Sett of Anatomical Tables (Smellie), 28
sex for money, 137, 225
sexual abuse, 193, 242
sexual function, 38, 41, 133, 134, 137
Sheehan's syndrome, 40
Shiffman, Jeremy, 204
Shirress, Janet, 94
Shona people, Mozambique, 164
Sierra Leone, 162, 176
Sigault, Jean-René, 63–67
silver nitrate, 91, 118
Simmons, William, 62
Simpson, James Young, 89
Sims, J. Marion, 96–116, 120–22, 250; attempts by, to cure vesico-vaginal fistula, 108–12; background and education of, 96–100; encountering a vesico-vaginal fistula, 103–7; key to surgical success of, 112–16; medical practice of, 100–101; opening Woman's Hospital of New York, 116; reconstructive surgery in 1840s and, 101–2
Sims position, 106, 112, 114
Sims speculum, 107, 112
Singer, Peter, 199
Smellie, William, 28, 57
Smith, Adam, 215, 216, 221
social factors, 3–4, 35, 38, 44, 161, 163; in Burkina Faso, 170; compassion, 215, 216, 217; contraceptive agency and, 166; in Ethiopia, 254, 266, 272; in Hausaland, 122, 123, 127–28, 130, 132–39, 142, 147, 148, 150, 154; social costs of emergency services, 174
social responsibility, 137, 242
social vulnerability, 236, 237
Somalia, 37, 258
South Asia, 2, 18, 37, 160
specificity of test, 158, 180, 181, 303
sphygmomanometer, 202, 303
splenomegaly, 141, 303
Sri Lanka, 159, 175
St. George's Hospital, London, 88
stigma, 4, 36, 44, 126, 148, 149, 167, 168, 193, 228, 238, 264
stillbirth, 1, 301; obstetric fistula and, 33, 41–42, 94, 103, 119, 147, 249, 251, 261, 262, 269; obstructed labor and, 31, 38, 49, 64, 67, 220, 257; of Queen Henhenit's child, 14, 16; reduction of, by Cesarean section, 197
St. Luke's Hospital, New York, 120
Storeng, K. T., 170

Story of My Life, The (Sims), 250
structural violence, 210, 228–29, 275, 276, 303; in Hausaland, 127–30, 145; and vulnerabilities of poor women, 231–38
studies, prospective, 58, 202, 241, 302
sub-Saharan Africa: Cesarean section rate in, 191; education of women in, 156; emergency obstetric services in, 18, 46, 190; lack of healthcare personnel in, 191; maternal mortality in, 2, 57, 142, 144, 191; persistence of obstetric fistula in, 122; "sisterhood of suffering" in, 111–12; unrepaired obstetric fistulas in, 3, 37, 160
Sudan, 37, 130
suffering, sisterhood of, 111, 276–77
Sukuma people, Tanzania, 164
Sundari, T. K., 185
surgery. *See* vesico-vaginal fistula surgery
symphysiotomy, 48, 63–69, 303

Tanzania, 164, 169, 172, 179, 194, 201–3, 207, 210
Tazhib, Farhang, 186–87
tenesmus, 105, 303
Thaddeus, Sereen, 159, 160, 186
Theory of Justice, A (Rawls), 225
Theory of Moral Sentiments, The (Smith), 215
therapeutic pluralism, 161, 207
Thomas, T. Gaillard, 78
Thompson, Grant, 217
transportation infrastructure, 159, 175, 206, 209, 252, 276; communication, planning, and, 174–79; delays in getting to place of care and, 171–83; in Ethiopia, 251, 252, 266; in the Gambia, 172; in Hausaland, 150, 152; in Malawi, 177; in Nigeria, 176–77
Treatise on the Theory and Practice of Midwifery (Smellie), 57
Trevitt, Lorna, 139
Trevor, Jean, 134
triage, 179, 303
trust, 206–8

Uganda, 36, 166–67
Umeora, O. U. J., 197
Unknown Famine, The (documentary), 254
UN Millennium Development Goals, 204
ureteral injury, 38, 39, 87
uretero-vaginal fistula, 39, 297–98, 303
urethral injury, 12, 32, 38, 39, 40, 65, 66, 67, 90, 141, 165, 198, 262, 271
urinary catheterization, 91, 93, 94–95, 107, 108–10, 112, 113, 115, 120, 122, 190, 198–99, 224–25, 244, 245, 250, 277
urinary diversion, 263–64, 267, 272